Ortonville Library

P9-DHQ-666

# How to Make Almost Any Diet Work

*Repair Your Disordered Appetite*
*and Finally Lose Weight*

Anne Katherine

Pioneerland Library System
P. O. Box 327
Willmar, MN 56201

**HAZELDEN®**

Hazelden
Center City, Minnesota 55012-0176

1-800-328-9000
1-651-213-4590 (Fax)
www.hazelden.org

©2006 by Anne Katherine
All rights reserved. Published 2006
Printed in the United States of America

This published work is protected by copyright law. Unless a statement on the page grants permission to duplicate or permission has been obtained from the publisher, duplicating all or part of this work by any means is an illegal act.

To request permission, write to Permissions Coordinator, Hazelden, P.O. Box 176, Center City, MN 55012-0176. To purchase additional copies of this publication, call 1-800-328-9000 or 1-651-213-4000.

ISBN-13: 978-1-59285-357-1
ISBN-10: 1-59285-357-9


Library of Congress Cataloging-in-Publication Data
Katherine, Anne.
    How to make almost any diet work : repair your disordered appetite and finally lose weight / Anne Katherine.
        p. cm.
    Includes bibliographical references (p. 363).
    ISBN-13: 978-1-59285-357-1
    ISBN-10: 1-59285-357-9
1. Reducing diets.    2. Reducing—Psychological aspects.    3. Compulsive eating.
4. Food habits.  I. Title.
    RM222.2.K362 2006
    613.2'5—dc22
                                    2006016698

This book is for educational purposes. It is not intended to replace medical advice. This publication is intended to provide authoritative and accurate information, and is up to date and timely as of its date of publication; however, it is not meant to replace the services of a trained professional, physician, support group, or recovery group. This book is sold with the understanding that the publisher and author are not rendering individual psychological or medical services, or individual services of any kind, to the reader. Should such services be necessary, please consult an appropriate professional.

### Author's Note

The author's evaluations of diet plans and books are entirely independent, and she has received no consideration or reward from any author or publisher. Her comments do not imply endorsement by this publisher, or endorsement of this book by any other author or publisher.

Any charts presented as examples in this book either have been released to the author and publisher with explicit permission provided (although to provide anonymity, in all cases, people's names have been changed) or, in a few cases, have been created by the author for illustrative purposes.

Be sure to consult a qualified medical professional before making any changes to your eating.

10   09   08   07   06   6   5   4   3   2   1

Cover design by David Spohn
Interior design and typesetting by Kinne Design
Illustrations by Patrice Barton

*Dedicated to Two Sherrys*

Sherry A
and
Sherry B

Thank you Sherry Ascher for profound support—for championing my missions, washing thousands of dishes, and handling the sharp tools.

Thank you Sherry Buckner for being the archetype for thinking beyond the perimeter, for supporting my recovery, for sculpting a true-hearted friendship, and for giving me the best of reasons to rededicate myself to this work.

IN MEMORIAM:

Charles Wolflin

1927–2005

*Take my love with you to your shining new world.*

# Contents

# Illustrations

# IN GRATITUDE

Ahhh, friends, both the honey and spice of life:

> I am grateful every day for the community of precious people who enrich my life (listed in order of longevity): Dusty, Abe, Jabber, Cassie, Shirley, Dottie, Sandy, Bob, Jill, Kevin, Luann, Susan, Connie, Harry, Barbara, Wauneta, Gloria, Blaine, Joan, Jean, Marilyn, Katie, Zim, Milli, John, Pat, Doc, Rabbitt, Cliff, Linda, Ron, Don, John, Kate, Cindy, Lynn, Rick, Ande, Rod, Lynette, Sherry, Pat, Darl, Charlie, Susan, Yvonne, Jim, Lorrie, and, of course, Mary.

And family, the foundation that makes risk possible:

> Thank you to Fran, Sherry, my beloved foster daughter, my cherished daughter-in-spirit, Dan, Justina, Eli, Dylan, Jim and Carol, Tom and Susanne, and two demanding cats.

Thanks yet again, team:

> Scott Edelstein, honorable man, extraordinary agent, herald and warrior both,
>
> Becky Post, spectacular editor, drawbridge,
>
> Becky Aldridge, smart and gentle copy editor, fulcrum,
>
> Christine Lockhart, keeper of the keys, finder of the lost, and modest oracle.

I want to also pay tribute to two women and the thriving professional community they've fostered:

> Yvonne Agazarian, whose brilliant, life-giving processes have the potential to rescue this limping world,
>
> Susan Gantt, who has transfused my professional life and catalyzed a dazzling transformation of my interior landscape.

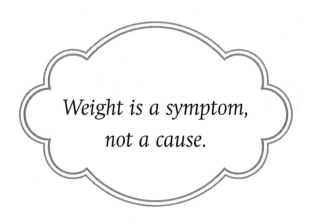

*Weight is a symptom,*
*not a cause.*

# How This Book Can Help

This book is for anyone who eats too much. That includes most Americans.

According to the National Center for Health Statistics, in a study conducted from 1999 to 2002, fully 64 percent of American adults were found to be obese or overweight.

Every year we are offered new diets, new books on dieting, and new weight-loss programs. Every week in supermarket checkout lines, we can find at least three magazine covers that offer new eating plans guaranteed to permanently take off those inches or pounds. But are these working?

Compare the 1994 national statistics on overweight and obesity for American women who were five feet, four inches tall. Figure 1 shows the percent who were thirty or more pounds overweight.[1]

FIGURE 1

**Overweight and Obese Americans 1994**

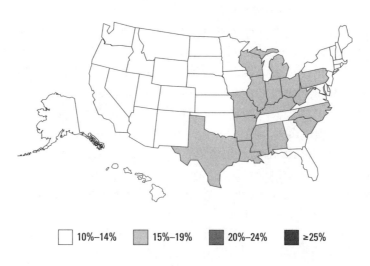

Now let's look at the data for 2002.

FIGURE 2

**Overweight and Obese Americans 2002**

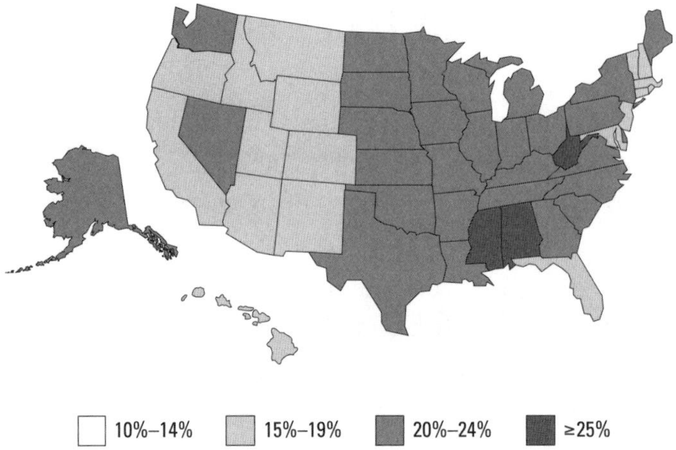

| | 10%–14% | | 15%–19% | | 20%–24% | | ≥25% |

In just eight years, the nation got 5 percent heavier, with every state showing a rise in obesity. In nine states, the incidence of obesity jumped 10 percent. Clearly, the increase in diet plans is not decreasing obesity. Here's why.

Many Americans, including health care professionals and citizens alike, continue to gaze in the wrong direction. Diets continue to be pursued as the solution to extra weight when weight is a symptom, not a cause.

From my work with hundreds of women, evidence from recent studies, and my own experience as a large woman, it's clear to me that *no* diet can be sustained over time unless the causes of overeating are attended to first. After all, a diet can be fabulous, but if you can't stay on it, what good is it?

For most people, diets can't work as the first line of defense. Instead, we need to turn our attention in a different direction. Once the causes of overeating have been tackled, then and only then can a specific diet plan be effective. Even then, a diet can work for you only if it is adapted to your specific body chemistry. Not even the best diet plan can be followed verbatim; it must always be filtered through intelligent awareness of the real causes of extra weight.

Another book that I've written can serve as a companion to this one. *When Someone You Love Eats Too Much: What You Need to Know—and How to Help\** is for the people who care about you and want to help: your sister, best friend, mother, daughter, husband, partner, mate, brother, son, father, and so on. It is also for the professionals who provide you with health care: your doctor, counselor, therapist, nurse practitioner, dentist, etc. The book explains what they should and shouldn't do to support you in your effort to lose weight and develop a healthier relationship with food.

The two books together form a complementary set. Together they put everyone on the same page and give them a shared foundation regarding the real causes of overweight and the necessities for dealing with them.

With *this* book, I intend to liberate you from the enormous weight you've been carrying—the weight on your shoulders. If you have felt weak, guilty, ashamed, humiliated, or out of control with regard to eating or weight, this book will help set you free. You'll see that the problem has not been a personality flaw or lack of willpower. You'll realize that you've been struggling against some extremely powerful chemical forces that an entire country has not wanted to name. Best of all, you'll learn an approach to healthier eating—and a lighter body—that will finally work.

So read this book and follow its step-by-step guidance. You will learn to change your relationship with food and eating. Then you will select a diet plan and custom-tailor it for you and your circumstances.

Your life is about much more than your size or appearance. With your struggles over food and eating managed, you can turn attention to your life's real mission—whatever has been resting in your heart.

. . .

* To be published. Check www.annekatherine.org for availability.

# 1

# Sit Down with the Dragon

THE FAMILY drew near the old farmhouse in high spirits. Before Uncle Harry even pushed his car door shut, Papa Blaine called quips from the porch. Joan reached down to help her sister Gloria lug a huge basket of exotic fare up the porch steps. Meanwhile, Aunt Barbara leaned out of the doorway to wave people indoors, admitting a few bright leaves as well. They skittered along the polished floor, and Cousin Milli grabbed them for the centerpiece.

Three people—Grandma, Caroline, and Gerald—faced this event with anxiety. Grandma was fighting a battle with diabetes—and the sugary foods she could no longer have; Caroline had started and stopped more times than she wanted to count; and Gerald had been in solid recovery for five years. They'd have been better off not attending, but this autumn tradition was an important family event, and they didn't want to miss a chance to be with people they loved.

Finally, all was ready, and the whole crowd gathered at the large oak table. Everyone took a seat and, one by one, each selection was passed around.

Grandpa introduced his gift first. "This is a perky little cabernet I found in the Robe Valley. It's from a small family vineyard that doesn't even have a label, but I pried this out of them. It's as smooth as syrup. Everyone have a taste."

Grandma, wanting to show support for her husband, lifted the wineglass to her lips and took a small sip. Caroline pretended to sip and tried not to inhale the full-bodied scent of the wine. The three glasses in front of Gerald stayed empty; he planned to drink coffee.

Papa Blaine bounced to his feet. "Listen, everybody, I can't wait. You've got to try mine next. It looks like an ordinary claret, but it's much more."

Cousin Ed protested, "No, no. Try these instead." He gestured to his wife who began passing a fancy bowl filled with orange capsules. "I found these at a little market in Colombia. Take these and the rest of the day will be unbelievably vivid."

Linda, just back from her first year at college, interrupted, "Try my pot first. It's the favorite of everyone on campus."

Great-Grandma's authoritative wheeze cut through the chaos. "Now children, you know we drink the wines first, before we have the pills and pot."

Everyone subsided with little murmurs of apology.

Grandma watched as Grandpa filled her row of glasses with each new wine that came by. How was she going to get through this day without drinking? No matter how many times she tried to explain to her husband that she was a diabetic, he didn't seem to get it. True to form, he continued to describe each new wine glowingly, wanting her to have a taste of each one.

Caroline had been sober just three months. She looked at her filled wineglasses, thinking she wasn't going to get through this afternoon with her sobriety intact. She didn't want to seem different or call attention to herself. She wished she could be like the others who could drink all these wines and then just stop, but she knew that if she had even a little bit, she'd fall back into a nonstop binge.

Gerald gritted his teeth and sipped his coffee. Years of solid recovery didn't protect him from the scent of the wine. Although he jovially passed each bottle, joining in with the jokes and laughter, this get-together was not easy for him. He used to be a secret drinker, so he knew the most dangerous time for him would be after the event, during cleanup, when his relatives' backs were turned and he was tempted to pick up their glasses and swallow the little mouthfuls of wine that remained.

**Sitting Down with the Dragon**

Of course, this scene is ludicrous. Alcoholics and drug addicts who are clean and sober aren't usually forced to sit at a family table while attractive liquors and pills are passed around in an endless parade of temptation. But if you give this scenario just a moment's thought, you can see that the food addict or compulsive overeater has to face something that no other addict does— ongoing, insistent contact with her addictive substance.

A recovering pot smoker doesn't have to hold a toke in his mouth on a daily basis. The sober alcoholic isn't invited into a bar three times a day. A pill addict gone clean isn't offered bowls of tablets and capsules morning, noon, and night.

However, a binge eater, compulsive overeater, or food addict sits down with the dragon three times a day. She sees, smells, tastes, and handles her triggering substance recurrently. No wonder recovering from an eating disorder is so dang hard.

*Hold on,* you might be thinking. *I just want to lose weight. Why are you bringing up eating disorders and food addiction?*

Because, if you haven't found a diet that works by now, there's a good reason. A diet *can't* work if you aren't first treating your disordered appetite.

I propose that we've all been looking at the wrong aspect of the problem: eating. Even the phrase *eating disorder* is misleading. The real question is, *What* causes eating to be disordered? Most people aren't willfully choosing the wrong foods and eating too much. Most of us overeat unhealthy foods because we're driven to consume them. They call to us with seductive smells and images, and we can't resist.

## Appetite and Addiction

A common definition of the word *appetite* is a natural desire for food. But to scientists, the word has a more specific meaning—*appetite* is the brain's trigger for eating. It is stimulated by a switch deep inside the brain. When the switch is on, you think of little else other than acquiring and eating particular foods. When the switch is off, you have no interest in food.

Numerous factors influence appetite, but the strongest are the physical changes that can lead to food addiction. In this book, we will deal with the chief and most powerful triggers for appetite that are known—but to have true long-term success with weight loss, we must also address your food addiction.

*Whoa,* you might be thinking, *who said I was addicted to food? I just have these pounds to shed.*

Okay, but why do you have pounds to shed? And how many times have you tried to lose them? Just how many diets have you consumer tested?

Even taking into account a genetic propensity toward heaviness and the fact that society has become more sedentary, the reason many of us have trouble losing weight is that it's hard to change the way we eat. And why is it hard to change the way we eat? Because we are, many of us, addicted to food.

Food is very much like alcohol. Most adults enjoy drinking alcohol, do it in moderation, and don't have any problem with it. But millions of Americans are alcoholics, and once they have even a tiny amount of alcohol, their addiction is triggered and they can't stop drinking. Similarly, almost everyone likes food. But many of us—millions of us—are food addicts too.

## Where Do You Stand?

I'd like to ask you a few questions.

Yes No     Are there times when you don't really taste the food you're eating?

Yes No     Do you sometimes head for food with a single-mindedness or desperation that has more to do with relief and comfort than hunger?

Yes No     Do you ever purposefully delay eating—sometimes not eating until late afternoon or evening—so that once you sink into the food, you won't have to be pulled away?

Yes No     Do you orchestrate your eating to bring about maximum relief?

Yes No     Are mealtimes like stepping-stones that help you get through the day?

Yes No     Or, do you nibble more or less nonstop all day in order to get through it?

Yes No     Do you have private rituals around eating? For example, do you save the best for last? Do you always eat the filling first and the crust last or vice versa? Are you careful to balance the dip and chips so they come out even? Do you save your favorite foods to eat during your favorite television show?

Yes No     When you eat, do you feel a sense of relief, comfort, or dreaminess?

Yes No     Is food one of your best friends?

Yes No     Once you have a little sugar or chocolate or some high-fat nibbles, is it hard for you to stop eating?

All of these questions refer to classic symptoms of food addiction. If you answered yes to four or more of them, there's no need to be worried or ashamed. In fact, you're in very good company. Literally millions (and, I suspect, tens of millions) of Americans of all ages and backgrounds are food addicts. (I'm one myself, though I've been in recovery for more than twenty-four years.)

The good news is that food addiction can be overcome, but not by following the regimen in a diet book or an off-the-rack weight-loss program. What you need instead is a customized recovery plan for your food addiction.

Once you've devised such a plan—and this book will show you how—then, and only then, will you be in a position to select a diet that can work for you. Like an off-the-rack garment, that diet will need to be altered to suit your unique body—something else this book will show you how to do.

### The Power of Food

For a food addict, eating is about the fix more than the flavor. For her, food provides far more than taste and nutrition. It brings comfort and relief. It alters her mood, helps her relax, lets her forget the day's stresses, and soothes any hurts and slights.

*It's not the flavor, it's the fix.*

How can food do this much?

Food can do all this for an addict because it initiates a chain reaction in her body. This chain reaction eventually triggers compelling brain chemicals that control mood, memory, judgment, sedation, and relief. These are not merely psychological reactions, but actual changes in brain and body chemistry.

How can any diet plan stand up against all this? It can't. And that's why, for food addicts, standard diets simply don't work.

I'm not knocking diets here. Almost any reasonable diet plan can work for a small percentage of people—provided they're not food addicts. In a country of 300 million people, a diet with only a 4 percent success rate can help 12 million people lose weight and keep it off. That's a lot of people. And that's why, for any sensible diet program, you can find a large number of people who will say, "It worked great for me."

But even the most successful diet plan won't work straight off the shelf for food addicts. The reason is simple: A diet is an eating plan designed to help people lose weight. However, the extra weight carried by a food addict is a *consequence* of her addiction. When a food addict goes on a diet, she's trying to treat that consequence. Clearly, for anything to really work, it has to be aimed at the cause.

## Working toward a Lighter You

*How to Make Almost Any Diet Work* is the companion book, even the instruction manual, for any diet you want to try. This book offers solutions aimed at the root of eating patterns that cause weight gain. It will show you, step by step, how to take care of your need for food in a way that makes dieting possible.

With it, you will be able to choose a diet that can work for you, because it will help you determine what adaptations will make the difference between a diet plan that works and one that disappoints you yet again.

> *You didn't fail at diets. Diets failed you.*

You *can* have a lighter body, and this book will help you make that happen. Along the way, you will make changes that improve the quality of your life remarkably. Beyond the health benefits and greater energy you will gain, you'll deepen your understanding of yourself, stand stronger in the world, and bolster your capacity for connection—and, yes, even joy.

• • •

# 2

# Don't Change a Hair on Your Head

 ❧ YOU ARE going to start doing something important almost immediately. Still, what I'm about to say may surprise you—I *don't* want you to stop eating sugar or start eating less. For now, please don't change a thing about what, how, when, where, or how much you eat.

Before we start changing things, I want you to do some research on your own body chemistry. I want you to examine how you feel before and after you eat, every hour of the day, for one week. My ulterior motive is to show you that, in the past, you didn't fail at dieting. Instead, diets failed you.

**STEP 1**

Learn your body's language.

I plan to prove to you that appetite, hunger, fullness, and satiety all result from chemicals operating inside of you. Plus, I want you to have before-and-after snapshots of your body's reaction to this program. Ultimately, you'll see for yourself that if you respect your body's chemistry, rather than push against it (as many diets cause you to do), you can maintain an eating plan for as long as necessary. The result will be a healthy, fit, energetic body that can carry you where you want to go and let you do what you want to do.

Because your body operates differently from anyone else's, only you can generate the data on your body's chemical functioning. From this information we can diagnose which of the seven causes of appetite disorder are affecting you. This identification will ultimately help you discriminate between diet advice you can follow, and advice to avoid like scalding doorknobs.

**A Special Thirty-Step Process**

You have probably heard the word *step* used in many programs. Alcoholics Anonymous and Overeaters Anonymous both have Twelve Steps. There's also a spiritual process called The 15th Step. The plan I'm giving you piece by piece is different from these programs; it is neither sponsored by them nor directly aligned with them. (Of course, they are excellent programs and could be good support to what I offer you here.)

So Step 1 of this plan is not the same as the first step of Food Addicts Anonymous. Instead, it is the first step of a unique thirty-step process that you will learn in this book. You can think of each step as one pace toward emancipation from food, or as one tread up a stairway toward a freer life.

If you feel daunted by the idea of thirty steps, remember this: Not everyone will have to take every step. And the reason for having so many steps is to make each step as easy as possible.

Each time you've tried a diet that failed you, you've taken too big a step. These thirty steps protect you from making an impossible leap. They make the process gradual enough to be successful.

Here's a peek at the first nine steps:

Step 1: Learn your body's language.

Step 2: Make a commitment to yourself.

Step 3: Make your first eating change and start following a map.

Step 4: Prepare to have the comfort you need.

Step 5: Begin eating change two: Eat snacks that are 50/50.

Step 6: Understand the chemistry of comfort.

Step 7: Improve your satiety through serotonin.

Step 8: Decode your body's signals.

Step 9: Determine which track to follow.

**Pas de Deux—A Dance for Two**

Let's begin by talking about two forces in the human body: appetite and satiety. These are like internal switches that turn your desire to eat on and off. When appetite becomes disordered, seven situations make it worse, and seven significant signals can repair it. As we work together, I will describe each of these fourteen influences on your eating.

Hunger and fullness are counterparts to appetite and satiety. Hunger, like appetite, leads to eating. Fullness, like satiety, can lead you away from food. Hunger and fullness counterbalance each other, just as appetite and satiety do.

However, each system can operate independently from the other. You can be driven to eat (appetite) without being hungry. And you can be driven away from eating (satiety) without being full.

FIGURE 3

**The Hunger-Fullness, Appetite-Satiety Relationship**

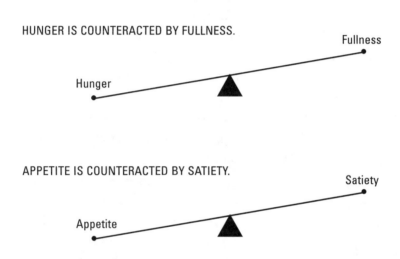

HUNGER IS COUNTERACTED BY FULLNESS.

Fullness

Hunger

APPETITE IS COUNTERACTED BY SATIETY.

Satiety

Appetite

## About Hunger

True hunger is the result of coordinated messages from your stomach and blood sugar level. When your stomach is empty, a chemical called ghrelin is released in various places, but primarily from the stomach. Ghrelin is a type of peptide that contains twenty-eight amino acids. It stimulates eating by prodding the arcuate nucleus of the hypothalamus.

Don't be scared by the technical jargon. It's important for you to know that when it comes to changing your pattern of eating, what you've been taking as personal failure is actually the result of powerful chemical reactions inside your body.

Hunger is what you feel when your stomach is empty. As the emptiness progresses and becomes a hollowness, you feel hungrier. When the stomach is empty, the brain receives a message that this situation needs to be remedied, and the suggested remedy is eating. As the stomach feels more hollow, the urge to eat increases.

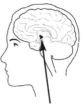

FIGURE 4

The Hypothalamus

HYPOTHALAMUS

Low blood sugar is also a condition that demands correction. Low blood sugar alarms the body, because without sufficient blood sugar, the brain quickly runs out of the fuel needed to function well. Thinking becomes cloudy, mental acuity drops, and normal mental tasks take longer to accomplish.

We experience low blood sugar differently from hunger. We feel hunger in the stomach, but we feel low blood sugar in our energy level and our ability to focus and think. It may cause a headache, a tightening of the forehead, or a darkening of vision.

When hunger accompanies low blood sugar, the hollowness seems to involve our whole body, and we are pointed toward eating. Our focus switches from other thoughts and narrows on food.

### DEFINITIONS

**Peptide**
• A chain of amino acids

**Amino Acid**
• The primary component of protein

**Protein**
• What a steak is made of. Proteins are comprised of amino acids and peptides.

**Orexins**
• Neuropeptides that stimulate eating

Hunger is initially stopped by fullness, which is what we experience when our stomachs are distended. Sensors in the stomach wall note the stretching, warmth, and heaviness caused by food and send this information to the brain.

For normal eaters, this feedback is enough to stop their eating. However, for food addicts or people with other appetite disorders, fullness may not carry enough force to stop them from eating.

Even after a meal, new hunger signals can override fullness if either ghrelin or blood sugar levels are *influenced* by the *content* of your meal. For example, we can know that we've eaten plenty, and yet an hour after eating, while still feeling full, we may begin to feel hungry again. Ghrelin is the likely culprit in this scenario. Usually an hour after eating, your ghrelin level falls, causing hunger to disappear—but if your meal was high in fat, ghrelin can rebound and cause false hunger.

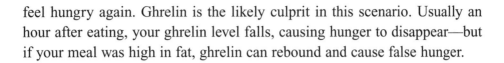

Hunger + Low Blood Sugar → Need to Eat

Eating → Fullness and Blood Sugar Rise

If you've eaten a meal high in simple sugars and carbs—such as pasta, bread, and dessert—your blood sugar may rise so quickly that your body responds with an outpouring of insulin to prevent your blood sugar level from becoming dangerously high. Thus, even if you feel stuffed, high insulin can make your blood sugar drop, causing hunger, light-headedness, and cloudy thinking. (Incidentally, insulin gets rid of extra sugar in the blood by shoving it into fat cells. If a fat cell gets too full, it divides into two fat cells. You don't want that to happen because that makes more hungry little mouths inside of you.)

No matter what combination of foods you eat at a meal, the sugars in that food are extracted first and converted to blood sugar. If you eat simple sugars and carbohydrates, such as candy or crackers, that conversion starts in the mouth and the sugars are rapidly absorbed. Alcohol also moves quickly into your system, especially when your stomach is empty.

So, you can be truly hungry because your stomach is empty. You can also feel hungry, even though you've recently eaten, if you've had a meal that was high in fat and/or simple sugars or carbs.

## Appetite and Satiety

Appetite and satiety result from the operation of other chemicals, and they are different from hunger and fullness in an interesting way. Hunger and fullness occur across a continuum based on your own internal sense of the state of your stomach. You can be mildly hungry, really hungry, or starving. You can be nearly full, full enough, very full, or stuffed.

Satiety, instead, operates like a light switch. It is either on or off. You are satiated, or you are not. Appetite is similar. It is usually either on or off. (Although appetite *can* be amplified by one factor: food addiction.) If the appetite switch is thrown, you may still appear to be working or driving or tending the children, but inside of you, a mechanism is pointing you toward food.

When appetite is driving you, you can eat and eat and eat some more. It doesn't taper off. It stays in forward gear until it is turned off by satiety, or until food consumption causes sleepiness, shame, or an end to the food supply.

### Satiety

Whereas fullness can stop hunger, satiety stops appetite. Satiety results from certain chemical signals—different signals from those that indicate fullness. If you're eating when these signals fire, they tell you to stop eating. You immediately lose your desire for food and your attention goes elsewhere.

Generally, a person who is overweight has a defect in reaching satiety. This is not the whole story, but it is a significant part of the story. We'll talk more about this shortly.

### Appetite

Appetite is another line of chemical communications about eating. When particular bundles of nuclei in the hypothalamus are stimulated, they cause appetite, or the urge to eat.

Numerous conditions can stimulate appetite and some of these have nothing to do with hunger. Thus you can have a strong urge to eat or even crave certain foods without being hungry.

*Whereas hunger is a function of immediate energy needs, appetite is a function of survival.* Appetite is concerned with the survival of the body as a whole, and it makes adjustments in response to threats to survival, such as fasting and danger.

> **Hypothalamus**
>
> The hypothalamus is located on the underside of the brain. It regulates sleep, thirst, sex drive, body temperature, mood, and appetite.

### Hunger vs. Appetite and Fullness vs. Satiety

You can have an appetite without being hungry, which means you can crave food desperately even though your blood sugar is fine and your stomach is comfortable.

Similarly, you can be full and not satiated. Your tummy can be stuffed to the hurting point, and yet you want to keep on eating. Your first task will be to discriminate among these four forces.

**Energy Needs**

What are *your* body's signals to eat? How do *you* know when you are hungry? In the list below, check any of the signals that you sometimes experience. If you like, add any other signal you've noticed.

**Hunger Signals**

☐   Your stomach feels empty or hollow.

☐   Your stomach growls.

☐   Your stomach demands your attention.

☐   Your stomach feels like it's caved in.

☐   _____

☐   _____

☐   _____

**Low Blood Sugar Signals**

☐   You have trouble concentrating.

☐   You have to do the same mental task over and over. (For example, you reread the same words two or three times and still don't understand them.)

☐   You struggle with mental tasks that are usually easy for you.

☐   You start losing the big picture.

☐   You feel light-headed.

☐   Your thinking feels cloudy or imprecise.

☐   Your head starts aching.

☐   Your vision clouds or darkens.

☐   You feel hungry.

☐   You say, "I need to eat."

☐   Your energy level drops.

☐   You lose alertness.

☐   You find it difficult to make decisions.

☐    You feel irritable, snappy, or grouchy.

☐    _____

☐    _____

☐    _____

## Catching Your Appetite Switch in Action

True hunger means you just need food, period. Appetite makes you want a particular kind of food. The following signals indicate that you are experiencing appetite rather than hunger.

*Appetite Signals*

- Feeling excited about an opportunity to eat
- Anticipation of eating eclipsing other aspects of a situation, such as the company or the occasion
- Having intrusive thoughts of food
- Making a hidden plan to eat
- Picturing a food or a restaurant almost unconsciously
- Appearing to function well, yet at the back of your mind being preoccupied with food pictures, restaurant routes, or plans to eat
- Making arrangements to get a particular food even if it requires you to manipulate people or circumstances
- Giving yourself (or others) legitimate reasons for going to a certain place, when in fact your goal is a particular food source
- Wanting a certain food very, very much
- Feeling driven to eat or to get a particular food
- Eating without being able to stop
- Eating, or wanting to eat, larger portions than other people
- Getting preoccupied with someone else's serving if it looks bigger than yours
- Feeling anger toward a server or restaurant if your portion is smaller than someone else's

- Getting preoccupied with another person's unfinished dessert or starch
- Choosing your entrée based on the starches that are included with it (e.g., choosing the spaghetti because it is served with garlic bread, rather than the quiche because it is served with fruit)
- Having difficulty listening to the conversation at your table because you want seconds or are thinking about going back to the buffet table
- Making plans, while still eating your first serving, to get your next serving
- Eating for a longer time span than a meal usually lasts
- Eating quickly
- Eating lots of simple carbs or sugars
- Eating even though you feel full

Over the next few days, when you feel an urge to eat, examine the urge closely. When is hunger growling at you, and when is appetite driving your thoughts?

**Fullness or Satiety?**

Fullness is experienced in the stomach. It is a physical sensation. Satiety is much more difficult to recognize because it's the absence of appetite. Many overeaters have so little acquaintance with satiety that they don't begin to recognize it until they've been on this program for a few weeks.

Satiety is the absence of food thoughts, the disappearance of appetite, and a complete lack of interest in eating. An analogy would be the feeling you have ten minutes after a headache is gone. You're suddenly released and alive—your headache forgotten. When you are satiated, food is forgotten. The following lists can help you differentiate between fullness and satiety.

*Fullness Signals*

- Your stomach no longer feels empty.
- Your stomach feels comfortable.
- Your stomach feels satisfied, warm, or heavy.
- Your stomach feels too full or on the edge of being uncomfortably full.
- You feel stuffed.

*Satiety Signals*

- Your appetite disappears.
- You have no interest in food.
- You're interested in something other than eating.
- You're ready, even impatient, to leave the table to do something else.
- The food on your plate loses all appeal.
- You want to push your plate away.
- Food seems repugnant or offensive.
- You can't make yourself eat.

**It's Not Your Fault**

Many of my clients with appetite disorder, before embracing a recovery program, report that they haven't felt hunger in years. Lots of factors drive their eating, but hunger is not one of them.

If this is true for you too, then know that you are not alone. Millions of us eat for reasons other than hunger—primarily we eat to soothe ourselves.

Sometimes it seems as if everything connected with food or eating is shameful. If you do feel shame about your relationship with food or about your body, that shame may make it hard for you to look at yourself and what you eat.

But let's look deeper. What is shameful about needing to be soothed? Life *is* too hard at times. Sometimes eating is the only way we are able to give ourselves a break. You are not to blame because life has hurt you, and you are not wrong for needing to stop the hurt.

Obviously, if you learned to turn to food for relief, you weren't taught other ways to soothe yourself. Over the years, you learned that food made you feel better. Good for you. You found a way to survive.

Soon I'm going to teach you what you need to know so that you'll have other options besides eating when you need relief.

I'm asking you to trust me here because once you begin to understand the degree to which your eating is chemically driven—way beyond your conscious control—you'll start to see that overeating is not your fault.

Later in this book, you'll discover ways to take responsibility for your appetite and free yourself from its control. In the meantime, I'm a witness testifying that you didn't knowingly choose to have an appetite disorder. The problem snuck up on you slowly and had you in its clutches long before you knew what was going on.

## You Deserve to Eat

Sadly, for you, one of the most natural acts for all living creatures—eating— has become one of dread and shame. But we all must eat, even turtles and rhododendrons. It couldn't be more basic—to feed yourself, to be nurtured.

You deserve to eat, and you deserve to eat without feeling guilty about it. So bear with me. In the pages to come, you'll slowly learn what you need to make a pivotal life change: the information, the skill training, and the step-by-step alterations. You'll also develop a new relationship with your own fine self.

One of the reasons we overeat is so that we can, for a time, lose ourselves. We have an inner pain that we don't think we can bear getting close to. The act of eating drops a curtain in front of that pain. Yet here I am, asking you to look inside, which is, I know, asking a lot. I'm inviting you to raise the curtain and to start feeling what is going on inside your body in relation to hunger and eating.

At first, this will seem hard. Many of us who are now in recovery thought, at the beginning, *Maybe this can change for other people, but it won't work for me.* I understand that discouragement. When we've been defeated by food and appetite over and over, we have trouble believing we could stop being victimized by it.

I won't ask you to change anything yet. For now, just draw back enough of the curtain to notice the interplay of appetite, hunger, fullness, satiety, and blood sugar in your own body.

I'll be with you every step of the way, with help, concern, encouragement, and understanding. Remember, many others, including me, have walked this same path and come out the other side happier, healthier, more relaxed, and lighter. You can walk it too.

On your journey, willingness will be your most important asset. If you can find the willingness to let go of what hasn't been working and give this program your best shot by following each of its steps, it will move your life powerfully.

Thousands of others (including myself) have taken this same plunge. We've had to develop our own willingness, to let go of ineffective ideas, and to trust others who have gone before us. Join us. We welcome you.

**Your Body Signals Chart**

You'll start by keeping a record of your body signals. This exercise has several purposes:

- To provide practice detecting the difference between appetite and hunger signals, and between fullness and satiety signals.
- To give a visual representation of the relationship between the foods you eat and your physical states.
- To give you a "before" record that will help you see and appreciate the progress you make as your body's chemical functioning changes.
- To diagnose the causes of your appetite disorder.
- To begin your "willingness" training.

The following Body Signals Chart* is really four minicharts in one, arranged along a timeline.

- Top chart: the chemical composition of the foods you eat.
- Chart above the middle timeline: your fluid intake.
- Chart under the middle timeline: your fullness, hunger, appetite, and satiety levels.
- Bottom chart: your blood sugar and energy indicators.

Let's look at how to use each one of these four minicharts.

*Food*

If you've ever been on a diet (like we haven't field-tested nearly every diet to come along!), you've probably been asked to keep a food diary. This is a record of all the foods you eat each day. My experience with this, both personally and with clients, is that we record what we are eating when we think we are being good, and we neglect to write down foods when we think we are being bad. Soon the diary becomes a tyrant, scrutinizing us with drawn brows. We resent it, feeling both controlled and confined by it. That's a lot of power to give a piece of paper.

---

* This chart and all upcoming Body Signals Charts can also be found in Appendix E.

# Body Signals Chart, Week 1

Date: _____

| CATEGORY | DESCRIPTIONS | BASELINE DATA—NO CHANGES | | | | | | | | | | | | | | | | | | | | | | |
|---|---|---|---|---|---|---|---|---|---|---|---|---|---|---|---|---|---|---|---|---|---|---|---|---|---|
| Timeline | Circle Wake-up | 6AM | 7 | 8 | 9 | 10 | 11 | 12PM | 1 | 2 | 3 | 4 | 5 | 6 | 7 | 8 | 9 | 10 | 11 | 12AM | 1 | 2 | 3 | 4 | 5 |
| **Food**<br>*Numbers go in this section* | Proteins | | | | | | | | | | | | | | | | | | | | | | | | |
| | Complex carbs | | | | | | | | | | | | | | | | | | | | | | | | |
| | Simple carbs | | | | | | | | | | | | | | | | | | | | | | | | |
| | Fats | | | | | | | | | | | | | | | | | | | | | | | | |
| Check | **Equal/NutraSweet** | | | | | | | | | | | | | | | | | | | | | | | | |
| **Drink**<br>*Dots go in this section* | Water | | | | | | | | | | | | | | | | | | | | | | | | |
| | Pop | | | | | | | | | | | | | | | | | | | | | | | | |
| | Diet pop | | | | | | | | | | | | | | | | | | | | | | | | |
| | Coffee | | | | | | | | | | | | | | | | | | | | | | | | |
| | Herbal drink | | | | | | | | | | | | | | | | | | | | | | | | |
| | Milk | | | | | | | | | | | | | | | | | | | | | | | | |
| | Juice | | | | | | | | | | | | | | | | | | | | | | | | |
| | Alcohol | | | | | | | | | | | | | | | | | | | | | | | | |
| | Tea | | | | | | | | | | | | | | | | | | | | | | | | |
| Check | **Caffeine** | | | | | | | | | | | | | | | | | | | | | | | | |
| Timeline | | 6AM | 7 | 8 | 9 | 10 | 11 | 12PM | 1 | 2 | 3 | 4 | 5 | 6 | 7 | 8 | 9 | 10 | 11 | 12AM | 1 | 2 | 3 | 4 | 5 |
| **Fullness** | Stuffed | | | | | | | | | | | | | | | | | | | | | | | | |
| | Comfortable | | | | | | | | | | | | | | | | | | | | | | | | |
| | Empty | | | | | | | | | | | | | | | | | | | | | | | | |
| **Hunger** | Starving | | | | | | | | | | | | | | | | | | | | | | | | |
| | Really hungry | | | | | | | | | | | | | | | | | | | | | | | | |
| | Mildly hungry | | | | | | | | | | | | | | | | | | | | | | | | |
| | Not hungry | | | | | | | | | | | | | | | | | | | | | | | | |
| **Appetite** | Craving food | | | | | | | | | | | | | | | | | | | | | | | | |
| | Food focused | | | | | | | | | | | | | | | | | | | | | | | | |
| | Quiet | | | | | | | | | | | | | | | | | | | | | | | | |
| **Satiety** | Satiated | | | | | | | | | | | | | | | | | | | | | | | | |
| | Not | | | | | | | | | | | | | | | | | | | | | | | | |
| **Energy** | High | | | | | | | | | | | | | | | | | | | | | | | | |
| | Medium | | | | | | | | | | | | | | | | | | | | | | | | |
| | Low | | | | | | | | | | | | | | | | | | | | | | | | |
| **Thinking** | Very sharp | | | | | | | | | | | | | | | | | | | | | | | | |
| | Clear | | | | | | | | | | | | | | | | | | | | | | | | |
| | Cloudy | | | | | | | | | | | | | | | | | | | | | | | | |
| **Blood Sugar Reaction** | Headache | | | | | | | | | | | | | | | | | | | | | | | | |
| | Light-headed | | | | | | | | | | | | | | | | | | | | | | | | |
| | Even | | | | | | | | | | | | | | | | | | | | | | | | |
| | Sugar daze | | | | | | | | | | | | | | | | | | | | | | | | |
| | Sleepy | | | | | | | | | | | | | | | | | | | | | | | | |
| **Mood** | Optimistic | | | | | | | | | | | | | | | | | | | | | | | | |
| | Okay | | | | | | | | | | | | | | | | | | | | | | | | |
| | Depressed | | | | | | | | | | | | | | | | | | | | | | | | |
| **Stressed?** | Highly | | | | | | | | | | | | | | | | | | | | | | | | |
| | Mildly | | | | | | | | | | | | | | | | | | | | | | | | |
| | No | | | | | | | | | | | | | | | | | | | | | | | | |
| **Seeking Comfort?** | | | | | | | | | | | | | | | | | | | | | | | | | |
| Timeline | | 6AM | 7 | 8 | 9 | 10 | 11 | 12PM | 1 | 2 | 3 | 4 | 5 | 6 | 7 | 8 | 9 | 10 | 11 | 12AM | 1 | 2 | 3 | 4 | 5 |

Duplicating this page for personal use is permissible.

The chart I'm asking you to fill in is different. It isn't about being good or bad; it is simply about what you eat and how you feel. I want you to pay attention to what you eat—not as a form of control or embarrassment, but to help you notice that certain foods lead to chemical changes that, in turn, influence your physical state. You'll begin to see foods as the chemicals that compose them and relate how these chemicals create positive and negative changes in your body.

The system taught here may seem a little awkward at first, but it's quick and easy to use once you learn it. Here's how it works:

You don't have to write down everything you eat. Instead, look at the food you eat in an hour's time as a bunch of chemicals that can be divided into proportions of proteins, complex carbs, simple carbs, and fats. Notice that you don't need to record the amount you eat. The quantity might be a little or a lot, but we're not looking at that.

| Timeline | | 6AM | 7 | 8 | 9 | 10 | 11 | 12PM |
|---|---|---|---|---|---|---|---|---|
| **Food** | Proteins | | | | | | | |
| | Complex carbs | | | | | | | |
| *Numbers go in this section* | Simple carbs | | | | | | | |
| | Fats | | | | | | | |

In any given hour, consider the total of all the food you eat as ten units. Then decide how many of those ten units are fats, how many are proteins, how many are simple carbs, and how many are complex carbs. (More on carbs in a moment.)

For example, if from 9 to 10 a.m., you ate nothing but a pat of butter, you would put a ten in the fats box below 9 a.m. If you ate nothing but a cup of mayonnaise, you'd still put a ten in the fats box. Again, it's not the quantity, but the proportion that you are measuring.

*Pat of butter or cup of mayonnaise*

| Timeline | | 6AM | 7 | 8 | 9 | 10 | 11 | 12PM |
|---|---|---|---|---|---|---|---|---|
| **Food** | Proteins | | | | | | | |
| | Complex carbs | | | | | | | |
| *Numbers go in this section* | Simple carbs | | | | | | | |
| | Fats | | | | 10 | | | |

Now, let's suppose that, instead, you eat an apple and a slice of cheese at 9 a.m. You would put a five in the complex carbs box for the apple and a five in the proteins box for the cheese. (Most cheese is primarily protein, so you'd list it as a protein.) Perfect accuracy isn't the point; you're trying to paint a general portrait here, not design a computer chip. Measure individual foods according to their predominant category. For example, you would count bacon and cream as fats, and milk, eggs, and most meat as protein.

*Apple and cheese*

| Timeline | | | 6AM | 7 | 8 | 9 | 10 | 11 | 12PM |
|---|---|---|---|---|---|---|---|---|---|
| **Food** | | Proteins | | | | 5 | | | |
| | | Complex carbs | | | | 5 | | | |
| *Numbers go in this section* | | Simple carbs | | | | | | | |
| | | Fats | | | | | | | |

If you eat a peanut butter sandwich on multigrain bread, that would count as a five in the fats box and a five in the simple carbs box. (Peanut butter contains more fat than protein, and most commercial multigrain breads have more simple than complex carbs.)

*Peanut butter sandwich*

| Timeline | | | 6AM | 7 | 8 | 9 | 10 | 11 | 12PM |
|---|---|---|---|---|---|---|---|---|---|
| **Food** | | Proteins | | | | | | | |
| | | Complex carbs | | | | | | | |
| *Numbers go in this section* | | Simple carbs | | | | 5 | | | |
| | | Fats | | | | 5 | | | |

At the bottom of the food section, there's a row labeled NutraSweet and Equal. Make a check mark any time you have a food or drink that contains these artificial sweeteners.

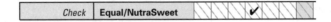

| *Check* | **Equal/NutraSweet** | | | | ✔ | | | |
|---|---|---|---|---|---|---|---|---|

## Simple vs. Complex Carbs

For now, list any sugary product as a simple carb. This includes honey, molasses, maple syrup, dried fruit, and fruit juice. You'll learn why later. White bread (including French and Italian bread, focaccia, pizza crust, etc.), multigrain bread, restaurant-quality wheat bread, pita bread, white rice, corn chips, tortillas, pasta, and other ethnic starches should all be counted as simple carbs.

Only 100 percent whole-grain products (breads, pastas, rolls, etc.), brown and wild rice, whole fruits, and all vegetables should be listed as complex carbs.

If you're saying, *Wait a minute, I know my food groups and it's not that simple,* relax. Please don't focus on categorizing foods perfectly. You need to resist that tendency because it distracts from the value of this exercise. It's far more important that you begin the practice of looking into your body, the food you put into it, and the effect that food has on your mood, energy, and mental clarity. Throughout this book, you'll find lots of examples to use as guidelines.

## Fluids

In the second minichart—the one right above the middle timeline—you'll put a dot for each cup (eight ounces) of fluid that you drink. For example, if you drink three eight-ounce glasses of water between 10 and 11 a.m., you will mark three dots in the water box below 10 a.m. If, at noon, you drink one cup of herbal tea and a sixteen-ounce Sprite, you'll put one dot in the herbal box and two dots in the pop box below 12 p.m.

| Timeline | | 6AM | 7 | 8 | 9 | 10 | 11 | 12PM |
|---|---|---|---|---|---|---|---|---|
| **Drink** | Water | | | | | ••• | | |
| | Pop | | | | | | | •• |
| *Dots go in this section* | Diet pop | | | | | | | |
| | Coffee | | | | | | | |
| | Herbal drink | | | | | | | • |
| | Milk | | | | | | | |
| | Juice | | | | | | | |
| | Alcohol | | | | | | | |
| | Tea | | | | | | | |
| *Check* | Caffeine | | | | | | | |

Any time you drink something that contains caffeine, such as a Pepsi, coffee, or nonherbal tea, then *in addition* to the dot in the appropriate box, place a check mark in the caffeine box for that hour as well. Don't worry about recording a splash of milk in your coffee, but if you have an eight-ounce latte, half dots should go in both the milk and coffee boxes.

*Cola*

| Timeline | | 6 AM | 7 | 8 | 9 | 10 | 11 | 12 PM |
|---|---|---|---|---|---|---|---|---|
| **Drink** | Water | | | | | | | |
| | Pop | | • | | | | | |
| *Dots go in this section* | Diet pop | | | | | | | |
| | Coffee | | | | | | | |
| | Herbal drink | | | | | | | |
| | Milk | | | | | | | |
| | Juice | | | | | | | |
| | Alcohol | | | | | | | |
| | Tea | | | | | | | |
| *Check* | Caffeine | | ✔ | | | | | |

Milk is both a drink and a protein, so eight ounces of milk gets a dot in the milk box *and* a number in the proteins box. Cocoa made with milk gets a dot in the milk box, numbers in the simple carbs and proteins boxes, and a check in the caffeine box. (Cocoa is illustrated below at 9 a.m. on the timeline.)

*Milk      Cocoa*

| Timeline | | 6 AM | 7 | 8 | 9 | 10 | 11 | 12 PM |
|---|---|---|---|---|---|---|---|---|
| **Food** | Proteins | 10 | | | 5 | | | |
| | Complex carbs | | | | | | | |
| *Numbers go in this section* | Simple carbs | | | | 5 | | | |
| | Fats | | | | | | | |
| **Drink** | Water | | | | | | | |
| | Pop | | | | | | | |
| *Dots go in this section* | Diet pop | | | | | | | |
| | Coffee | | | | | | | |
| | Herbal drink | | | | | | | |
| | Milk | • | | | • | | | |
| | Juice | | | | | | | |
| | Alcohol | | | | | | | |
| | Tea | | | | | | | |
| *Check* | Caffeine | | | | ✔ | | | |

Again, don't worry about being perfect, and allow yourself a learning curve. Remember that you're in training. You are building a foundation that will save you from having to keep a food diary later on.

### Stimulation to Eat or to Stop Eating

Beneath the timeline is a minichart for measuring appetite, hunger, fullness, and satiety. These boxes need only a dot to record how you're feeling. Once an hour, pause and pay attention to the inside of your body. Feel what's happening in your stomach. If it's empty, place a dot in the empty box found in the fullness category. If you are hungry, how hungry are you—mildly hungry, really hungry, or starving? Put a dot in the appropriate hunger box. (See 6 a.m. on the timeline below for an example.)

| Timeline | | | 6AM | 7 | 8 | 9 | 10 | 11 | 12PM | 1 | 2 | 3 | 4 |
|---|---|---|---|---|---|---|---|---|---|---|---|---|---|
| **Fullness** | Stuffed | | | | | | | | | | • | • | |
| | Comfortable | | | | • | • | • | | | | | | • |
| | Empty | | • | • | | | | • | • | • | | | |
| **Hunger** | Starving | | | • | | | | | | | • | | |
| | Really hungry | | • | | | | | | | • | | | |
| | Mildly hungry | | | | | | | • | | | | • | |
| | Not hungry | | | | • | • | • | | | | | • | • |
| **Appetite** | Craving food | | | • | | | | | | | • | | |
| | Food focused | | • | | | | | • | • | • | | • | |
| | Quiet | | | | • | • | • | | | | | | • |
| **Satiety** | Satiated | | | | • | • | • | | | | | | |
| | Not | | • | • | | | | • | • | • | • | • | |

Next, notice what's happening with your appetite. (You may want to reread the appetite signals list on page 18.) Are you having any signs of appetite, such as thoughts about food or a desire for a particular food? If so, put a dot in the food focused box in the appetite category. (See 6 a.m. on the timeline above.)

Or is your appetite more intense? Are you craving food, feeling driven to eat, or willing to manipulate your current situation to set up eating? Then put a dot in the craving food box. (See 7 a.m. on the timeline above.)

Next it's time to examine your fullness. Is your stomach full? If so, how full is it? If you feel stuffed, then the stuffed box gets a dot. (See 2 p.m. on the time-line above.)

Many overeaters feel satiety so infrequently that at first they may not recognize it. Still, we often have one moment of satiety—when we first get up in the morning. (I'll explain why very soon.) If that's a time when you feel divorced from food, or are even confident that you won't overeat for the day, that's satiety. Satiety is a complete lack of interest in food, even a feeling of revulsion at the idea of eating.

### Body Chemistry Indicators

The bottom minichart is where you pay attention to various indicators of your energy, thinking, blood sugar, mood, and stress levels. Track these levels in the same way you tracked your feelings about eating earlier.

| Timeline | | 6 AM | 7 | 8 | 9 | 10 | 11 | 12 PM | 1 | 2 | 3 | 4 |
|---|---|---|---|---|---|---|---|---|---|---|---|---|
| **Energy** | High | | • | | | | | | | | | |
| | Medium | • | | • | • | | | | | | | |
| | Low | | | | | • | • | | | | | |
| **Thinking** | Very sharp | | • | | | | | | | | | |
| | Clear | • | | • | • | | | | | | | |
| | Cloudy | | | | | • | • | | | | | |
| **Blood Sugar Reaction** | Headache | | | | | | • | | | | | |
| | Light-headed | • | | | | • | | | | | | |
| | Even | | | • | • | • | | | | | | |
| | Sugar daze | | | | | | | | | | | |
| | Sleepy | | | | | | | | | | | |
| **Mood** | Optimistic | | | | | | | | | | | |
| | Okay | • | • | • | • | | | | | | | |
| | Depressed | | | | | • | • | | | | | |
| **Stressed?** | Highly | | | | | | | | | | | |
| | Mildly | | | | • | • | • | | | | | |
| | No | • | • | • | | | | | | | | |

### What to Do

Please make seven photocopies of the blank chart on page 23. For one week, carry a new blank copy with you each day. Circle the time you wake up and fill in the boxes once each hour, beginning when you first get up and ending just before you go to sleep. Please do not look back at the previous days' charts to compare.

If you miss an hour, think back and fill in the chart as best you can. (I've noticed that if I wait even two hours before filling in my chart, I have trouble recalling my body states for the previous hours. Our body states are transient. We know the now of them much better than we know their past.)

**Please do not skip this exercise.** I know it's tempting to dash ahead when you've been longing for an answer, but I want to prove to you something important about your body.

When the first week is over, save your seven daily charts because the following week I'm going to give you an experiment to do. Then you'll make new charts that you'll compare to your charts from this week. (You'll keep daily charts for four weeks, as you make three eating changes, one per week. At the end of that time, we'll be able to diagnose most of the causes of your disordered appetite.)

*Again, please don't change anything* about the way you normally eat. Resist the tendency to "be good" (or to "be bad"), so that your chart does not look as it typically would for you. You will discover much more if you have an accurate baseline of what is normal for you. Don't cheat yourself out of the impact of this demonstration by changing your eating habits this week.

---

### WHY DO THIS EXERCISE?

1. You will learn to use a tool that you'll need several times throughout this book.

2. You will learn to discriminate between appetite and hunger.

3. You will watch for moments of satiety.

4. You will observe the impact eating and not eating have on other important body functions.

5. You will notice how these important indicators change after you try some of the suggestions in this book.

6. You will exercise your "willingness" muscles.

7. You will practice doing something splendid for yourself.

8. You will discover that you can influence the chemical processes inside your body.

9. You will use your daily charts to diagnose the causes of your appetite disorder.

---

*Food Proportions*

Probably the most difficult aspect of the chart is figuring out the proportions of proteins, fats, and simple and complex carbs in the foods you eat. You may be asking, *Is this about calories or portion size? Is this about measuring or weighing?*

My answer is this: You can be precise if it's important to you. It isn't important to me. A good guess makes me happy.

I know this about you: You already know a lot about food.

| FOOD PROPORTIONS SPELLED OUT |
|---|
| 10 = Entire meal or only ingredient |
| 9 = Most of meal or nearly all of the ingredients |
| 8 = Large portion |
| 7 = Two-thirds of the meal or ingredients |
| 6 = More than half, but less than two-thirds of the meal or any other ingredient |
| 5 = Half of the meal or ingredients |
| 4 = Almost half of the meal or ingredients |
| 3 = One-third of the meal or ingredients |
| 2 = Small portion or amount of ingredients |
| 1 = Tiny part of the meal or ingredients |

You probably know the approximate calorie counts of a variety of foods. You probably know that a gram of fat has more than twice the calories of a gram of carbohydrate or protein.

You may find that if you start by figuring out what number goes into the fats category, the others are easier to estimate.

For example, a snack of cheese and crackers may look like this:

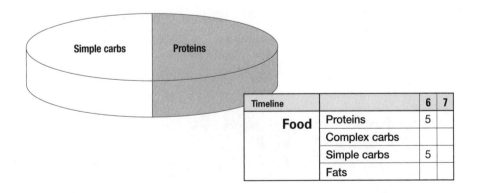

| Timeline | | 6 | 7 |
|---|---|---|---|
| **Food** | Proteins | 5 | |
| | Complex carbs | | |
| | Simple carbs | 5 | |
| | Fats | | |

31

Whereas a more complex meal of meat, salad, potatoes, butter, and salad dressing could look like this:

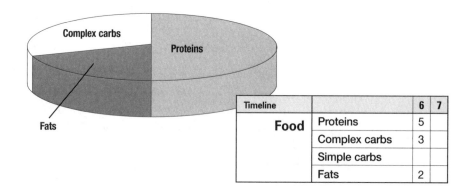

| Timeline | | 6 | 7 |
|---|---|---|---|
| Food | Proteins | 5 | |
| | Complex carbs | 3 | |
| | Simple carbs | | |
| | Fats | 2 | |

How did I get these figures? The salad dressing and butter are fats. Their volume is tiny, which would give them a value of 1; however, fats are doubled because their caloric value is twice that of the foods in other categories. Therefore, I assign the fats category with a value of 2.

The meal contains no simple carbs. Salad and potatoes make up less than half the meal, and meat is dense. So I assign the meat a value of 5, half the meal, which leaves 3 as the value for the complex carbs.

Add a roll, and the picture changes yet again, especially if you add more butter. The butter for the roll increases the fat portion from 2 to 2.5. The roll is still a smaller portion than the salad and potato, so the value assigned to it is smaller—1.5. This causes the proportions of the meat and complex carbs to shift.

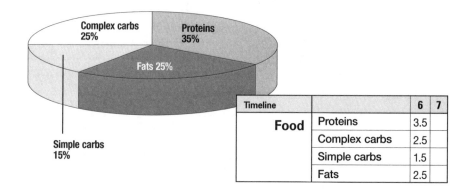

| Timeline | | 6 | 7 |
|---|---|---|---|
| Food | Proteins | 3.5 | |
| | Complex carbs | 2.5 | |
| | Simple carbs | 1.5 | |
| | Fats | 2.5 | |

Now add a rich dessert. The rich dessert increases the fat portion yet again. Now the fat portion increases from 2.5 to 3, becoming a third of the meal. The rest of the dessert is comprised of simple carbs. Now the simple carbs—the roll and the dessert—are a larger portion than the salad and potato. They trade proportions. Taken together, the fats and carbs are now two-thirds of the meal, reducing the meat portion to a third.

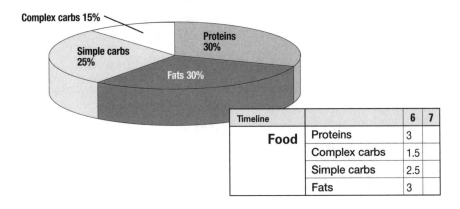

| Timeline | | 6 | 7 |
|---|---|---|---|
| **Food** | Proteins | 3 | |
| | Complex carbs | 1.5 | |
| | Simple carbs | 2.5 | |
| | Fats | 3 | |

## Sample Meals

*Meal: Plain omelet*

| **Food** | Proteins | 10 | |
|---|---|---|---|
| | Complex carbs | | |
| | Simple carbs | | |
| | Fats | | |

*Meal: Sausage omelet*

| **Food** | Proteins | 6 | |
|---|---|---|---|
| | Complex carbs | | |
| | Simple carbs | | |
| | Fats | 4 | |

*Meal: Cream cheese omelet, restaurant wheat toast, butter*

| **Food** | Proteins | 4 | |
|---|---|---|---|
| | Complex carbs | | |
| | Simple carbs | 3 | |
| | Fats | 3 | |

*Meal: Cream cheese omelet, potatoes, sourdough toast, butter*

| **Food** | Proteins | 3 | |
|---|---|---|---|
| | Complex carbs | 1 | |
| | Simple carbs | 2 | |
| | Fats | 4 | |

*Snack: Hard candy*

| Food | | | |
|------|------|------|---|
| | Proteins | | |
| | Complex carbs | | |
| | Simple carbs | 10 | |
| | Fats | | |

*Meal: Hamburger on a bun and fries*

| Food | | | |
|------|------|------|---|
| | Proteins | 3 | |
| | Complex carbs | 1 | |
| | Simple carbs | 2 | |
| | Fats | 4 | |

*Meal: Green salad with assorted veggies and blue cheese dressing*

| Food | | | |
|------|------|------|---|
| | Proteins | 1 | |
| | Complex carbs | 7 | |
| | Simple carbs | | |
| | Fats | 2 | |

*Meal: Fish and chips*

| Food | | | |
|------|------|------|---|
| | Proteins | 4 | |
| | Complex carbs | 2 | |
| | Simple carbs | | |
| | Fats | 4 | |

*Meal: Vegetable soup and green salad with oil and vinegar dressing*

| Food | | | |
|------|------|------|---|
| | Proteins | | |
| | Complex carbs | 9 | |
| | Simple carbs | | |
| | Fats | 1 | |

*Meal: Fish and chips, coleslaw, and garlic bread*

| Food | | | |
|------|------|------|---|
| | Proteins | 2 | |
| | Complex carbs | 2 | |
| | Simple carbs | 1 | |
| | Fats | 5 | |

*Meal: Clam chowder and green salad with Italian dressing*

| Food | | | |
|------|------|------|---|
| | Proteins | 1 | |
| | Complex carbs | 5 | |
| | Simple carbs | 2 | |
| | Fats | 2 | |

*Meal: Steak and green salad with ranch dressing*

| Food | | | |
|------|------|------|---|
| | Proteins | 6 | |
| | Complex carbs | 1 | |
| | Simple carbs | | |
| | Fats | 3 | |

*Meal: Hamburger on a bun and green salad with dressing*

| Food | | | |
|------|------|------|---|
| | Proteins | 4 | |
| | Complex carbs | 2 | |
| | Simple carbs | 2 | |
| | Fats | 2 | |

*Meal: Steak, potato, sour cream, butter, and green salad with vinegar and oil*

| Food | | | |
|------|------|------|---|
| | Proteins | 4 | |
| | Complex carbs | 2 | |
| | Simple carbs | | |
| | Fats | 4 | |

*Meal: Salmon, wild rice, and steamed veggies*

| Food | | |
|------|------|---|
| | Proteins | 8 |
| | Complex carbs | 2 |
| | Simple carbs | |
| | Fats | |

*Meal: Fettuccini alfredo, green salad with Italian dressing, garlic breadsticks*

| Food | | |
|------|------|---|
| | Proteins | 1 |
| | Complex carbs | 1 |
| | Simple carbs | 5 |
| | Fats | 3 |

*Meal: Sausage pizza*

| Food | | |
|------|------|---|
| | Proteins | 1 |
| | Complex carbs | 1 |
| | Simple carbs | 4 |
| | Fats | 4 |

*Snack: Apple and cheese*

| Food | | |
|------|------|---|
| | Proteins | 5 |
| | Complex carbs | 5 |
| | Simple carbs | |
| | Fats | |

You now have the tools you need to observe your eating and your body's reactions for one week. When you're ready, please begin. Feel free, during this next week, to read the next four chapters.

. . .

# Body Signals Chart, Week 1

Date: _____

| CATEGORY | DESCRIPTIONS | BASELINE DATA—NO CHANGES | | | | | | | | | | | | | | | | | | | | | | | |
|---|---|---|---|---|---|---|---|---|---|---|---|---|---|---|---|---|---|---|---|---|---|---|---|---|---|
| Timeline | Circle Wake-up | 6AM | 7 | 8 | 9 | 10 | 11 | 12PM | 1 | 2 | 3 | 4 | 5 | 6 | 7 | 8 | 9 | 10 | 11 | 12AM | 1 | 2 | 3 | 4 | 5 |
| **Food** | Proteins | | | | | | | | | | | | | | | | | | | | | | | | |
| *Numbers go in this section* | Complex carbs | | | | | | | | | | | | | | | | | | | | | | | | |
| | Simple carbs | | | | | | | | | | | | | | | | | | | | | | | | |
| | Fats | | | | | | | | | | | | | | | | | | | | | | | | |
| *Check* | **Equal/NutraSweet** | | | | | | | | | | | | | | | | | | | | | | | | |
| **Drink** | Water | | | | | | | | | | | | | | | | | | | | | | | | |
| *Dots go in this section* | Pop | | | | | | | | | | | | | | | | | | | | | | | | |
| | Diet pop | | | | | | | | | | | | | | | | | | | | | | | | |
| | Coffee | | | | | | | | | | | | | | | | | | | | | | | | |
| | Herbal drink | | | | | | | | | | | | | | | | | | | | | | | | |
| | Milk | | | | | | | | | | | | | | | | | | | | | | | | |
| | Juice | | | | | | | | | | | | | | | | | | | | | | | | |
| | Alcohol | | | | | | | | | | | | | | | | | | | | | | | | |
| | Tea | | | | | | | | | | | | | | | | | | | | | | | | |
| *Check* | **Caffeine** | | | | | | | | | | | | | | | | | | | | | | | | |
| Timeline | | 6AM | 7 | 8 | 9 | 10 | 11 | 12PM | 1 | 2 | 3 | 4 | 5 | 6 | 7 | 8 | 9 | 10 | 11 | 12AM | 1 | 2 | 3 | 4 | 5 |
| **Fullness** | Stuffed | | | | | | | | | | | | | | | | | | | | | | | | |
| | Comfortable | | | | | | | | | | | | | | | | | | | | | | | | |
| | Empty | | | | | | | | | | | | | | | | | | | | | | | | |
| **Hunger** | Starving | | | | | | | | | | | | | | | | | | | | | | | | |
| | Really hungry | | | | | | | | | | | | | | | | | | | | | | | | |
| | Mildly hungry | | | | | | | | | | | | | | | | | | | | | | | | |
| | Not hungry | | | | | | | | | | | | | | | | | | | | | | | | |
| **Appetite** | Craving food | | | | | | | | | | | | | | | | | | | | | | | | |
| | Food focused | | | | | | | | | | | | | | | | | | | | | | | | |
| | Quiet | | | | | | | | | | | | | | | | | | | | | | | | |
| **Satiety** | Satiated | | | | | | | | | | | | | | | | | | | | | | | | |
| | Not | | | | | | | | | | | | | | | | | | | | | | | | |
| **Energy** | High | | | | | | | | | | | | | | | | | | | | | | | | |
| | Medium | | | | | | | | | | | | | | | | | | | | | | | | |
| | Low | | | | | | | | | | | | | | | | | | | | | | | | |
| **Thinking** | Very sharp | | | | | | | | | | | | | | | | | | | | | | | | |
| | Clear | | | | | | | | | | | | | | | | | | | | | | | | |
| | Cloudy | | | | | | | | | | | | | | | | | | | | | | | | |
| **Blood Sugar Reaction** | Headache | | | | | | | | | | | | | | | | | | | | | | | | |
| | Light-headed | | | | | | | | | | | | | | | | | | | | | | | | |
| | Even | | | | | | | | | | | | | | | | | | | | | | | | |
| | Sugar daze | | | | | | | | | | | | | | | | | | | | | | | | |
| | Sleepy | | | | | | | | | | | | | | | | | | | | | | | | |
| **Mood** | Optimistic | | | | | | | | | | | | | | | | | | | | | | | | |
| | Okay | | | | | | | | | | | | | | | | | | | | | | | | |
| | Depressed | | | | | | | | | | | | | | | | | | | | | | | | |
| **Stressed?** | Highly | | | | | | | | | | | | | | | | | | | | | | | | |
| | Mildly | | | | | | | | | | | | | | | | | | | | | | | | |
| | No | | | | | | | | | | | | | | | | | | | | | | | | |
| **Seeking Comfort?** | | | | | | | | | | | | | | | | | | | | | | | | | |
| Timeline | | 6AM | 7 | 8 | 9 | 10 | 11 | 12PM | 1 | 2 | 3 | 4 | 5 | 6 | 7 | 8 | 9 | 10 | 11 | 12AM | 1 | 2 | 3 | 4 | 5 |

Duplicating this page for personal use is permissible.

# 3

# Come into My Parlor

WITH MOST ADDICTIONS, people have moments when they can just say "No!" When someone offers us that first cigarette, joint, or pill, we usually know that what they're giving us is addictive. We have a moment when we make a choice.

Not so with food addiction. It creeps up subtly. A person gets set up and drawn into food addiction in hidden stages so that she doesn't realize it when she's finally hooked.

Let's use satiety as an example. Katie is a normal eater. When she eats two-thirds of the food on her plate, a chemical in her stomach called cholecystokinin shoots a telegram up her spinal cord that lands in a little section of the hypothalamus called the satiety center. As soon as the satiety center gets the message, it's as though a lever is flipped. Katie loses all interest in eating further. She pushes her plate away and starts thinking of something else.

Not so with Janka. Janka has delayed satiety. Her cholecystokinin doesn't pass on messages until forty-five to ninety minutes after she starts eating. Absent of an internal message to stop, Janka could well continue chewing and swallowing for a couple of hours.

When she eats around others, she stops because they stop, or because her plate is empty. But when she gets up from the table, she's not satiated, so she leaves the table unsatisfied, regardless of the amount she has eaten.

This unconsciously sets her up to be food-aware. She'll have subtle thoughts about food, be susceptible to treats around the office, and be hyperaware of the candy machine and food smells on the street. At her first opportunity to eat without being witnessed, she'll binge, trying to achieve satiety.

This creates a new problem because we reach satiety separately on each food we eat. For example, if your meal consisted of a platter of steaming, fresh-picked green beans tossed lightly with olive oil and Italian herbs, you'd eat for a while and then you'd stop. Even if waitstaff passed a parade of green bean platters before you, your interest in green beans would be gone. You could even still be a bit hungry, but entirely incapable of placing one more bean in your mouth. That's satiety.

But then, if the waitstaff suddenly came forth with platters of planked salmon in a beurre caper sauce, the salmon just slightly crisped at the edges, you could eat that. You could eat salmon to your heart's content, but again, then you would stop. You wouldn't want one more bite of salmon even if it were fresh-caught Copper River king salmon flown in seconds ago. Now you would be satiated with both salmon and green beans.

But lo, here come the waitstaff again! This time they bear bamboo skewers with cherry tomatoes, onion leaves, asparagus tips, water chestnuts, and basil, all grilled over a mesquite fire and finished with balsamic vinegar droplets. Surprise! Suddenly, you are interested in eating again. (By the way, are you feeling hungry? Colorful descriptions of food, as well as food pictures, commercials, food smells, and people eating in front of you can all stimulate appetite, which you now know is the opposite of satiety.)

 *Most overeaters and food addicts have a defect in satiety.*

Because we reach satiety separately on each food item, we can ordinarily be satisfied with a chicken Caesar salad for lunch, yet eat a great deal more on Thanksgiving or at a buffet.

So, back to Janka, who has left the table unsatiated and is wandering the world food-aware. If she takes herself somewhere that has an array of different foods, she'll be drawn to most of them. After she eats one food and reaches satiety with it, she'll still be reactive to the others. On her own, Janka will keep eating and eating.

Most food addicts and overeaters have a satiety defect. Their satiety is long delayed, so they are not signaled to stop eating. Satiety may not kick in until much later, perhaps even into the early morning hours.

Many overeaters awaken to a feeling of confidence that they will not overeat, that now they can resist food. Unfortunately, this feeling may make them skip breakfast, which will set them up, chemically, to eat too much later.

The vicious cycle of food addiction can thus be, in part, laid down because of a defect in satiety. I'll explain the relationship between defective satiety and addiction later. For now, this defect explains why the food addict, unlike most other addicts, doesn't get a chance to *just say no.* Her addiction has snuck up on her—the result of a combination of chemical reactions, brain alterations, and, possibly, genetic propensity and family problems.

Many food addicts get started on their addiction when young, as early as six years old. If their addiction showed up on their little bodies as weight gain, they may have been treated in the opposite way than would have helped them. They may have been subjected to strict diets, diet pills, humiliation, or ferocious teasing, or they may have been set apart or treated differently from other children. All of these only make the addiction worse. For example, cruel teasing or ostracism only drives these children to seek comfort in more food.

As you'll soon see for yourself, certain diets only worsen the condition of delayed satiety. And diet pills create a false satiety that the body soon adjusts to and overrules with rebound appetite. From then on it's a spiral trap: Taking more diet pills creates a stronger false satiety, which is trumped by yet more appetite.

As you can see, ignorant treatment of children who are heavier than most simply gives them a hearty push toward lifelong problems with eating and builds a foundation for food addiction. Remember, the body always puts survival first. Appetite is essential to survival, so the body will defend all direct assaults on it. What works instead is to support real satiety, not generate an illusion of it. That is the goal of this book.

### An Obscure Obsession

Food addicts can be controlled by their addiction for twenty, thirty, even forty years, oblivious that an addiction is calling the shots. Each time they turn to a diet to save them from the pain of being visibly different, the diet fails them. But each time, what they believe is that *they* failed.

If you are a food addict, a diet plan won't be successful unless you prepare for it and tailor it to respect your food addiction. And certain things you won't be able to do at all, even if the diet says you can.

A diet *can* work for you if you can be discriminating about its advice and know what to accept and what to reject. Most important, the ability to stay on a diet and sustain weight loss depends entirely on keeping a recovery mentality. This will all be explained as the chapters of this book unfold. But first, some good news. If you follow the advice you find here, your satiety will improve.

Meanwhile, commit this principle to memory:

*Don't swallow diets whole boar.*

. . .

# 4

# A Rose by Any Other Name

FOOD ADDICTION, compulsive overeating, binge eating—we hear phrases like these all the time, but how are they different? Want to challenge yourself? Try filling in the definition for each term below.

Compulsive overeating:

_____

Food addiction:

_____

Binge eating:

_____

Bulimia:

_____

Eating disorder:

_____

Appetite disorder:

_____

Let's take a look at each of these.

**Compulsive Overeating**

This phrase was in use long before the others. For many years, before the world gained a wider understanding of addiction, it was the only way we food addicts knew how to describe ourselves. Believe it or not, twenty-five years ago there wasn't even a term for food addiction, let alone treatment centers for it. (A weight-loss clinic or the charmingly named "fat farm" is a different animal entirely.)

Compulsive overeating is something quite specific: excessive, uncontrollable eating. A compulsive overeater can't stop herself from eating beyond her nutritional needs. She eats more calories each day than are necessary. Strangely enough, she may also be malnourished. While she's eating excessive amounts of sweets, carbs, or fats, she's likely neglecting to eat enough fruits and vegetables. Each morning she may tell herself she's going to change the way she eats, but each afternoon or evening, the urge to eat overwhelms any promises or decisions she made earlier.

**Food Addiction**

Food addiction is a biochemical dependence on certain foods that alter a person's mood or feelings. Like other addictions, food addiction is a neurochemical process that includes alterations in the mind's physiology, cravings, an inability to control use, an increasing tolerance to the substance, increasingly negative consequences, and distorted, narcissistic thinking. Most compulsive overeaters are addicted to specific foods.

While addiction to drugs or alcohol is now well recognized and viewed as serious, addiction to food is not understood as well and is often (incorrectly) perceived as trivial. This was vividly illustrated for me this week at a recovery meeting. As a food addict, I was in the minority, the other attendees being in recovery from drug or alcohol addiction. Nearly everyone there understood addiction as thoroughly as breathing, and most had at least a decade of recovery. In the meeting, I clearly stated that I'm a food addict—yet after the meeting, a woman in long-term alcohol and drug recovery offered me a box of sweets. I recoiled from the box, putting my hands in front of me, and she offered them again, suggesting that I carry them with me to give to others.

Never in a million years would this same woman have offered a bottle of scotch to a recovering alcoholic to tote about, just in case a friend might want a drink. This, in a nutshell, describes the difference between our culture's attitude toward food addiction versus attitudes toward alcohol or drug addiction.

The consequences of drug use or excessive alcohol use are often immediate and obvious when a drunk driver maims an entire family, or a meth addict pummels his wife. A person who is high or drunk can cause harm not only to his brain or his liver, but to innocent bystanders and family members. Thus, addiction to alcohol and other drugs is taken seriously.

The consequences of food addiction may take years or decades to show up, typically as diabetes, heart disease, or high blood pressure. Consequences that affect others, such as a decrease in our attention or enthusiasm, may be so subtle or gradual that our close family and friends may not be aware of what they are missing. Most people don't think they are losing much if a family member is a food addict; hence food addiction recovery is not necessarily protected or valued.

## Binge Eating

Binge eating is gradually becoming the official medical and psychiatric term for overeating. To clinicians, it describes the observable behavior of excessive eating. When used by those who do it, however, the term means out-of-control eating, usually of sweets, fats, and/or carbs.

Officially, a binge is an episode that involves eating a large quantity of food in a relatively short period of time. However, grazing—a term not included in a medical dictionary—is also a form of binge eating. Food is eaten in bits and pieces over several hours and can look minor, even to the person doing the eating, but a sizable amount can still be consumed. In either case, the person is only halfway present. Some part of her mind is almost continually focused on getting food.

With a food binge, a person seeks and finds sedation. Grazing brings a milder result—a dulling of alertness. Clearly, these strategies work, or they wouldn't be repeated. Eating proves to be an effective way to obtain relief and sedation. But it can only provide such comfort by stimulating brain chemicals that alter consciousness. Because this is the same process that brings about and sustains addiction, most binge eaters are also food addicts.

### Bulimia

Officially classified as bulimia nervosa, bulimia refers to binge eating that is followed by some compensatory action designed to rid the body of the food or avoid the weight gain it can cause. Such action may include vomiting, fasting, taking laxatives or diuretics, getting enemas, and overexercising.

### Eating Disorder

An eating disorder is a general classification under which certain diagnoses fall. Bulimia nervosa and anorexia nervosa (not eating enough to sustain health) have official medical status as eating disorders. The other terms defined in this chapter are also types of disordered eating even though they are not officially recognized as such.

Eating is the last act in the chain reaction triggered by appetite. Calling the problem an "eating" disorder causes focus on the behavior or the result, instead of the cause.

### Appetite Disorder

The true cause of overeating is disordered appetite. Seven different factors cause appetite to malfunction, and each of these factors must be addressed in order to restore appetite to its normal function—that of prodding a person to eat normal amounts of healthy food at appropriate intervals.

Appetite disorder and food addiction have a reciprocal relationship. Food addiction is one of the causes of appetite disorder. And some of the other causes of appetite disorder can lead to food addiction. A person with a genetic propensity for food addiction may have an immediate reaction to addictive foods early in life. This, then, will lead to the collapse of other normal appetite regulators. Of the various factors that sustain disordered appetite, the most powerful is food addiction.

### The Term That Leads to Solutions

I prefer to use the terms *food addiction* and *appetite disorder* for several reasons.

- An appetite disorder is the underlying cause of most excessive eating.
- Food addiction is the reason bingeing works to alter alertness.
- Using the right term leads us to more effective solutions.

• Looking at any of these disorders as aberrant behavior tempts us
to blame ourselves for it. (Heaven knows, others already blame us
with impunity.)

How often have you said to yourself, *Just stop eating!* or *Divide the food on the plate in half and just eat one half,* or *Push yourself away from the table*—and kept on eating? This is the danger of looking at binge eating as a behavioral problem. We believe it ought to be simple to change our behavior, and when we can't, we blame ourselves.

The behavior of overeating, no matter which term we use for it, is the consequence of a largely unconscious, internal process. This process is usually an active, but hidden, addiction. The right label leads us to the proper focus. We concentrate our attention on the areas that *can* make a difference and that can lead us through the delicately powerful healing process that allows us to change.

• • •

# 5

# Don't Get Me Started

  LET'S SEE. We have a diagnosis for you if you don't eat enough: anorexia. We have a diagnosis if you try to get rid of food after you've eaten it: bulimia. We have a diagnosis for you if you're carrying more weight than is considered healthy: obesity. Yet we don't have a medical diagnosis for you if you eat too much.

So, according to the medical community, obesity is a serious problem; getting rid of food after bingeing is a serious problem; but bingeing itself is not. Doesn't this sound like a *Seinfeld* plot?

### A Stunning Lack of Logic

As of now, neither compulsive overeating nor food addiction has the status of an official medical diagnosis. However, it looks like binge eating has won the race. In the newest bible of the American Psychiatric Association, the *Diagnostic and Statistical Manual of Mental Disorders, 4th Edition*, known in the trade as the *DSM-IV,* binge eating gets a minor mention as an "eating disorder not otherwise specified."

It seems strange to me. In a country where type 2 diabetes is appearing at ever-younger ages due to massive consumption of sugar and carbs, heart disease is the number-one killer, and obesity is considered the second most preventable disease, overeating doesn't even get a mention in the *DSM-IV.*

At a recent, well-planned professional workshop on low-carb diets, I was amazed that we went through the entire event without one mention of food addiction. It's time for our culture, and our health professionals, to wake up.

### A River in Egypt

It seems to be a cultural phenomenon to pretend that we aren't a nation of addicts. Most Americans seem to be in a pervasive state of denial as we supersize our portions and fill our gullets with foods that research has deemed poisonous.

*Denial isn't just a river in Egypt.*

All this denial, even at the professional level—which affects both professional training and health care policy making—has a huge effect on you. It's hard enough to have a disorder that isn't widely understood, but it's even harder if professionals are looking at it from the wrong perspective.

The national (un)consciousness is working against you. You can't count on every doctor to support you in ways that could make an actual difference. Most research money isn't going toward truly significant help for you. And your insurance probably won't cover forms of treatment that could actually work.

No wonder it's been so hard to stay on a food program. It wasn't because of any weakness on your part; you've been bucking a cultural phenomenon in addition to your own internal chemicals.

You *cannot* rely on the American culture to support you. So it is all the more important to become part of a society of people who truly understand food addiction.

**Wake Up and Smell the Distraction**

Consider that the very sight or smell of food can trigger appetite. This means that the external pressure to eat is extraordinary. Let's examine how conducive your environment is to helping you make a change in your eating.

1. For one day, tally the number of times you are exposed to food, food ads, eating, or discussions about food.
2. List the places where you can go without being exposed to any food, eating, or food smells.
3. List all the holidays and celebrations during the calendar year that do not involve eating.
4. Write down how many minutes it takes to be confronted with an opportunity for eating after you leave the house.

* An in-joke among people in recovery—de Nile (denial).

5. List how many times in a normal day you must buy food, be exposed to food, handle food, sit down with food, or clean up food.

The unfortunate reality is that our culture will relentlessly encourage you (and everyone else) to eat. Fortunately, there's a lot you can do to avoid, deflect, and move beyond these messages. Stay with me and you'll see.

. . .

# 6

# What! Me, Addicted?

🐝 MAYBE. By keeping track every day of what your body is telling you, you've already started gathering the information that will make it possible for you to answer that question, yea or nay.

It's not surprising that many Americans are addicted to food. Today America offers a wider range of addictive foods in more venues than ever before. Getting addicted to something in America is easy. We have evolved to a way of living that pushes people toward addiction.

For example, when we get sick, we put ourselves back to work as soon as possible. Many of us work even when we are sick. If we cross a major life threshold, such as the death or birth of a loved one, again we go back to work prematurely, amputating our grief or joy. We don't get enough sleep and end up fatigued. Our very lifestyle pushes us in the direction of more eating.

Addictive foods become a way to get comfort, slow down, forget, and remove ourselves from our stressful world. In particular, they give us comfort without making us so drunk or high that we put ourselves or others in acute danger. Few food addicts steal purses, rob banks, or extort money from others to feed our addiction. Among the many addictions we could have fallen prey to, we got one that causes the least damage to others.

Good for you. You found a way to survive and to comfort yourself without bringing much harm to others. Now, let's take care of that one little irritating detail—the fact that food addiction is harmful to you. For food addiction isn't benign. It has very real negative health effects.

When these health problems first show up, we may still have the option of reversing them. But if we ignore the wake-up call, a time may come when we lose our power of choice, when we've crossed the line into fewer options.

Here are the common dangers of leaving a food addiction untreated:

- **Danger 1—Diabetes.** Losing weight can make us much less vulnerable to diabetes and its attendant miseries. Certain kinds of food abstinence can also help delay the onset of diabetes.

   If we have early signs of diabetes, we can sometimes still turn things around by exercising, changing our eating, and losing weight. But diabetes can progress quickly if we don't make those changes. And once people have to start using insulin, they often gain weight. It's very hard to lose weight on insulin.

- **Danger 2—Loss of mobility.** Extra weight can add wear to our skeletal frame, and a point can come when we are no longer able to exercise. We then lose a valuable tool for maintaining our health and weight.

- **Danger 3—Heart disease.** The types of food that cause us to gain weight are usually the same foods that are harmful to our hearts. Few people gain weight by bingeing on broccoli. Fatty and starchy foods are the culprits that clog arteries and plump up fat cells, causing decreased energy and increased resistance to moving—both of which circle back to promote weight gain.

You still have time to make a difference for yourself. The important thing to remember, however, is that we only have so long to put off taking care of ourselves. We are given a grace period, sometimes lasting years, before the more drastic consequences of food addiction capture us. But eventually time runs out.

Today you have a choice. You have the power to make a difference for yourself by making the decision to continue with the healing and recovery process in this book.

A lot is resting on your willingness to pursue recovery. If you'll keep good records on your Body Signals Charts for four weeks, I'll show you how to use them to diagnose the causes of your appetite disorder, and then we can construct your personalized recovery program together.

• • •

# 7

# The Plan

❧ YESTERDAY I was in line at the supermarket and picked up a magazine that enticed me with this headline: "Exercises for Women with No Time to Spare."

That sounded good, so I flipped to the article. They wanted me to move! I was still going to have to do leg lifts and sit-ups. I thought the article would feature some new, special invention that could help me build muscles while I was driving to work.

You might be hoping for something just as magical here.

Unfortunately, I don't have magic, but I do have a plan that can work if you'll work it. It's not a diet. It's a step-by-step preparation that can help you choose the right kind of diet, stay on that diet, and keep progressing once you leave the diet behind.

I won't go into details about diets yet; there are important steps for you to take before dieting can work. Most of the steps are small ones, and with each, you'll build a foundation for the one that follows.

You won't have to give up a lot of foods at once. Instead, you'll rearrange how you eat and your approach to eating. You'll slowly acquire ways to soothe yourself that will eventually work better than food.

## STEP 2

### Make a commitment to yourself.

Each step really matters, so please don't skip a step or fast-forward through one. I wouldn't give you a step without a reason. Sometimes the purpose of a step will be to improve your brain chemistry. Sometimes a step will make later steps possible.

You might feel that a certain step is too hard, and you'll be tempted to either skip it or stop working the plan. Please don't do either. I encourage you to make the following commitment to yourself right now: *Even if a step is hard or challenging, I will try it for one week.*

I will give each step,

No matter how hard,

My very best effort

For one week.

I am going to make this process as easy for you as I can. But sometimes it *is* hard. For those times, here's your backup plan:

> *If I want to put off a step or give up altogether,*
> *I promise to talk about this idea with*
> *someone outside my home whom I trust.*

The following are people you can consider:

- A trusted friend, someone who wants the best for you
- Your minister, priest, rabbi, imam, pastor, or shaman
- A counselor or therapist
- A safe and trusted mentor, teacher, or leader

By the way, if you skipped the exercise in Chapter 2, now would be a good time to go back and do it. That was your first step. Setting these intentions is your second step. Now we'll move on toward the third.

• • •

# 8

# An Iota That Makes You Eat

AS YOU LEARNED in Chapter 2, if you are eating when you are not hungry, you are being controlled by your appetite. If you are eating too much on a regular basis, then your appetite is not working correctly.

We will look at seven major causes of appetite disorder. As you follow the eating maps I provide and fill out your Body Signals Charts for the next three weeks, you'll be gathering the data that will make it possible for us to diagnose the causes that are affecting you.

You are about to embark on your first eating changes. These changes have two purposes:

1. To diagnose the causes of your appetite disorder

2. To remove the barriers to weight loss

Each cause of appetite disorder is related to an imbalance of the brain chemicals that control eating. One of the most potent of these is also the simplest to fix: excessive neuropeptide Y (NPY).

NPY is a chain of thirty-six amino acids. When it is released in the hypothalamus, it makes a person eat—a lot. An unpleasant side effect is that it also tells the body to stop burning calories.

Great. Under the influence of NPY, we're eating more and burning less. Then it won't come as a surprise that if you have too much NPY, you'll gain weight. If you are being flooded with NPY on a regular basis, guess what? It will make you obese.

Every time you skip a meal, miss breakfast, or even delay a meal too long (once your body has become sensitive to missed meals), your body produces more NPY.

*Your body is so logical.* You aren't eating when you should, so it does something to make you eat.

Cleverly, NPY doesn't kick in until you start eating again. So, while you're skipping meals all day, it leaves you alone. It figures you must not have access to food; else why are you missing your mealtime? However, once you start eating, NPY influences you to eat more. Now that you have finally restored your food supply with a woolly mammoth, NPY wants you to have a really big portion.

After all, you've been demonstrating to your body that your food supply is unstable. It wants to make sure you store enough for tomorrow's famine.

Can you see the vicious cycle you perpetuate every time you skip a meal?

So I say to you, and if I could say it louder, I would: *Never skip a meal.* One more time: *Never, ever skip a meal.* Eat breakfast. Eat lunch. Eat supper. Don't skip a meal.

Is repairing your disordered appetite beginning to sound more doable?

Never skip a meal.

Never skip a meal.

Never skip a meal.

Never skip a meal.

Never skip a meal.

Never skip a meal.

. . .

# 9

# Stepping toward Recovery

CONGRATULATIONS! You're already on the third step. You now have a "before" picture of your body chemistry from one week of eating as you normally do, while recording your body's reactions on your Body Signals Charts. This will be very important later as we compare your body chemistry from this week to the changes in your chemistry as you progress through the steps. You've also made a commitment to continue for one more week, and you've promised yourself to get help if the process gets tough and you feel like quitting.

## Your First Eating Change

Now that you've filled out Body Signals Charts for seven days, you are ready to make your first eating change. For this second week, as well as for weeks three and four, I want you to continue filling out a Body Signals Chart every hour. Each week the chart will be a little different, to reflect the eating change for that week.

STEP 3

Make your first eating change and start following a map.

Beginning with this week, you'll get an eating map, and each week thereafter we'll add one change. It's important to give yourself one week for each change and not scrunch changes together. Here's why:

- We'll use each weekly change to diagnose the causes of your appetite disorder.

- At the end of your fourth week on this program, we'll have data from each of the three weeks of food changes, plus the baseline from your first week. From this data, we can identify five of the seven causes of appetite disorder. (We'll get to the other two later.)

- To correctly interpret your data, you'll need one full week of daily charts that reflect each change.

- The changes work cumulatively. When you add the second eating change, you will also continue with the first eating change. The eating map will summarize these changes for you.

Do you remember how you used to rush headlong into a diet, investing it with all your hopes and dreams? That didn't work out, did it? Most of the time, the diet was too alien to your normal eating patterns. It required too much change at once to be sustainable.

Give yourself a genuine chance to let this new program work for you. Get used to each change, one week at a time. This means you'll have to find a way to handle that part of your mind that has a diet mentality. You know what I mean—the part that drives you to jump on the scale every three minutes, the part that starts comparing your body to others, the part that will sabotage this program for you if you let it call the shots.

Remember, what you and I are doing together is slowly removing the barriers to weight loss. We are preparing you to be successful with a diet. Our strategy is to build up your satiety and to remove, slowly, the things that trigger your appetite. Once you have a calm appetite and a rebuilt satiety, you will be ready for your diet.

*Making the First Change*

Throughout this week, starting with breakfast, eat every two to three hours during the time that you're awake, for a total of five or six snacks or meals each day. I'm not telling you what to eat or how much—with one exception. Do not have any simple carbs as a snack. Want them with a meal? No problem. But for snacks, stay away from crackers, candy, bread, fruit juice, and sugar. I think you'll be interested to see your chemical patterns three weeks from now as you make these small, weekly changes.

Ready? Begin by making seven copies of the Body Signals Chart on page 59. It's almost—but not quite—identical to the previous one you used.

**Sound Simple?**

The curious thing about this week's eating map is that it sounds simple. What could be easier than asking a food addict to eat? Especially now that you

# Body Signals Chart, Week 2

Date: _____

| CATEGORY | DESCRIPTIONS | CHANGE: EAT EVERY 2–3 HOURS | | | | | | | | | | | | | | | | | | | | | | |
|---|---|---|---|---|---|---|---|---|---|---|---|---|---|---|---|---|---|---|---|---|---|---|---|---|---|
| Timeline | Circle Wake-up | 6AM | 7 | 8 | 9 | 10 | 11 | 12PM | 1 | 2 | 3 | 4 | 5 | 6 | 7 | 8 | 9 | 10 | 11 | 12AM | 1 | 2 | 3 | 4 | 5 |
| **Food** | Proteins | | | | | | | | | | | | | | | | | | | | | | | | |
| | Complex carbs | | | | | | | | | | | | | | | | | | | | | | | | |
| *Numbers go in this section* | Simple carbs | | | | | | | | | | | | | | | | | | | | | | | | |
| | Fats | | | | | | | | | | | | | | | | | | | | | | | | |
| *Check* | **Equal/NutraSweet** | | | | | | | | | | | | | | | | | | | | | | | | |
| **Drink** | Water | | | | | | | | | | | | | | | | | | | | | | | | |
| | Pop | | | | | | | | | | | | | | | | | | | | | | | | |
| *Dots go in this section* | Diet pop | | | | | | | | | | | | | | | | | | | | | | | | |
| | Coffee | | | | | | | | | | | | | | | | | | | | | | | | |
| | Herbal drink | | | | | | | | | | | | | | | | | | | | | | | | |
| | Milk | | | | | | | | | | | | | | | | | | | | | | | | |
| | Juice | | | | | | | | | | | | | | | | | | | | | | | | |
| | Alcohol | | | | | | | | | | | | | | | | | | | | | | | | |
| | Tea | | | | | | | | | | | | | | | | | | | | | | | | |
| *Check* | **Caffeine** | | | | | | | | | | | | | | | | | | | | | | | | |
| Timeline | | 6AM | 7 | 8 | 9 | 10 | 11 | 12PM | 1 | 2 | 3 | 4 | 5 | 6 | 7 | 8 | 9 | 10 | 11 | 12AM | 1 | 2 | 3 | 4 | 5 |
| **Fullness** | Stuffed | | | | | | | | | | | | | | | | | | | | | | | | |
| | Comfortable | | | | | | | | | | | | | | | | | | | | | | | | |
| | Empty | | | | | | | | | | | | | | | | | | | | | | | | |
| **Hunger** | Starving | | | | | | | | | | | | | | | | | | | | | | | | |
| | Really hungry | | | | | | | | | | | | | | | | | | | | | | | | |
| | Mildly hungry | | | | | | | | | | | | | | | | | | | | | | | | |
| | Not hungry | | | | | | | | | | | | | | | | | | | | | | | | |
| **Appetite** | Craving food | | | | | | | | | | | | | | | | | | | | | | | | |
| | Food focused | | | | | | | | | | | | | | | | | | | | | | | | |
| | Quiet | | | | | | | | | | | | | | | | | | | | | | | | |
| **Satiety** | Satiated | | | | | | | | | | | | | | | | | | | | | | | | |
| | Not | | | | | | | | | | | | | | | | | | | | | | | | |
| **Energy** | High | | | | | | | | | | | | | | | | | | | | | | | | |
| | Medium | | | | | | | | | | | | | | | | | | | | | | | | |
| | Low | | | | | | | | | | | | | | | | | | | | | | | | |
| **Thinking** | Very sharp | | | | | | | | | | | | | | | | | | | | | | | | |
| | Clear | | | | | | | | | | | | | | | | | | | | | | | | |
| | Cloudy | | | | | | | | | | | | | | | | | | | | | | | | |
| **Blood Sugar Reaction** | Headache | | | | | | | | | | | | | | | | | | | | | | | | |
| | Light-headed | | | | | | | | | | | | | | | | | | | | | | | | |
| | Even | | | | | | | | | | | | | | | | | | | | | | | | |
| | Sugar daze | | | | | | | | | | | | | | | | | | | | | | | | |
| | Sleepy | | | | | | | | | | | | | | | | | | | | | | | | |
| **Mood** | Optimistic | | | | | | | | | | | | | | | | | | | | | | | | |
| | Okay | | | | | | | | | | | | | | | | | | | | | | | | |
| | Depressed | | | | | | | | | | | | | | | | | | | | | | | | |
| **Stressed?** | Highly | | | | | | | | | | | | | | | | | | | | | | | | |
| | Mildly | | | | | | | | | | | | | | | | | | | | | | | | |
| | No | | | | | | | | | | | | | | | | | | | | | | | | |
| **Seeking Comfort?** | | | | | | | | | | | | | | | | | | | | | | | | | |
| Timeline | | 6AM | 7 | 8 | 9 | 10 | 11 | 12PM | 1 | 2 | 3 | 4 | 5 | 6 | 7 | 8 | 9 | 10 | 11 | 12AM | 1 | 2 | 3 | 4 | 5 |

Duplicating this page for personal use is permissible.

know that this is the best way to prevent an accumulation of NPY.

If I hadn't been working with food addicts for more than twenty years, I'd put a period on this chapter and go on to the next one. But this eating change strikes immediately at one of a food addict's key issues—we tend to neglect ourselves. We aren't the best at self-care. This is in part due to the general pattern of avoidance that we live in almost constantly. We try not to let ourselves feel too much. We're rarely fully present. We try not to open up too much. We rarely fall all the way into a true belly laugh. We cut off our tears. We hold back sobs. We use words like *irritated* or *frustrated* instead of stating or feeling our full red-hot anger. We are more likely to stay busy than grieve.

For now, I just want you to eat every two or three hours. This will take some planning. You'll need to carry food with you and stash some food in your car and workplace. You'll need to shop with snacks in mind. (At the end of the chapter, you'll find some healthy snack ideas.)

> **EATING MAP, WEEK 2**
>
> - Eat every two or three hours.
> - Do not have simple carbs (e.g., flour, fruit juice, sugar) as snacks.

As a food addict in recovery, I know how we usually operate. We skip meals. We delay eating and use that to justify a big meal later. We may put most of the nutrition for the day into a single minibuffet.

Why would we do this? If we so love to eat, why miss meals? Why resist eating every two or three hours? Because, as food addicts, we aren't using food as nutrition. We are using it like a drug—for relief, comfort, solace, sedation, and reward.

So we need relief. And we live in a world that doesn't get food addiction. Next chapter, please.

• • •

**Remember, if you are receiving treatment or taking medicine for a medical condition, check with your doctor before making any eating changes this book recommends.**

## HEALTHY SNACK IDEAS

- Soup
- Half a sandwich
  (on 100 percent whole-grain bread)
- Cheese and veggies
- Cheese and fruit
- Fresh fruit
- Almonds
- Veggies and dip
- Nuts and raisins
- Hard-boiled egg
- Gazpacho
- Veggies and salsa
- Cream cheese and salsa
- Cheese
- Yogurt
- Jerky
- Meat slices
- Milk
- Smoked fish
- Baked potato

- Baked sweet potato
- Squash
- Celery filled with cheese or nut butter
- Yogurt sprinkled with granola
- Sugar-free granola
- Sugar-free trail mix
- Sliced turkey or chicken
- Meat roll-ups
  (sliced meat spread with mayo or cream cheese, topped with lettuce, and rolled into a cigar shape)
- Meat roll-ups with salsa
- Olives
- Pickles
- Pickled peppers

# 10

# Relief

WHY IS IT HARD for us food addicts to eat regularly? Because we like to save eating for later.

Whether we are conscious of what we are doing or not, by waiting until day's end to eat, we are setting up a binge. Over time, we have discovered that eating specific foods in certain quantities gives us relief, so we opt for the scenario that will give us maximum relief.

Here's the crux of food addiction: We overeat *only* because it works to bring relief. If it didn't work, we wouldn't do it. So why does it work?

Here's the simple answer: Particular foods, certain quantities, or even chewing itself can cause a chain of chemical reactions that culminate in the parts of the brain that regulate pain relief, sedation, and sleepiness, as well as a decrease in vigilance or hyper-concern about others.

> *We overeat only because it works.*
> *If it didn't bring us relief, we wouldn't do it.*

It's possible to learn to manipulate your own brain by activating certain switches that change your physical and emotional states. Eating is the tool that controls these switches.

You can learn this type of manipulation very early in life—even by the age of five, before you are a fully conscious person—especially if your brain is genetically predisposed to addiction.

The more you manipulate your brain chemicals to give yourself relief, the more dependent you become on that relief. Eventually, you can become addicted to your own body's relief chemicals.

Once that happens, you lose control, and your nervous system, not you, starts calling the shots. Your nervous system starts craving a regular flow of the relief chemicals, so it instigates food-seeking behavior that operates beneath the radar of your conscious thought. In other words, your nervous system points you toward food or eating. It will even support you in skipping meals, setting you up unconsciously for a really big eating session later in the day.

This massive system is a food addiction, which is the major cause of appetite disorder. And it is a true addiction, as I'll explain later.

Overruling this complex and massive system requires extreme consciousness. I will give you tricks that can help you stay conscious of your eating for a day, a week, or a month. But, for a lifetime, you'll need more than tricks. I tell you now: You can't be conscious enough in the long run to beat a food addiction by yourself. You need companions who understand the complexity of the problem. You and they need to be partners in overcoming food addiction.

• • •

# 11

# Comfort

LET'S GET the most difficult reality out in the open right away. *You cannot do this alone.* If you could, you'd have done it by now.

You've tried thinking yourself out of eating. You've tried bribes and threats. You've tried self-hate, self-love, prayer, spiritual power, and signs on the refrigerator. You're an expert on nutrition. You've bought an entire library of self-help books with hearty sections on diets and healthy eating. If intelligence were enough, you would be done.

I am soon going to tell you a simple way to help yourself enormously, a change that will begin to slowly improve the signals your brain sends to you about eating. This little trick works like a wonder.

But will you do it?

That's the catch, isn't it? No matter how much we want to stop eating, we don't want to stop eating.

How many times have you bought the fat-free mayo and then not finished the jar? How about the bottles of pills for only $19.95 that would help you, only you stopped taking them? You've tried simple, but supposedly effective, remedies before and lost interest. Right?

**STEP 4**

Prepare to have the comfort you need.

Why?

Here's why:

Eating is our safety net. It's our warm embrace, our dependable relief, our reward for self-sacrifice. Our need to eat is bigger than we are. We can't, by ourselves, be strong enough to stand up to it—at least not for any sustained period of time.

Remember, you live in a world that doesn't even recognize food addiction, let alone support recovery from it. You've already made an inventory of the many ways food confronts you every single day. And you can't even be sure that health care professionals really understand food addiction and the true causes of binge eating.

Plus, any time you run into someone who is diet focused (such as some health care professionals, many women, and possibly your mother), that person may make comments that get your mind off track—comments that make you forget that a diet is a tool, not an answer.

Most of all, to sustain healthy eating day after day, you've got to be able to find relief from a source other than food. If food has been your best friend, you need a new best friend.

What you need is at least one special person to work with you on this project. The two of you will talk to each other frequently, meet together at least once a week to discuss the exercises, share some of the thoughts that make you turn to food, and cheer each other over rough spots.

And, guess what? As much as you need the support, wisdom, tolerance, and encouragement of another person, someone in your neighborhood needs your support just as much. This person, who has been struggling alone with this same issue, will have her life changed for the better by working with you. You will help each other.

Not just any buddy will do. If you are a woman, you need to work with another woman. A man should work with another man. This has nothing to do with gender roles, sexuality, or boundaries. The fact is men tend to lose weight faster, and they tend to dwell in their left-brains. There's nothing wrong with either of these, but the result is often that a man provides insufficient support for a woman. (An exception is a man, often gay, who is comfortable with right-brain thinking.)

Your partner in this endeavor should not—and, in fact, cannot—be your partner or spouse. You need to work with someone who has no investment in your outcome. A partner with a secret agenda for you to look thinner, a spouse with control issues, or a mate who is fearful of losing you to the health risks of extra weight will not have the detachment you need when it comes time to report that you want to eat outside of the eating map.

This person probably can't be your sister, either. Unless there's never been a smidgeon of rivalry between you, the chances are that one or both of you will begin competing, and one of you will win. As I'll explain later, this kind of competition absolutely forces your biochemistry to instigate bingeing.

The partner you choose also needs to be someone who knows what it is like to be driven to eat. You need someone who is also facing her own binge eating, overeating, or food addiction. If you partner with someone who isn't, it will be harder for you to expose your secret thoughts and longings for food.

Even partnering with someone who is in recovery from another addiction won't cover enough bases. Folks in recovery from drug or alcohol addiction can offer tremendous wisdom about the recovery process, and they are good people for you to hang out with *if* they can respect your need to have limited exposure to *your* drug—food. However, many recovering alcohol and drug addicts end up as sugar addicts, and many are in denial about it. Thus they can unwittingly sabotage you. There is also a tendency for them to see food addiction as a less serious addiction than theirs, and that attitude won't serve you.

Therefore, your recovery partner should be

- Your gender
- A compulsive overeater, binge eater, or food addict
- A peer, not someone with more or less power in the relationship than you (not a boss, parent, child, or employee)
- Someone willing to face her own appetite disorder through a program for recovery
- Someone willing to put this recovery program before any diet
- Someone willing to keep confidential everything you say about your own process, your eating, your struggles, and your needs
- Someone trustworthy and honest, so you can be safe in her commitment to confidentiality

Ideally, this person should live nearby, so you can meet face to face. But if this isn't possible, a long-distance relationship—though less than ideal—can work, provided you can reach each other easily by phone and/or e-mail.

**What About Joining a Support Group?**

There are ready-made support groups with decades of experience that will welcome you, such as Overeaters Anonymous and Food Addicts Anonymous. In a later chapter, I'll talk about these various groups and their strengths and limitations.

Attending group meetings *in addition* to meeting with your recovery partner can be quite beneficial. However, for some, groups can be intimidating, at least at first.

*A diet is a tactic; a program is a strategy.*

The advantage of a group is this: Sooner or later, issues will arise between you and your partner. In part, these issues will be straw men created by the addiction to get you back under its control. Using the guidelines in Chapter 34 will be your best protection against such problems. Still, a group provides alternate warm hearts when you end up on the outs with someone.

**Finding a Recovery Partner**

Whether you choose to become part of a group or not, you must find a recovery partner for the program in this book to work. Here's the step-by-step process for finding one:

1. Make a list of the people you know who fit the qualifications listed on page 67.

2. Of the people on your list, which ones feel safest? For which ones do you have the warmest feelings? Feel free to rank several people according to these two criteria.

3. Consider whether each of these people is genuinely trustworthy and honorable. If someone is not or is in question, remove that person from your list.

4. Call the person, explain a bit about this book, and propose working together. You may want to use the script on page 69.

5. If she's not interested or available, try the next person on your list. Keep trying until you find someone who says yes.

## SAMPLE SCRIPT

### An Invitation for Mutual Support

"Hi, _____ . It's _____ . I'm calling because I've been reading a book that I think can really help me with my problem with overeating. But the author, Anne Katherine, insists that I can't do it alone. She suggested that I make a list of people I feel comfortable with, and you are at the top of my list. Are you interested in going through her book, *How to Make Almost Any Diet Work,* with me? We could help each other.

"The main thing is to get started. She's got a meeting agenda for us to use, guidelines, and scripts to help us, so that we can get started in the right direction. She's also pretty firm about us each needing our own copy of the book.

"Would you be able to get together on _____ ? Great. Let's pick a time.

"I should mention that she has a beginning exercise that I'm already doing. It's a chart to help us be aware of our body chemistry before we start changing anything about the way we eat. If you want, I could drop off a chart for you while you're waiting to get your copy of the book.

"Thank you so much."

Now you're ready for Step 4: Prepare to have the comfort you need by finding a recovery partner. Therefore, your task this week is to look for a good recovery partner—and to keep looking (for longer than a week, if necessary) until you find one who agrees to take this journey with you. It's okay to continue reading while you search for a partner.

• • •

# 12

# 50/50

❧ READY FOR your next step? With the first eating change, you have already removed barriers to weight loss, and this next change will take you even further. You will start to increase your levels of peptide YY (PYY). Sound good?

In Chapter 8, you learned about neuropeptide Y (NPY) and how it stimulates extreme appetite. If someone injected you with NPY, you couldn't stop yourself from eating.

PYY counteracts the effects of NPY. It lets you fight fire with fire. You combat NPY with PYY. They are both peptides, so they understand each other.

Peptide YY is a chain of thirty-six amino acids that (usually) inhibits appetite. PYY promotes satiety. It is a chemical stop sign that says, "Stop eating."

How do you get some of this PYY? It doesn't come in a pill; you have to get your body to manufacture it.

The odds are that you are deficient in PYY, and that this contributes to your appetite disorder. Want to know how you became deficient in PYY? By skipping meals.

Whenever you've fasted or eaten below your energy requirements for any length of time, your body suppressed the manufacture of PYY. So if you've been on some severe diets or fasts, you are almost certainly PYY deficient.

FIGURE 5

**The PYY Effect**

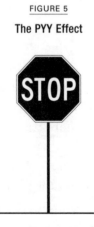

It makes sense. When you scared your body into thinking the food supply was dwindling, it had to guarantee you'd tank up when the food wagon returned. Therefore, when you started eating after a fast, your body held back on the PYY so that you would consume extra food.

Now here's what's supposed to happen. Fifteen minutes after you begin eating, the PYY in your bloodstream should rise, reaching a plateau about seventy-five minutes later. At this point, you wouldn't eat if someone paid you to. For people who don't have an appetite disorder, the more food they eat, the more PYY enters their system.

But if your PYY is restricted, a bigger meal doesn't make much difference in your PYY levels until long after you eat. So imagine you've saved your eating for later in the day. The long fast suppresses PYY so that you can eat and eat without ever reaching satiety. Then PYY finally peaks sometime in the night, causing you to wake up satiated. Finally, your appetite is suppressed— but at the beginning of the day, when you should be eating breakfast.

In this state of satiety, you want to skip breakfast; but by missing a meal, the whole vicious cycle starts over again. If you don't break your fast in the morning, NPY will build up and PYY will be suppressed, stimulating you to eat too much again later.

There's only one way out of this trap. Never skip a meal; and *never, ever* skip breakfast, no matter how satiated you feel. By not skipping meals, you deliberately build up your PYY.

You've got to get your body to trust you. You've got to prove to it that you are not beset by famine. You can do this by eating every two to three hours (food change one) and by eating snacks that promote brain repair. (That's eating change two, which is coming up.)

Continue eating this way long enough, and your PYY levels will slowly start to recover. And you definitely want your PYY back. Once your body receives its regular dose of PYY, your food intake could naturally be reduced by 33 percent every day, with no further effort on your part.[1]

Protein is the raw material for peptides, and frequent feedings of protein give your brain a steady

**STEP 5**

Begin eating change two: Eat snacks that are 50/50.

supply of the materials it needs to repair itself. So at snack times, eat 50 percent protein and 50 percent complex carbs. Any complex carb qualifies except for foods made with sugar, wheat, or flour.

Carry these 50/50 snacks with you at all times, replenishing your home and work supplies before you'll need them. Don't set back the progress you've made in your body's chemical balance by missing a snack or meal.

| 50/50 SNACKS | |
|---|---|
| **Protein Snacks** | **Some 50/50 Combinations** |
| • Cheese | • Yogurt and granola (sugar-free) |
| • Meat | • Celery with cheese or nut butter |
| • Yogurt | |
| • Milk | • Apple and cheese |
| • Nuts or nut butter | • Pineapple and cottage cheese |
| • Eggs | • Banana and nuts |
| • Jerky | • Hard-cooked egg and dill pickles |
| • Fish | |
| • Smoked fish | • Milk and applesauce |
| • Soy nuts | • Tuna and grapes |
| • Tofu (tofu burgers, cold cuts, etc.) | • Soy nuts |
| | • String cheese and pear |
| **Complex Carb Snacks** | • Tomato and chicken slices |
| • Fresh fruit | • Smoked salmon and asparagus |
| • Vegetables | • Ricotta cheese and strawberries |
| • Dill or sour pickles | |
| • Sugar-free granola | • Oatmeal and nuts |
| • Oatmeal | • Sugar-free granola with milk or soy milk |

This week you'll keep records with Body Signals Chart, Week 3. You are making an important change this week, and it should be interesting to see what happens to your chemical markers.

If you make this change correctly, your chart could look something like this:

| Timeline | Circle Wake-up | 6AM | 7 | 8 | 9 | 10 | 11 | 12PM | 1 | 2 | 3 | 4 | 5 | 6 | 7 | 8 | 9 | 10 | 11 |
|---|---|---|---|---|---|---|---|---|---|---|---|---|---|---|---|---|---|---|---|
| **Food** | Proteins | | 6 | | 5 | | | 5 | | | 5 | 4 | | 5 | | | | | |
| | Complex carbs | | 3 | | 5 | | | 3 | | | 5 | 3 | | 5 | | | | | |
| | Flour | | | | | | | 1 | | | | 2 | | | | | | | |
| | Sugar | | 1 | | | | | 1 | | | | 1 | | | | | | | |
| | Fats | | | | | | | | | | | | | | | | | | |

Why no sugar, wheat, or flour at snack times? You can still eat carbs at your regular meals, but having crackers, sweets, or bread for snacks creates a risk of bingeing. I want you to get used to healthy snacking now because when you make some significant changes in your eating later on, 50/50 snacking will make future transitions easier. The idea is to boost your PYY without triggering your food addiction.

This change is so important that your Body Signals Chart for this week has three new items. Instead of a single simple carbs row, there are now two separate rows for flour and sugar. If you are snacking appropriately, your chart should not have a number entered into either the flour or sugar lines at the snack times between meals.

And what about wheat? Granted, 100 percent whole wheat flour is a complex carb. But from now on, since 100 percent whole grain bread or crackers are made from flour, they must be counted in the flour row.

---

**EATING MAP, WEEK 3**

- Eat every two to three hours, for as long as you are awake.

- Eat snacks that are 50/50— 50 percent protein and 50 percent complex carbs.

- Do not eat snacks made from flour, wheat, or sugar, or other simple carbs.

- Bring 50/50 snacks wherever you go.

# Body Signals Chart, Week 3

Date: _____

| CATEGORY | DESCRIPTIONS | CHANGE: EAT 50/50 SNACKS | | | | | | | | | | | | | | | | | | | | | | |
|---|---|---|---|---|---|---|---|---|---|---|---|---|---|---|---|---|---|---|---|---|---|---|---|---|---|
| Timeline | Circle Wake-up | 6AM | 7 | 8 | 9 | 10 | 11 | 12PM | 1 | 2 | 3 | 4 | 5 | 6 | 7 | 8 | 9 | 10 | 11 | 12AM | 1 | 2 | 3 | 4 | 5 |
| **Food** | Proteins | | | | | | | | | | | | | | | | | | | | | | | | |
| | Complex carbs | | | | | | | | | | | | | | | | | | | | | | | | |
| *Numbers go in this section* | Flour | | | | | | | | | | | | | | | | | | | | | | | | |
| | Sugar | | | | | | | | | | | | | | | | | | | | | | | | |
| | Fats | | | | | | | | | | | | | | | | | | | | | | | | |
| Check | **Equal/NutraSweet** | | | | | | | | | | | | | | | | | | | | | | | | |
| **Drink** | Water | | | | | | | | | | | | | | | | | | | | | | | | |
| | Pop | | | | | | | | | | | | | | | | | | | | | | | | |
| *Dots go in this section* | Diet pop | | | | | | | | | | | | | | | | | | | | | | | | |
| | Coffee | | | | | | | | | | | | | | | | | | | | | | | | |
| | Herbal drink | | | | | | | | | | | | | | | | | | | | | | | | |
| | Milk | | | | | | | | | | | | | | | | | | | | | | | | |
| | Juice | | | | | | | | | | | | | | | | | | | | | | | | |
| | Alcohol | | | | | | | | | | | | | | | | | | | | | | | | |
| | Tea | | | | | | | | | | | | | | | | | | | | | | | | |
| Check | **Caffeine** | | | | | | | | | | | | | | | | | | | | | | | | |
| Timeline | | 6AM | 7 | 8 | 9 | 10 | 11 | 12PM | 1 | 2 | 3 | 4 | 5 | 6 | 7 | 8 | 9 | 10 | 11 | 12AM | 1 | 2 | 3 | 4 | 5 |
| **Fullness** | Stuffed | | | | | | | | | | | | | | | | | | | | | | | | |
| | Comfortable | | | | | | | | | | | | | | | | | | | | | | | | |
| | Empty | | | | | | | | | | | | | | | | | | | | | | | | |
| **Hunger** | Starving | | | | | | | | | | | | | | | | | | | | | | | | |
| | Really hungry | | | | | | | | | | | | | | | | | | | | | | | | |
| | Mildly hungry | | | | | | | | | | | | | | | | | | | | | | | | |
| | Not hungry | | | | | | | | | | | | | | | | | | | | | | | | |
| **Appetite** | Craving food | | | | | | | | | | | | | | | | | | | | | | | | |
| | Food focused | | | | | | | | | | | | | | | | | | | | | | | | |
| | Quiet | | | | | | | | | | | | | | | | | | | | | | | | |
| **Satiety** | Satiated | | | | | | | | | | | | | | | | | | | | | | | | |
| | Not | | | | | | | | | | | | | | | | | | | | | | | | |
| **Energy** | High | | | | | | | | | | | | | | | | | | | | | | | | |
| | Medium | | | | | | | | | | | | | | | | | | | | | | | | |
| | Low | | | | | | | | | | | | | | | | | | | | | | | | |
| **Thinking** | Very sharp | | | | | | | | | | | | | | | | | | | | | | | | |
| | Clear | | | | | | | | | | | | | | | | | | | | | | | | |
| | Cloudy | | | | | | | | | | | | | | | | | | | | | | | | |
| **Blood Sugar Reaction** | Headache | | | | | | | | | | | | | | | | | | | | | | | | |
| | Light-headed | | | | | | | | | | | | | | | | | | | | | | | | |
| | Even | | | | | | | | | | | | | | | | | | | | | | | | |
| | Sugar daze | | | | | | | | | | | | | | | | | | | | | | | | |
| | Sleepy | | | | | | | | | | | | | | | | | | | | | | | | |
| **Mood** | Optimistic | | | | | | | | | | | | | | | | | | | | | | | | |
| | Okay | | | | | | | | | | | | | | | | | | | | | | | | |
| | Depressed | | | | | | | | | | | | | | | | | | | | | | | | |
| **Stressed?** | Highly | | | | | | | | | | | | | | | | | | | | | | | | |
| | Mildly | | | | | | | | | | | | | | | | | | | | | | | | |
| | No | | | | | | | | | | | | | | | | | | | | | | | | |
| **Seeking Comfort?** | | | | | | | | | | | | | | | | | | | | | | | | | |
| **Body Conscious?** | | | | | | | | | | | | | | | | | | | | | | | | | |
| Timeline | | 6AM | 7 | 8 | 9 | 10 | 11 | 12PM | 1 | 2 | 3 | 4 | 5 | 6 | 7 | 8 | 9 | 10 | 11 | 12AM | 1 | 2 | 3 | 4 | 5 |

Duplicating this page for personal use is permissible.

The bottom of the chart also has a new row: Body Conscious. Each time you realize you are paying attention to what's going on inside of you in terms of hunger, appetite, stress level, emotions, and so on, make a check mark.

| Body Conscious? | | ✔ | | | ✔ | | ✔ | ✔ | | | | ✔ | ✔ | ✔ | | | ✔ | | |
|---|---|---|---|---|---|---|---|---|---|---|---|---|---|---|---|---|---|---|---|

. . .

# 13

# The Chemistry of Comfort

EVERY CELL in your body is aware. Although you perceive awareness as coming from your mind—and it does—your entire body is also tuned in, listening and attending. We are so conscious of our consciousness that we tend to discount the power of our other self, our animal body.

Alert as a lizard and swift as a hummingbird, your animal body constantly registers changes in your vicinity and discriminates among them on the basis of threat or nonthreat, advantage or disadvantage, reward or punishment.

An addiction to food comes from your animal body. It operates out of its own consciousness: deeper, more automatic, and less articulate than the consciousness you are aware of. It is a relief-seeking mechanism. It has the capacity to orchestrate a whole series of actions that will culminate in relief while you're only vaguely conscious of being directed.

Here's a typical scenario.

[9:00 a.m.] Your boss: "I need to speak to you, but not now. Come to my office at 4:30 this afternoon."

[9:01 a.m.] You sort of blank out. You may move papers or appear to work, but in reality you feel disconnected.

What's going on inside of you? Your amygdala, a little oval-shaped bundle on each side of your deep brain, is checking to see if your boss's message constitutes a threat. It does this by checking with the hippocampus, another little bundle located close by.

Your hippocampus searches your memory banks to compare your boss's words and tone to past

**STEP 6**

Understand the chemistry of comfort.

77

experiences. Together the amygdala and the hippocampus decide that your boss sounded threatening. Immediately the reticular activating system (RAS) and the locus coeruleus pass the threat on, and parts of the brain, particularly your hypothalamus, are flooded with norepinephrine (NE). As a result, your heart rate increases, your breathing quickens, and you become hyperalert.

You notice that two co-workers are whispering to each other by the coffee machine. You are convinced that they know what's going on and that they are talking about you. You notice that no one in the office has e-mailed you or left you voice messages. You become certain that you've made some terrible mistake that everyone knows about.

You try to figure out what you did wrong. All your past mistakes suddenly become very vivid and you try to think of how to fix things. You may dive into some project to appease the boss or impress your co-workers. You may come up with a plan to treat or surprise your co-workers, so they'll be on your side. Instead of eating lunch, you go to the flower vendor and get flowers for everyone, or you go to the grocery store and buy a box of treats to share.

Finally, 4:30 arrives and you are at your boss's door. He says, "Come in, come in. I wondered if you would be willing to organize the staff party next month. You did such a good job last year."

Weak with relief, you agree enthusiastically, not even thinking about how much work it will require and what short notice this is. When you leave work, your brain is burned out.

The flood of NE has overstimulated your brain, which now needs to do something to regulate itself

---

### PARTS OF THE BRAIN—DEFINITIONS

**Amygdala**
- Checks all incoming stimulation for the possibility of a threat.

**Hippocampus**
- Keeps archives on all previous experiences and searches its database for comparative experiences when e-mailed by the amygdala.

**Reticular Activating System (RAS)**
- Alerts the body.

**Locus Coeruleus**
- Passes on the alert to the sympathetic nervous system, focuses attention externally, and increases paranoia.

**Sympathetic Nervous System**
- Prepares to fight or flee.

back to a soothed level. The result is you turn your car into a drive-through where you are barely conscious of ordering large sizes, extra food, and two desserts. You may even go to more stores to gather products made from flour, fat, sugar, and, possibly, salt.

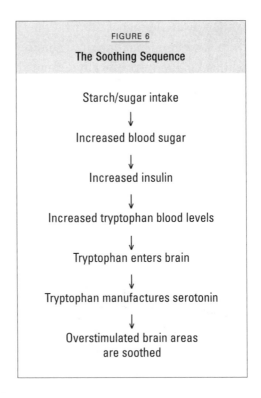

FIGURE 6

**The Soothing Sequence**

Starch/sugar intake
↓
Increased blood sugar
↓
Increased insulin
↓
Increased tryptophan blood levels
↓
Tryptophan enters brain
↓
Tryptophan manufactures serotonin
↓
Overstimulated brain areas
are soothed

Once home, you consume these. As a consequence, your blood sugar becomes elevated, which causes a flood of insulin. The insulin then converts the sugar into fat and pushes it into fat cells. It also causes the amino acid tryptophan to enter the brain in greater than normal concentrations.

Tryptophan is rapidly transported to the ends of certain neurons and immediately converted to serotonin. Within twenty minutes of your sugar and flour consumption, serotonin is released in your brain.

Serotonin soothes your locus coeruleus, which then stops its hypervigilance. The serotonin acts on your hypothalamus and you become calmer. Your breathing slows. You feel more relaxed, possibly sleepy. You become less alert, less focused on others.

Meanwhile, another part of your brain is becoming activated—the pleasure center. We'll trace that chain reaction in a future chapter. For now, keep in mind that soothing results from one chemical pathway, pleasure is the result of another, and both are activated by eating sugar and starch.

Stress, fear, threat, and uncomfortable feelings are, therefore, the second major cause of appetite disorder. As with NPY, the appetite becomes disordered as a result of a chemical chain reaction—one that, in this case, is triggered by stress.

Once the dominoes start falling, they can be stopped most successfully with something that produces comfort. Many of the tools you'll learn to use in this book are specifically designed to interrupt this soothe-seeking chain reaction.

Remember two things about this chain reaction:

1. In the early stages of your learning process, you will rarely be aware that the relief-seeking sequence has been activated.

2. Once the sequence starts, it will proceed relentlessly toward relief until some sort of relief has been achieved.

### Finding a Safe Place

You are already an expert on how to use food to soothe yourself. Relief-seeking proceeds so automatically that it operates on its own, below your radar.

So the question is: Are you willing to take some small steps, one at a time, to build an alternative system that can, eventually, be more effective than food at giving you relief?

Food comforts, no question. But other sources of comfort can be just as powerful. If you aren't used to them, it takes some time to *get* used to them. Can you make a decision, right now, to give yourself that time?

You and your recovery partner can build a place of safety, creating a new system for finding relief. It's enormously comforting to be understood and accepted. As you begin to care about each other's well-being, you may also feel the unmatched relief of being truly known.

Because the food-seeking system is already solidly in place, you can imagine that it will take some persistence before your new alternative system can compete. Make room for yourself and your friend to have a learning curve. Try to accept that you'll both make mistakes and will need practice at giving and receiving support.

• • •

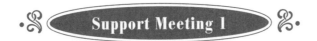

## Support Meeting 1

### Exercise: Building Support

Schedule an initial meeting with your recovery partner. Plan to meet from an hour to ninety minutes. Then, use the guidelines below to get your meeting started in the right direction.

**TIP**

Start and end on time. Keeping time boundaries strengthens the meeting.

*Opening*

(See Appendix A for an opening you and your recovery partner can read aloud at the beginning of each meeting.)

*Today's Agenda*

1. Get to know each other better by talking about any or all of the following. (Time: all but the last fifteen minutes of the meeting.)

   • What are your feelings about starting this program?

   • How does it feel to be doing this program with your recovery partner?

   • What has it been like to keep the Body Signals Charts?

   • Are there times when you don't want to fill out your daily chart? How is that related to the foods you are choosing to eat that day?

   • What is your reaction to the five principles described in the opening of the sample meeting in Appendix A?

2. Planning support. (Time: ten minutes.)

   Discuss how to support each other in filling out your Body Signals Chart every day. For example, you might decide to check in with each other at the end of each day with an e-mail or phone call, just to say, "I get credit! I filled in my chart today." A lovely response would be a verbal pat on the back, such as, "Attagirl, you rock!"

**TIP**

Keep these phone calls short (absolutely no longer than five minutes) and on topic.

3. (Optional) If you are really curious to see what your charts can tell you, you may start interpreting them now. To do so, skip to Chapter 15. Start with the beginning of that chapter and help each other follow the instructions until you get to the heading "Week 3 Charts." At that point, come back and continue with Chapter 14.

### Closing

(See Appendix A for additional information on bringing the meeting to a close.)

**LIKES AND LEARNINGS**. You may want to close all of your meetings with "likes and learnings." The technique of using learnings as a way to quickly assess the value of an experience while also creating a transition for leaving that experience comes from Systems-Centered Training. (See Appendix C.)

Talk about either or both of the following:

- What did you like about today's meeting?
- What did you learn?

Close with an optional simple prayer *if* both (or all) of you would like. Many people use the Serenity Prayer.

> *God, grant me the serenity*
>
> *to accept the things I cannot change,*
>
> *the courage to change the things I can,*
>
> *and the wisdom to know the difference.*

# 14

# Reverse a Cause of Appetite Disorder

☙ IF YOU DROP a live electric wire into water, the water will carry the charge to anything that can conduct it. Neurotransmitters are chemicals found at the ends of neurons that act in a similar fashion. A neuron is like an electric wire, and a neurotransmitter is like a puddle at the end of the wire that allows the charge to bridge the gaps to adjacent neurons.

The billions of neuron connections in your body are all bridged by various neurotransmitters. Serotonin is one of these. It is the relief neurotransmitter. When you feel naturally soothed, relaxed, or mellow, serotonin is responsible. Serotonin soothes appetite as well, promoting satiety.

The third major cause of appetite disorder is deficient serotonin. Two biochemical cycles that involve serotonin affect appetite.

### Cycle One

Inadequate serotonin causes a person to be extra vulnerable to harsh conditions, criticism, ridicule, sarcasm, mild neglect, isolation, and physical pain. Inadequate serotonin can even cause clumsiness, which can provoke ridicule by others or loss of self-esteem. If you are deficient in serotonin, you will have difficulty being soothed because your natural, internal soothing mechanisms will be sluggish.

You're probably ahead of me now. The setup is obvious. Make any being vulnerable to pain, and then prevent it from being soothed. Worse, give it an attribute,

**STEP 7**

Improve your satiety through serotonin.

like clumsiness, which often results in ridicule and exposes it to social distress. What do you think happens?

This creature will track down relief. Once it finds it, it'll go there again when needed.

Your animal body, if serotonin is malfunctioning, will be superalert to any mechanism that delivers relief. It will catch on quickly when it discovers that eating sugary or starchy foods boosts serotonin levels.

But, guess what happens when you do eat sugary foods and artificially boost serotonin by, say, eating a lot of candy? You soon become deficient in serotonin again. And then, due to a lack of supply, your serotonin delivery system malfunctions.

*This is the exact mechanism that leads to binge eating and appetite disorder.* A lack of serotonin causes the increase in appetite that results in binge eating.

This mechanism explains what happens in mildly dysfunctional families in which one child has eating or addiction problems while her sibling handles life smoothly. The addicted or appetite-disordered child has a serotonin malfunction. The other child's serotonin transmits well, so he is less vulnerable to stressors and more easily soothed from multiple sources. This cycle is illustrated below.

FIGURE 7

**The Serotonin Deficiency Cycle**

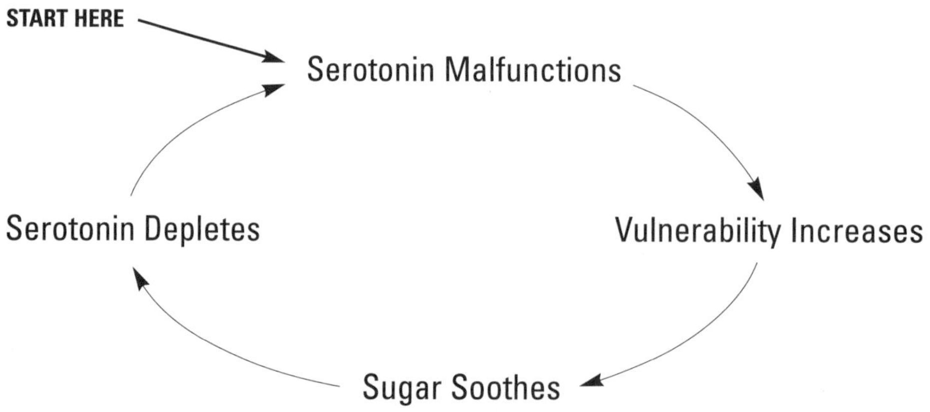

**START HERE**

Serotonin Malfunctions

Serotonin Depletes

Vulnerability Increases

Sugar Soothes

## Cycle Two

The other way to develop a defective serotonin system is to grow up in a harsh environment. Trauma has an extensive effect on the brain. Frightening situations, meanness, neglect, deprivation, and abandonment create imbalances in neurotransmitters and actual changes in neuron distribution, receptor sensitivity, receptor density, and dendrite concentration. (An example of stress-induced dendrite density is shown in Figure 8.)

These changes can be wrought by repeated trauma or by a single calamity. They can occur regardless of a person's age. However, while the brain is still developing and differentiating—through a person's midtwenties—trauma exerts a greater influence on the development of his or her neural networks.

## Neural Network

A neural network consists of integrated patterns of firing neurons. Once a pattern of nerve firing is established, a person's perceptions and reactions fall most easily into that pattern, making the person less likely to view a situation objectively. She may then misinterpret situations in the direction that matches her neural network, taking things personally that actually have nothing to do with her.

FIGURE 8

**Stress-Induced Dendrite Density** [1]

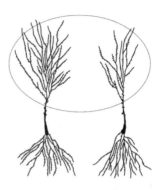

Above are neurons from two tree shrews. The circled fibers are dendrites. The shrew on the right was subjected to stress. Notice the decreased number of dendrites from this shrew.

If anyone has ever been mad at you just because you were sad—"STOP CRYING, or I'll give you something to cry about!"—that person was taking personally something that was actually your own business. Another example of taking something personally would be apologizing for bad weather, as if the weather could possibly be someone's fault. ("I'm sorry. I invited you all the way out here for a picnic, and now it's raining.") The chemistry behind such comments has to do, in part, with an imbalance between the distribution of serotonin and norepinephrine (NE), which is another neurotransmitter.

Like your car, in which water lines and oil lines run separately, each neuron works through a specific transmitter. Just as you wouldn't put oil in your radiator, a serotonin neuron wouldn't use NE.

Norepinephrine could be called the effort transmitter. Effort or trying hard stimulates NE firing in the neural network.

Trauma causes an increase in the branching of neurons that use NE in certain parts of the brain and a decrease in branching in other parts. The area in which the increase happens determines how this imbalance will manifest. For example, if trauma causes an increase in NE neurons such that the lateral hypothalamic area becomes overstimulated, a person's response to stress will be to binge eat. If trauma *decreases* NE branching in the feedback system of the locus coeruleus, it will cause a person to focus on others, be highly reactive to them, and be hypervigilant. The person will also have decreased awareness of his or her own internal processes.

Here's what will happen if one person has all three alterations in branching: When she is stressed, she will try hard; she will have difficulty accessing her internal states; and she will binge eat.

The body's natural response to this type of overfunctioning is to get the serotonin system in action, signaling to the person that it's time to take a break and relax. But a person deaf to her body's voice will miss the signal—and if she also happens to be deficient in serotonin, there won't even *be* a signal. Hence, she'll just keep overfunctioning ad infinitum.

Eating sugar will halt overfunctioning by flooding the brain with serotonin, but if the person is deficient in serotonin, she'll have to depend on a more powerful relief center—the addicted part of the brain. (We're not quite ready for that discussion yet. Just know that Super Soother is waiting in the wings.)

The brain tends to manufacture NE more readily than serotonin, partly because the ingredients for norepinephrine pass more easily into the brain (technically, through what is called the blood-brain barrier). When we're thinking survival, this makes sense. When a mastodon is charging, that's not a good time for a nap. It's more important to be able to fight than to relax.

In this world, we can feel threatened daily, even hourly. Worse, if our neural network developed in a scary home, then we have been programmed to view things as threatening, even when they aren't.

If all the children in a family have some sort of addiction or compulsive problem, there's a high probability that Cycle Two is at work. The addictions may vary—one child becomes an alcoholic, another has an appetite disorder, and the third has problems with rage—but all the children are affected, revealing that their neural networks developed in the presence of trauma. In contrast with families with a mix of children with and without addictions, the stressors in a Cycle Two family overwhelm even a healthy child's wiring and divert that child to Cycle Two problems.

Trauma influences the development of appetite disorder in the following sequence:

1. A neural network forms that expects and anticipates threat.
2. Over time, an overabundance of NE neurotransmitter receptors accumulates in the binge areas of the brain.
3. The person tends to respond to threat with extra effort, leading to ...
4. A demand for soothing, resulting in ...
5. Serotonin depletion, therefore ...
6. Triggering Cycle One, plus ...
7. Ongoing overfiring of NE leads to ...
8. Burnout and NE depletion.

This is illustrated in Figure 9, shown on the next page.

As you can see, Cycle Two can lead to Cycle One.

Fortunately, we can heal our brains. Many of the steps you are taking as you follow the program in this book will, if you keep going, start to alter your brain's wiring.

For the brain to heal, it needs regular nutrition and consistent blood sugar (eating change one), ample supplies of protein (eating change two), and practices that reduce the perception of threat (Step 6). Now, with the introduction of eating change three, you can intervene on Cycle One.

### Remedies

You may be wondering, *Is there a serotonin pill?* The answer is no. Even if we made one, it couldn't enter the brain. Your brain has a fence around it called the blood-brain barrier.

FIGURE 9

**The Influence of Trauma**

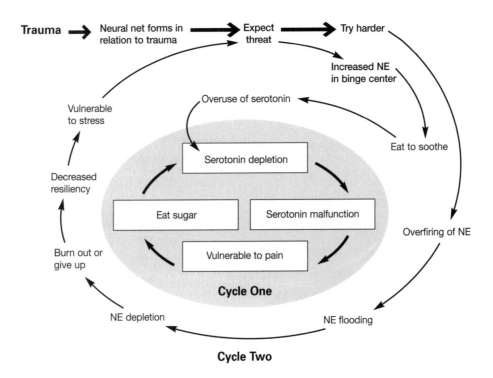

It's a good thing too. Otherwise, chemicals needed for the rest of the body would be too strong for the brain, and you could even be killed by some ordinary, familiar substance.

For a nutrient or chemical to enter the brain, it has to have some form of transportation across the barrier. For example, if you had a headache, eating willow bark would provide a lot of relief if it weren't for the blood-brain barrier. The salicylic acid in willow bark needs to undergo a chemical process—to be acetylized—to make a grand entrance into the brain. Voilà, aspirin—acetylsalicylic acid!

*Restore Serotonin Supplies*

To get more serotonin, you need to feed your brain the ingredients it uses to manufacture it. Tryptophan is the precursor, or main ingredient, of serotonin.

The easiest way to up your serotonin stores is to eat turkey or drink milk.

I can't tell you why turkey is a better source of tryptophan than other proteins. I once theorized it contained a greater percentage of tryptophan and then spent a day in the medical library disproving my theory. In fact, most proteins have about the same ratio of tryptophan to other amino acids. That means some other factor is involved, a factor we don't yet fully understand.

Regardless, satiety improves undeniably by eating turkey on a regular basis, which leads us to eating change three.

### Eating Change Three

For the next week, eat at least four ounces of turkey once a day. The week after, eat at least four ounces of turkey every other day. After that, eat turkey at least twice a week, unless you notice your appetite increasing. If that happens, add another serving of turkey per week, so that you are having turkey three times per week.

Milk is another superb source of active tryptophan. You can substitute three and a quarter glasses of milk for one turkey serving. In other words, instead of turkey, you could drink three and a quarter eight-ounce glasses of milk the appropriate number of times each week. For faster tryptophan delivery, warm your milk. You can also substitute two and a quarter ounces of mozzarella cheese or two and a half ounces of Parmesan cheese for one turkey serving.

For vegans, other effective sources of tryptophan are sesame and pumpkin seeds.

| TRYPTOPHAN FOODS | |
|---|---|
| *(milligrams of tryptophan per ounce of food)* | |
| **Turkey** | |
| • Light meat | 95 |
| • Dark meat | 65 |
| • Breast lunch meat | 54 |
| **Milk** | |
| • Whole | 21 |
| • Low-fat | 13.6 |
| • Yogurt | 9 |
| **Cheese** | |
| • Mozzarella | 170 |
| • Parmesan | 158 |
| • Cottage | 39 |
| **Seeds** | |
| • Sesame | 105 |
| • Tahini | 105 |
| • Sesame butter | 105 |
| • Pumpkin | 92 |
| • Sunflower | 74 |

Tryptophan pills are also available. These might be labeled tryptophan, 5-hydroxytryptophan, or 5-HTP. Tryptophan pills are not a good idea for people who are pregnant, nursing, or taking antidepressants. Check with your doctor before taking any artificial or concentrated source of tryptophan to be sure it won't interact negatively with your body or any medications you may be taking. Follow the dosage recommended on the label or your doctor's advice.

Any time your stress level increases, increase your turkey/tryptophan intake by at least one portion per week. (One portion is equivalent to four ounces of turkey (380 mg), four ounces of sesame seeds or sesame butter/tahini, or a little over two ounces of mozzarella cheese.)

**If you choose to up your tryptophan intake with pills, do not aim for 380 mg. Nutrients in food are natural and unconcentrated. The tryptophan in pills is much more concentrated, and the quantity cannot be compared to the amount in natural foods. So follow your doctor's advice or the label's directions.**

### Restore Serotonin Functioning

If, in addition to serotonin depletion, you have a malfunction in your serotonin delivery system, medication may be the answer. The most common indicator of this condition is depression.

The symptoms of depression include depressed mood, low energy, disordered sleep, low self-esteem, and a general expectation that things will go wrong. If you experience no change in these symptoms after two weeks of eating according to the guidelines in this chapter, see a specialist in depression medication. (Specialists include psychiatrists, psychiatric nurses, and nurse practitioners who have studied mood-altering medications.)

*Stress up? Up turkey!*

Antidepressants work in various ways to improve serotonin delivery or serotonin/norepinephrine balance. Even if you take an antidepressant, you still need to supply your brain with enough tryptophan so it can manufacture the needed neurotransmitter. When someone complains to me about their antidepressant not working, I check to see if they are feeding their hungry brain the tryptophan it needs.

*Resupply Norephinephrine Stores*

If you are following this program, you are already doing this. Your brain needs proteins to manufacture norepinephrine. Any protein will do. By eating your 50/50 snacks twice a day (eating change two), you've got this covered.

*Avoid Stressful Situations*

Oops. Asking too much. We'll come back to this subject later.

## Body Signals Chart, Week 4

This week the Body Signals Chart has one addition, a tryptophan row at the bottom of the food section. Each time you eat tryptophan, put a check mark in the appropriate box on the timeline. Soon you'll notice how tryptophan affects you.

Sometimes turkey makes people sleepy. If that happens to you, eat your turkey at a time of day when you don't mind sleepiness. Also, when people resupply themselves with tryptophan, they sometimes experience vivid dreaming. If you notice this effect, it's a signal that your body is finally getting a nutrient it needs.

• • •

---

### EATING MAP, WEEK 4

- Eat every two to three hours while you're awake.

- Eat snacks that are 50 percent protein/50 percent complex carbs.

- Do not eat snacks made from flour, wheat, sugar, or simple carbs.

- Take snacks with you wherever you go.

- Eat at least four ounces of turkey every day. You may substitute tryptophan from another source, such as milk, sesame seeds, or tahini, making sure your food intake is equivalent to about 380 mg of tryptophan.

- If your stress level goes up, increase the amount of tryptophan you eat.

Now is a good time to meet again with your recovery partner. You can use this meeting to continue to get to know each other and also to support each other with your new eating change and with keeping the Body Signals Charts for one more week.

### Opening

### Today's Agenda

Discuss:

1. What you noticed about following eating changes one and two.

2. What you noticed about filling out the charts this week.

3. If any old thinking about your body, eating, or dieting tried to clash with this new way of approaching a disordered appetite.

4. If you want to interpret your Week 3 charts now. (This is assuming you have already learned how to interpret your charts at your last meeting and are ready to advance to the section "Week 3 Charts" in Chapter 15.) When you get to the heading "Week 4 Charts: Assisted Serotonin," stop.

### Closing

# Body Signals Chart, Week 4

Date: _____

| CATEGORY | DESCRIPTIONS | CHANGE: ADD TRYPTOPHAN ONCE A DAY | | | | | | | | | | | | | | | | | | | | | | |
|---|---|---|---|---|---|---|---|---|---|---|---|---|---|---|---|---|---|---|---|---|---|---|---|---|---|
| Timeline | Circle Wake-up | 6AM | 7 | 8 | 9 | 10 | 11 | 12PM | 1 | 2 | 3 | 4 | 5 | 6 | 7 | 8 | 9 | 10 | 11 | 12AM | 1 | 2 | 3 | 4 | 5 |
| **Food** Numbers go in this section | Proteins | | | | | | | | | | | | | | | | | | | | | | | | |
| | Complex carbs | | | | | | | | | | | | | | | | | | | | | | | | |
| | Flour | | | | | | | | | | | | | | | | | | | | | | | | |
| | Sugar | | | | | | | | | | | | | | | | | | | | | | | | |
| | Fats | | | | | | | | | | | | | | | | | | | | | | | | |
| Check | **Tryptophan** | | | | | | | | | | | | | | | | | | | | | | | | |
| Check | **Equal/NutraSweet** | | | | | | | | | | | | | | | | | | | | | | | | |
| **Drink** Dots go in this section | Water | | | | | | | | | | | | | | | | | | | | | | | | |
| | Pop | | | | | | | | | | | | | | | | | | | | | | | | |
| | Diet pop | | | | | | | | | | | | | | | | | | | | | | | | |
| | Coffee | | | | | | | | | | | | | | | | | | | | | | | | |
| | Herbal drink | | | | | | | | | | | | | | | | | | | | | | | | |
| | Milk | | | | | | | | | | | | | | | | | | | | | | | | |
| | Juice | | | | | | | | | | | | | | | | | | | | | | | | |
| | Alcohol | | | | | | | | | | | | | | | | | | | | | | | | |
| | Tea | | | | | | | | | | | | | | | | | | | | | | | | |
| Check | **Caffeine** | | | | | | | | | | | | | | | | | | | | | | | | |
| Timeline | | 6AM | 7 | 8 | 9 | 10 | 11 | 12PM | 1 | 2 | 3 | 4 | 5 | 6 | 7 | 8 | 9 | 10 | 11 | 12AM | 1 | 2 | 3 | 4 | 5 |
| **Fullness** | Stuffed | | | | | | | | | | | | | | | | | | | | | | | | |
| | Comfortable | | | | | | | | | | | | | | | | | | | | | | | | |
| | Empty | | | | | | | | | | | | | | | | | | | | | | | | |
| **Hunger** | Starving | | | | | | | | | | | | | | | | | | | | | | | | |
| | Really hungry | | | | | | | | | | | | | | | | | | | | | | | | |
| | Mildly hungry | | | | | | | | | | | | | | | | | | | | | | | | |
| | Not hungry | | | | | | | | | | | | | | | | | | | | | | | | |
| **Appetite** | Craving food | | | | | | | | | | | | | | | | | | | | | | | | |
| | Food focused | | | | | | | | | | | | | | | | | | | | | | | | |
| | Quiet | | | | | | | | | | | | | | | | | | | | | | | | |
| **Satiety** | Satiated | | | | | | | | | | | | | | | | | | | | | | | | |
| | Not | | | | | | | | | | | | | | | | | | | | | | | | |
| **Energy** | High | | | | | | | | | | | | | | | | | | | | | | | | |
| | Medium | | | | | | | | | | | | | | | | | | | | | | | | |
| | Low | | | | | | | | | | | | | | | | | | | | | | | | |
| **Thinking** | Very sharp | | | | | | | | | | | | | | | | | | | | | | | | |
| | Clear | | | | | | | | | | | | | | | | | | | | | | | | |
| | Cloudy | | | | | | | | | | | | | | | | | | | | | | | | |
| **Blood Sugar Reaction** | Headache | | | | | | | | | | | | | | | | | | | | | | | | |
| | Light-headed | | | | | | | | | | | | | | | | | | | | | | | | |
| | Even | | | | | | | | | | | | | | | | | | | | | | | | |
| | Sugar daze | | | | | | | | | | | | | | | | | | | | | | | | |
| | Sleepy | | | | | | | | | | | | | | | | | | | | | | | | |
| **Mood** | Optimistic | | | | | | | | | | | | | | | | | | | | | | | | |
| | Okay | | | | | | | | | | | | | | | | | | | | | | | | |
| | Depressed | | | | | | | | | | | | | | | | | | | | | | | | |
| **Stressed?** | Highly | | | | | | | | | | | | | | | | | | | | | | | | |
| | Mildly | | | | | | | | | | | | | | | | | | | | | | | | |
| | No | | | | | | | | | | | | | | | | | | | | | | | | |
| **Seeking Comfort?** | | | | | | | | | | | | | | | | | | | | | | | | | |
| **Body Conscious?** | | | | | | | | | | | | | | | | | | | | | | | | | |
| Timeline | | 6AM | 7 | 8 | 9 | 10 | 11 | 12PM | 1 | 2 | 3 | 4 | 5 | 6 | 7 | 8 | 9 | 10 | 11 | 12AM | 1 | 2 | 3 | 4 | 5 |

Duplicating this page for personal use is permissible.

# 15

# Interpret Your Body's Language

IT'S FINALLY time to find out what causes your appetite disorder. Your Body Signals Charts provide you with a daily record of your appetite patterns since beginning this program, ideally for the last four weeks.

By looking at your charts, we can deduce what is happening in your brain to make you eat too much. Then we can create a program that fits your brain and your biology. Instead of trying to stop yourself from overeating, you can stop your unruly appetite.

> **STEP 8**
>
> Decode your body's signals.

You can do the work of this chapter on your own. However, it will be much easier and a lot more fun to do it with your recovery partner. Plus, it's good practice for using support.

Call your recovery partner to set up a meeting. Plan for it to last at least a couple of hours. In fact, you may need more than one meeting for each of you to learn all that your bodies are trying to tell you.

Start the meeting with the suggested opening (Appendix A), and then follow the agenda at the end of this chapter. Bring all your Body Signals Charts to the meeting, as well as pens or markers in several different colors, including two highlighting colors such as yellow or translucent pink.

## Learning to Read Your Charts—Week 1

You'll sort out the influence of various biochemicals on your appetite, one chemical at a time. To start, look at your daily charts for Week 1. Using a highlighter, trace the peaks and valleys shown below the timeline for each of the four indicators: fullness, hunger, appetite, and satiety. Use one highlighter color for the appetite and satiety lines, and the other highlighter color for the hunger and fullness lines. (See Example 1 on the next page.)

## Appetite Caused by NPY/Failure of PYY Satiety

First you are going to identify appetite that is caused by NPY. Look at the appetite line in Example 1.

EXAMPLE 1

Claire Week 1

### Body Signals Chart, Week 1

| CATEGORY | DESCRIPTIONS | BASELINE DATA—NO CHANGES | | | | | | | | | | | | | | | | | |
|---|---|---|---|---|---|---|---|---|---|---|---|---|---|---|---|---|---|---|---|
| Timeline | Circle Wake-up | 6AM | 7 | 8 | 9 | 10 | 11 | 12PM | 1 | 2 | 3 | 4 | 5 | 6 | 7 | 8 | 9 | 10 | 11 |
| **Food** | Proteins | | | | | | 3 | | | | | | | | 5 | | | | |
| | Complex carbs | *No Breakfast* | | | | | 2 | | | | | | | | | | | | |
| | Simple carbs | | | | | | 3 | 5 | | | | | | | 2 | 10 | 5 | | |
| | Fats | | | | | | 2 | 5 | | | | | | | 3 | | 5 | | |
| **Fullness** | Stuffed | | | | | | | | | | | | | | | | | | |
| | Comfortable | | | | | | | | | | | | | | | | | | |
| | Empty | | | | | | | | | | | | | | | | | | |
| **Hunger** | Starving | | | | | | | | | | | | | | | | | | |
| | Really hungry | | | | | | | | | | | | | | | | | | |
| | Mildly hungry | | | | | | | | | | | | | | | | | | |
| | Not hungry | | | | | | | | | | | | | | | | | | |
| **Appetite** | Craving food | | | | | | | | | | | | | | | | | | |
| | Food focused | | | | | | | | | | | | | | | | | | |
| | Quiet | | | | | | | | | | | | | | | | | | |
| **Satiety** | Satiated | | | | | | | | | | | | | | | | | | |
| | Not | | | | | | | | | | | | | | | | | | |

Notice that Claire craves food from 1 p.m. until 10 p.m. Do you also see that her appetite didn't get triggered *until* she'd actually eaten at noon? This is a classic NPY pattern—appetite rising *after* eating begins.

We don't have to look hard to find the cause. Claire skipped breakfast. As the morning progressed, her appetite remained quiet, but once she began eating, NPY kicked in, and for the rest of the day her appetite was driving her, troubling her with food thoughts all afternoon.

Satiety failed her. We see no evidence of PYY. Once she lost satiety, it was gone for the rest of the day, only kicking in overnight, so that she awakened with no appetite the next morning. (Notice that she felt satiated in the early morning.) With this pattern, Claire demonstrates a long-delayed onset of satiety.

She now has a PYY deficiency and has lost the benefit of one of the body's natural mechanisms to stop eating. Because of this, Claire ate more after her mealtime. Her lunch lasted two hours. Her dinner lasted three hours. This is what happens when someone has a long-standing pattern of skipping meals.

Now look at Arrie's chart, in Example 2 below. (By the way, the example charts have been donated through the generosity of actual people. Therefore, some charts may come from an earlier phase of this program and differ slightly from yours. Don't be concerned about variations in the chart. What matters is the points they illustrate.)

EXAMPLE 2

Arrie Week 1

### Body Signals Chart, Week 1

| CATEGORY | DESCRIPTIONS | BASELINE DATA—NO CHANGES | | | | | | | | | | | | | | | | | |
|---|---|---|---|---|---|---|---|---|---|---|---|---|---|---|---|---|---|---|---|
| Timeline | Circle Wake-up | 6AM | 7 | 8 | 9 | 10 | 11 | 12PM | 1 | 2 | 3 | 4 | 5 | 6 | 7 | 8 | 9 | 10 | 11 |
| **Food** | Proteins | | | | | | | | 4 | | | | | | | 3 | | | |
| | Complex carbs | | | | | | | | 1 | | | | | | | | | | |
| | Simple carbs | | | 10 | | | | | 2 | | | | | | | | 2 | 5 | 8 | |
| | Fats | | | | | | | | 3 | | | | | | | | 5 | 5 | 2 | |
| *Check* | Caffeine | | | ✔ | | | | | | | | | | | | | | | |
| **Fullness** | Stuffed | | | | | | | | | | | | | | | | | | |
| | Comfortable | | | | | | | | | | | | | | | | | | |
| | Empty | | | | | | | | | | | | | | | | | | |
| **Hunger** | Starving | | | | | | | | | | | | | | | | | | |
| | Really hungry | | | | | | | | | | | | | | | | | | |
| | Mildly hungry | | | | | | | | | | | | | | | | | | |
| | Not hungry | | | | | | | | | | | | | | | | | | |
| **Appetite** | Craving food | | | | | | | | | | | | | | | | | | |
| | Food focused | | | | | | | | | | | | | | | | | | |
| | Quiet | | | | | | | | | | | | | | | | | | |
| **Satiety** | Satiated | | | | | | | | | | | | | | | | | | |
| | Not | | | | | | | | | | | | | | | | | | |

Arrie started the day with an all-starch breakfast and a cup of coffee. For someone with an appetite disorder, that's like throwing gas on a fire. This meal triggered her appetite, plaguing her with cravings and thoughts of food for the rest of the day. She delayed lunch until 1 p.m., but it gave her appetite no relief. Then she put off dinner until 8 p.m., and once she started eating, she ate for three hours.

Her chart shows a complete failure of satiety. Arrie awakened in the morning wanting food, and satiety biochemicals failed to kick in at any point during the day. Eating did not abate her appetite. Because this is a typical eating pattern for Arrie—long gaps between meals, and many meals (such as this day's breakfast) with little true nutritional value—we can safely assume that her PYY is down and out.

Finally, look at Berthe's chart in Example 3 below.

EXAMPLE 3

Berthe Week 1

**Body Signals Chart, Week 1**

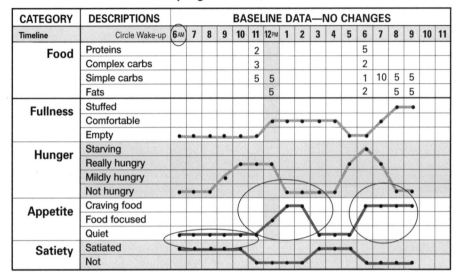

| CATEGORY | DESCRIPTIONS | BASELINE DATA—NO CHANGES | | | | | | | | | | | | | | | | | |
|---|---|---|---|---|---|---|---|---|---|---|---|---|---|---|---|---|---|---|---|
| Timeline | Circle Wake-up | 6AM | 7 | 8 | 9 | 10 | 11 | 12PM | 1 | 2 | 3 | 4 | 5 | 6 | 7 | 8 | 9 | 10 | 11 |
| **Food** | Proteins | | | | | | 2 | | | | | | | 5 | | | | | |
| | Complex carbs | | | | | | 3 | | | | | | | 2 | | | | | |
| | Simple carbs | | | | | | 5 | 5 | | | | | | 1 | 10 | 5 | 5 | | |
| | Fats | | | | | | | 5 | | | | | | 2 | | 5 | 5 | | |
| **Fullness** | Stuffed | | | | | | | | | | | | | | | | | | |
| | Comfortable | | | | | | | | | | | | | | | | | | |
| | Empty | | | | | | | | | | | | | | | | | | |
| **Hunger** | Starving | | | | | | | | | | | | | | | | | | |
| | Really hungry | | | | | | | | | | | | | | | | | | |
| | Mildly hungry | | | | | | | | | | | | | | | | | | |
| | Not hungry | | | | | | | | | | | | | | | | | | |
| **Appetite** | Craving food | | | | | | | | | | | | | | | | | | |
| | Food focused | | | | | | | | | | | | | | | | | | |
| | Quiet | | | | | | | | | | | | | | | | | | |
| **Satiety** | Satiated | | | | | | | | | | | | | | | | | | |
| | Not | | | | | | | | | | | | | | | | | | |

First Berthe skipped breakfast. She had a high-carb lunch at 11 a.m., and then didn't eat a meal or appropriate snack until 6 p.m. After lunch, her appetite increased until it finally went quiet at 3 p.m. You now recognize that as a sign of what? Answer: NPY, stimulating her appetite once food has been provided after a gap in eating. Satiety kicked in midafternoon—a four-hour delay.

After dinner, her appetite jumped and she craved food the rest of the evening. Yet she started the next day satiated even though she went to bed unsatiated after four hours of eating—a sign of much-delayed satiety.

Berthe's chart demonstrates an NPY/PYY imbalance—the result of maintaining irregular mealtimes and skipping breakfast.

Notice that for all three women, hunger and appetite are operating on different schedules. Even though Claire was stuffed after both lunch and dinner, she still wanted more to eat (appetite). Arrie was comfortably full after lunch and stuffed after dinner, but she still craved food. Berthe had no appetite before lunch or dinner even though she was hungry. After lunch, her hunger dropped while her appetite increased.

Now it's time for you to look at your own charts for Week 1. You are looking for the influence of NPY and PYY—for the interaction of appetite and satiety.

**Focus: Appetite and Satiety Rows**

Problems with NPY or PYY can be summarized as follows:

- Appetite increases during or after a meal.
- Satiety is delayed or occurs upon awakening.
- Meals are skipped, particularly breakfast.
- Eating continues following a meal.

Pick one color of marker and circle all peaks in appetite that *follow* a meal, whether the upward slope starts during the meal or just after. Notice also what happens to your eating. Does a meal stop your desire to eat (satiety)? Or do you eat more after you've had a meal? Do you go to bed wanting food, or is your appetite quiet? Do you wake up satiated or ready to eat?

*Your Patterns Related to NPY/PYY*

In the chart below, place a slash in the "Yes" box for each indicator of NPY influence on appetite as described in the list on the left. For example, as you look through your charts for Week 1, if you skipped breakfast three times, put three slashes in the "Yes" column next to "Skipped meals."

| SELF-DIAGNOSIS (NPY/PYY) | Yes | No |
|---|---|---|
| Delayed meals | | |
| Skipped meals | | |
| Appetite rises during a meal | | |
| Appetite rises after a meal | | |
| Eating continues after a meal | | |
| You awaken satiated | | |
| Totals | | |

Count up all the slashes in each column and put that number in the "Totals" row. If your "Yes" total is greater than four, an NPY/PYY imbalance is at least one cause of your appetite disorder.

### Ghrelin

When ghrelin rises, hunger rises. It's normal for hunger to rise before a regular mealtime, but feeling hungry soon after a plentiful meal means that some biochemical has been activated.

If your hunger spikes after you've had plenty of food, look at the proportion of fat contained in the meal. A meal high in fat can cause a rebound of the hunger-causing chemical ghrelin. See Example 4 below.

EXAMPLE 4

**Body Signals Chart, Week 1**

| CATEGORY | DESCRIPTIONS | BASELINE DATA—NO CHANGES | | | | | | | | | | | | | | | | |
|---|---|---|---|---|---|---|---|---|---|---|---|---|---|---|---|---|---|---|
| Timeline | Circle Wake-up | 6AM | (7) | 8 | 9 | 10 | 11 | 12PM | 1 | 2 | 3 | 4 | 5 | 6 | 7 | 8 | 9 | 10 | 11 |
| **Food** | Proteins | | | 6 | | | | 4 | | | | | 5 | | | | | | |
| | Complex carbs | | | | | | | | | | | | | | | | | | |
| | Simple carbs | | | 2 | | | | 3 | | | | | | | | | | | |
| | Fats | | | 2 | | | | 3 | | | | | 5 | 10 | | | | | |
| *Check* | **Equal/NutraSweet** | | | | | | | | | | | | | | | | | | |
| *Check* | **Caffeine** | | | | | | | | | | | | | | | | | | |
| **Fullness** | Stuffed | | | | | | | | | | | | | | | | | | |
| | Comfortable | | • | • | • | • | • | • | • | • | • | • | | | • | | | | |
| | Empty | | | | | | | | | | | | • | • | | | | | |
| **Hunger** | Starving | | | | | | | | | | | | | | | | | | |
| | Really hungry | | | | | | | | | | | | | | | | | | |
| | Mildly hungry | | | | | | | | | | | | | | | | | | |
| | Not hungry | | • | • | • | • | • | • | • | • | • | • | | | | • | • | | |

In this example, the 6 p.m. meal was 100 percent fat. Look at the ghrelin spike in the hunger row.

Now look at your own charts.

### Focus: Hunger Row

Problems:

- Hunger rising soon after a high-fat meal
- Eating right after a meal

Take another highlighter and circle all the peaks in hunger that *follow* a high-fat meal on each chart. Again, the upward slope may start during the meal or soon afterward. Do you find evidence of a ghrelin spike?

I'm going to save further discussion of ghrelin spikes until Chapter 35 because we won't be ready to look at this cause of disordered appetite until a lot of other ducks are lined up first. For now, just keep in mind that you may need to deal with them, but not until much farther down your recovery road.

**Week 2 Charts**

During Week 2, if you followed the eating map, you ate every two to three hours. Once again use highlighters to trace peaks and valleys below the time-line. Identify any NPY and ghrelin peaks, circling them with two different colors, just as you did on your Week 1 charts.

Now pick a new, third highlighter color. Use this color to indicate signs of progress. Anywhere on your Week 2 charts where you see an improvement—an increase in satiety; a decrease in appetite, hunger, or eating after a meal; an increase in energy; a more even blood sugar level; an increase or evenness in clarity of thought; or a decrease in stress—circle that improvement.

A comparison between energy and blood sugar indicators for Fania from Week 1 to Week 2 is shown on the next two pages.

You'll notice that just by making one change—adding meals every two to three hours—Fania did much better. Her energy level improved. Her blood sugar indicators became more even, and her thinking stayed clear throughout the day. She avoided food cravings, and she experienced increased satiety.

*Signs of Progress:*

- Comfortable fullness after meals
- Hunger that is stopped by meals
- Appetite that is stopped by meals
- Satiety that is reached after meals
- Lower hunger and appetite spikes
- Improved thinking, mood, and energy levels
- More even blood sugar and energy levels

EXAMPLE 5

Fania Week 1

## Body Signals Chart, Week 1

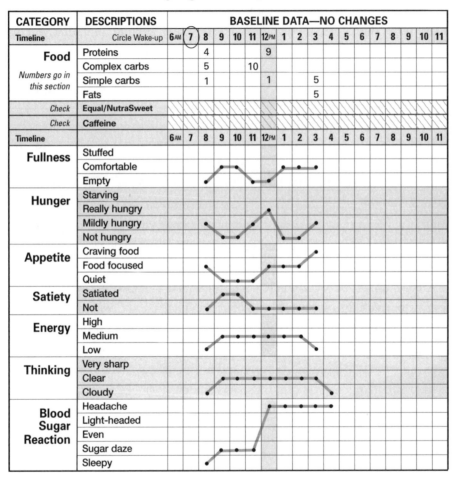

| CATEGORY | DESCRIPTIONS | BASELINE DATA—NO CHANGES |||||||||||||||||||
|---|---|---|---|---|---|---|---|---|---|---|---|---|---|---|---|---|---|---|
| Timeline | Circle Wake-up | 6AM | 7 | 8 | 9 | 10 | 11 | 12PM | 1 | 2 | 3 | 4 | 5 | 6 | 7 | 8 | 9 | 10 | 11 |
| **Food** | Proteins | | | 4 | | | | 9 | | | | | | | | | | | |
| | Complex carbs | | | 5 | | 10 | | | | | | | | | | | | | |
| *Numbers go in this section* | Simple carbs | | | 1 | | | | 1 | | | 5 | | | | | | | | |
| | Fats | | | | | | | | | | 5 | | | | | | | | |
| Check | **Equal/NutraSweet** | | | | | | | | | | | | | | | | | | |
| Check | **Caffeine** | | | | | | | | | | | | | | | | | | |
| Timeline | | 6AM | 7 | 8 | 9 | 10 | 11 | 12PM | 1 | 2 | 3 | 4 | 5 | 6 | 7 | 8 | 9 | 10 | 11 |
| **Fullness** | Stuffed | | | | | | | | | | | | | | | | | | |
| | Comfortable | | | | | | | | | | | | | | | | | | |
| | Empty | | | | | | | | | | | | | | | | | | |
| **Hunger** | Starving | | | | | | | | | | | | | | | | | | |
| | Really hungry | | | | | | | | | | | | | | | | | | |
| | Mildly hungry | | | | | | | | | | | | | | | | | | |
| | Not hungry | | | | | | | | | | | | | | | | | | |
| **Appetite** | Craving food | | | | | | | | | | | | | | | | | | |
| | Food focused | | | | | | | | | | | | | | | | | | |
| | Quiet | | | | | | | | | | | | | | | | | | |
| **Satiety** | Satiated | | | | | | | | | | | | | | | | | | |
| | Not | | | | | | | | | | | | | | | | | | |
| **Energy** | High | | | | | | | | | | | | | | | | | | |
| | Medium | | | | | | | | | | | | | | | | | | |
| | Low | | | | | | | | | | | | | | | | | | |
| **Thinking** | Very sharp | | | | | | | | | | | | | | | | | | |
| | Clear | | | | | | | | | | | | | | | | | | |
| | Cloudy | | | | | | | | | | | | | | | | | | |
| **Blood Sugar Reaction** | Headache | | | | | | | | | | | | | | | | | | |
| | Light-headed | | | | | | | | | | | | | | | | | | |
| | Even | | | | | | | | | | | | | | | | | | |
| | Sugar daze | | | | | | | | | | | | | | | | | | |
| | Sleepy | | | | | | | | | | | | | | | | | | |

EXAMPLE 5

Fania Week 2

## Body Signals Chart, Week 2

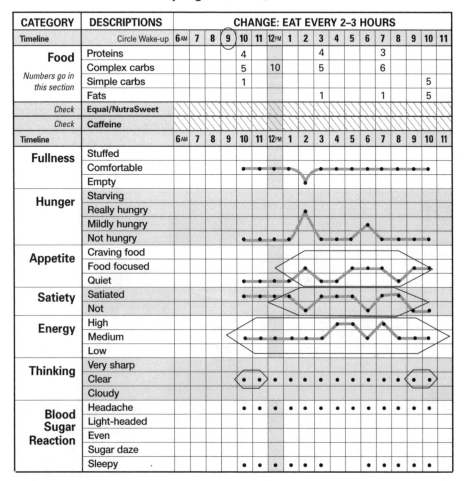

| CATEGORY | DESCRIPTIONS | CHANGE: EAT EVERY 2–3 HOURS | | | | | | | | | | | | | | | | | |
|---|---|---|---|---|---|---|---|---|---|---|---|---|---|---|---|---|---|---|---|
| Timeline | Circle Wake-up | 6AM | 7 | 8 | 9 | 10 | 11 | 12PM | 1 | 2 | 3 | 4 | 5 | 6 | 7 | 8 | 9 | 10 | 11 |
| **Food** Numbers go in this section | Proteins | | | | | 4 | | | | | 4 | | | | 3 | | | | |
| | Complex carbs | | | | | 5 | | 10 | | | 5 | | | | 6 | | | | |
| | Simple carbs | | | | | 1 | | | | | | | | | | | | 5 | |
| | Fats | | | | | | | | | | 1 | | | | 1 | | | 5 | |
| Check | **Equal/NutraSweet** | | | | | | | | | | | | | | | | | | |
| Check | **Caffeine** | | | | | | | | | | | | | | | | | | |
| Timeline | | 6AM | 7 | 8 | 9 | 10 | 11 | 12PM | 1 | 2 | 3 | 4 | 5 | 6 | 7 | 8 | 9 | 10 | 11 |
| **Fullness** | Stuffed | | | | | | | | | | | | | | | | | | |
| | Comfortable | | | | | | | | | | | | | | | | | | |
| | Empty | | | | | | | | | | | | | | | | | | |
| **Hunger** | Starving | | | | | | | | | | | | | | | | | | |
| | Really hungry | | | | | | | | | | | | | | | | | | |
| | Mildly hungry | | | | | | | | | | | | | | | | | | |
| | Not hungry | | | | | | | | | | | | | | | | | | |
| **Appetite** | Craving food | | | | | | | | | | | | | | | | | | |
| | Food focused | | | | | | | | | | | | | | | | | | |
| | Quiet | | | | | | | | | | | | | | | | | | |
| **Satiety** | Satiated | | | | | | | | | | | | | | | | | | |
| | Not | | | | | | | | | | | | | | | | | | |
| **Energy** | High | | | | | | | | | | | | | | | | | | |
| | Medium | | | | | | | | | | | | | | | | | | |
| | Low | | | | | | | | | | | | | | | | | | |
| **Thinking** | Very sharp | | | | | | | | | | | | | | | | | | |
| | Clear | | | | | | | | | | | | | | | | | | |
| | Cloudy | | | | | | | | | | | | | | | | | | |
| **Blood Sugar Reaction** | Headache | | | | | | | | | | | | | | | | | | |
| | Light-headed | | | | | | | | | | | | | | | | | | |
| | Even | | | | | | | | | | | | | | | | | | |
| | Sugar daze | | | | | | | | | | | | | | | | | | |
| | Sleepy | | | | | | | | | | | | | | | | | | |

*The five hexagons indicate improvements.*

Compare your own charts for Weeks 1 and 2. (If this seems complicated, pick a Week 1 chart that is fairly typical for the week and compare it one by one with each Week 2 chart.)

On the days you ate every two to three hours, compare your energy level, blood sugar indicators, and appetite and satiety profiles with days when you skipped or delayed meals.

*Changes Due to Eating Every Two to Three Hours*

Put a slash in each box that describes a positive change (sign of progress) during your own Week 2. Then count the number of slashes in each column and put the totals in the last line. Put the grand total in the last box.

**Changes Due to Eating Every Two to Three Hours**

| Indicator | Smaller Spikes | More Even | Stopped by Meals | Improved | Rises Appropriately |
|---|---|---|---|---|---|
| Fullness | | | | | * |
| Hunger | | | | | ** |
| Appetite | | | | | ** |
| Satiety | | | | | * |
| Energy | | | | | |
| Thinking | | | | | |
| Blood sugar | | | | | |
| Mood | | | | | |
| Stress | | | | | Grand Total |
| Progress Total | | | | | |

\* It's appropriate for fullness and satiety to rise during or immediately after a meal.

\*\* It's appropriate for hunger and appetite to rise before a normal mealtime.

◼ Shaded boxes above do not apply to this particular indicator.

Now let's look at Fania's summary, based on just one of her Week 2 charts.

EXAMPLE 6

Fania, Week 2

### Changes Due to Eating Every Two to Three Hours

| Indicator | Smaller Spikes | More Even | Stopped by Meals | Improved | Rises Appropriately |
|---|---|---|---|---|---|
| Fullness | | // | | /// | / * |
| Hunger | / | | // | | //// ** |
| Appetite | / | | // | | / ** |
| Satiety | | // | | //// | // * |
| Energy | | | | ///// | |
| Thinking | | // | | ////// | |
| Blood sugar | | | | | |
| Mood | | | | | |
| Stress | | | | | Grand Total |
| **Progress Total** | 2 | 6 | 4 | 18 | 8 | 38 |

\* It's appropriate for fullness and satiety to rise during or immediately after a meal.

\*\* It's appropriate for hunger and appetite to rise before a normal mealtime.

▇ Shaded boxes above do not apply to this particular indicator.

## Week 3 Charts

This is the week you gave yourself a wonderful gift. If you followed the eating map, you fed your brain healing doses of protein at frequent intervals.

Let's look at Fania's chart from Week 3, shown on the next page.

EXAMPLE 7

Fania, Week 3

## Body Signals Chart, Week 3

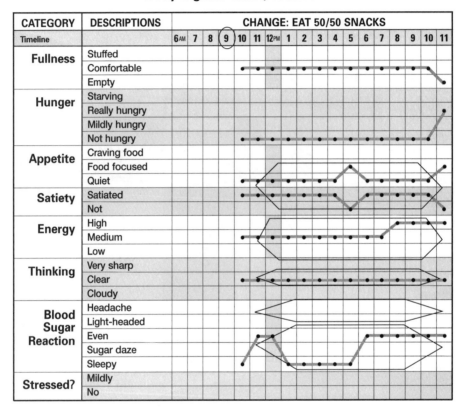

| CATEGORY | DESCRIPTIONS | CHANGE: EAT 50/50 SNACKS |
|----------|--------------|--------------------------|
| Timeline | | 6AM 7 8 9 10 11 12PM 1 2 3 4 5 6 7 8 9 10 11 |
| Fullness | Stuffed | |
| | Comfortable | |
| | Empty | |
| Hunger | Starving | |
| | Really hungry | |
| | Mildly hungry | |
| | Not hungry | |
| Appetite | Craving food | |
| | Food focused | |
| | Quiet | |
| Satiety | Satiated | |
| | Not | |
| Energy | High | |
| | Medium | |
| | Low | |
| Thinking | Very sharp | |
| | Clear | |
| | Cloudy | |
| Blood Sugar Reaction | Headache | |
| | Light-headed | |
| | Even | |
| | Sugar daze | |
| | Sleepy | |
| Stressed? | Mildly | |
| | No | |

During Week 3, Fania's indicators have improved yet again by becoming more even. Her energy level is higher and more even. Satiety and appetite levels have improved, and hunger isn't spiking the way it did previously. Interestingly, this week she also stopped having a persistent headache.

The following chart was recorded by Talia, a woman who follows the eating map daily. She has followed this pattern for months.

EXAMPLE 8

Talia

## Body Signals Chart, Week 3

| CATEGORY | DESCRIPTIONS | CHANGE: EAT 50/50 SNACKS | | | | | | | | | | | | | | | | | |
|---|---|---|---|---|---|---|---|---|---|---|---|---|---|---|---|---|---|---|---|
| Timeline | Circle Wake-up | 6AM | (7) | 8 | 9 | 10 | 11 | 12PM | 1 | 2 | 3 | 4 | 5 | 6 | 7 | 8 | 9 | 10 | 11 |
| **Food** | Proteins | | | 6 | | | 5 | | 5 | | | | 5 | 5 | | | | | |
| *Numbers go in this section* | Complex carbs | | | 4 | | | 5 | | 5 | | | | 5 | 5 | | | | | |
| | Simple carbs | | | | | | | | | | | | | | | | | | |
| | Fats | | | | | | | | | | | | | | | | | | |
| Check | **Equal/NutraSweet** | | | | | | | | | | | | | | | | | | |
| **Drink** | Water | | | | | • | • | | | | • | | | | | | | | |
| | Cola | | | | | | | | | | | | | | | | | | |
| *Dots go in this section* | Diet cola | | | | | | | | • | | | | | | | | | | |
| | Coffee | | | • | | | | | | | | | | | | | | | |
| | Herbal drink | | | | | | | | | | | | | • | | | | | |
| | Milk | | | • | | | | | | | | | | | | | | | |
| | Juice | | | | | | | | | | | | | | | | | | |
| | Alcohol | | | | | | | | | | | | | | | | | | |
| | Tea | | | | | | | | | | | | | | | | | | |
| Check | **Caffeine** | | | | | | | | | | | | | | | | | | |
| Timeline | | 6AM | 7 | 8 | 9 | 10 | 11 | 12PM | 1 | 2 | 3 | 4 | 5 | 6 | 7 | 8 | 9 | 10 | 11 |
| **Fullness** | Stuffed | | | | | | | | | | | | | | | | | | |
| | Comfortable | | | | | | | | | | | | | | | | | | |
| | Empty | | | | | | | | | | | | | | | | | | |
| **Hunger** | Starving | | | | | | | | | | | | | | | | | | |
| | Really hungry | | | | | | | | | | | | | | | | | | |
| | Mildly hungry | | | | | | | | | | | | | | | | | | |
| | Not hungry | | | | | | | | | | | | | | | | | | |
| **Appetite** | Craving food | | | | | | | | | | | | | | | | | | |
| | Food focused | | | | | | | | | | | | | | | | | | |
| | Quiet | | | | | | | | | | | | | | | | | | |
| **Satiety** | Satiated | | | | | | | | | | | | | | | | | | |
| | Not | | | | | | | | | | | | | | | | | | |
| **Energy** | High | | | | | | | | | | | | | | | | | | |
| | Medium | | | | | | | | | | | | | | | | | | |
| | Low | | | | | | | | | | | | | | | | | | |
| **Thinking** | Very sharp | | | | | | | | | | | | | | | | | | |
| | Clear | | | | | | | | | | | | | | | | | | |
| | Cloudy | | | | | | | | | | | | | | | | | | |
| **Blood Sugar Reaction** | Headache | | | | | | | | | | | | | | | | | | |
| | Light-headed | | | | | | | | | | | | | | | | | | |
| | Even | | | | | | | | | | | | | | | | | | |
| | Sugar daze | | | | | | | | | | | | | | | | | | |
| | Sleepy | | | | | | | | | | | | | | | | | | |
| **Stressed?** | Mildly | | | | | | | | | | | | | | | | | | |
| | No | | | | | | | | | | | | | | | | | | |

### EXAMPLE 8

#### Talia

Talia's thinking, energy, and blood sugar levels are even. She doesn't get starved. Hunger and appetite increase before a meal and then are stopped by the meal. She awakens hungry. (Being hungry in the morning before breakfast is a good sign.) Her appetite and satiety are in balance. PYY is working for her, and she isn't eating in a way that triggers excessive or uncontrollable appetite.

Now it's your turn. On your Week 3 charts, first highlight the peaks and valleys of all indicators below the timeline. Then identify and circle any NPY or ghrelin spikes.

*Signs of Progress:*

- Comfortable fullness after meals
- Hunger that is stopped by meals
- Appetite that is stopped by meals
- Satiety that is reached sooner after meals
- Hunger soon after waking
- Breakfast soon after waking
- Lower hunger and appetite spikes
- Improved thinking, mood, and energy levels
- More even blood sugar and energy levels
- Increased consciousness of what's going on in your body

Now compare your Week 3 charts with those of the previous weeks. Again, notice the differences between clarity of thinking, energy levels, and blood sugar levels. Also pay attention to the changes in your appetite, satiety, hunger, and fullness indicators. Use your improvement highlighter to circle your successes. Summarize these on the chart on the next page. (As before, put a slash in each box for each positive change; any box may contain multiple slashes. Then count the number of slashes in each column and put the totals in the last line. Put the grand total in the last box.)

## Changes Due to Addition of 50/50 Snacks

| Indicator | Smaller Spikes | More Even | Stopped by Meals | Improved | Rises Appropriately | |
|---|---|---|---|---|---|---|
| Fullness | | | | | * | |
| Hunger | | | | | ** | |
| Appetite | | | | | ** | |
| Satiety | | | | | * | |
| Energy | | | | | | |
| Thinking | | | | | | |
| Blood sugar | | | | | | |
| Mood | | | | | | |
| Stress | | | | | | |
| Consciousness | | | | | | Grand Total |
| **Progress Total** | | | | | | |

\* It's appropriate for fullness and satiety to rise during or immediately after a meal.

\*\* It's appropriate for hunger and appetite to rise before a normal mealtime.

▓ Shaded boxes above do not apply to this particular indicator.

If you see a general improvement, then you know you are on the right track toward repairing your disordered appetite. You are doing what can be done for your NPY/PYY levels. The longer you stay on the Week 3 regimen, the more these levels will improve. But every time you skip or delay a meal, you'll set yourself back a bit.

If your Week 3 charts are very even, you have no desire to binge, and you aren't craving foods, you may have already done everything you need to do to prepare yourself for dieting. In the next chapter, you'll choose your own personal track.

## Week 4 Charts: Assisted Serotonin

The last important change you made was to feed your brain the primary ingredient for manufacturing serotonin: tryptophan. If you've been deficient in serotonin or tryptophan, this modification may have made a pervasive improvement.

Some of the benefits of improved serotonin levels include the following:

• More stress-proof

• More relaxed

• Less vigilant

• Less paranoid

• Less pain

• More in touch with inner body states

• Decreased appetite

• Improved satiety

• Quicker fullness

• Slower eating

• Faster satiety

• Decreased drive to eat starches

• Improved sleep

As you can see, I'm sorta sweet on serotonin. What's not to like?

Cholecystokinin is a hormone that signals the brain that the stomach is full. When serotonin improves, cholecystokinin also improves. Hence, improved serotonin means faster delivery of a fullness message—and, therefore, an earlier message to stop eating.

Let's compare two of Krista's Body Signals Charts from Weeks 1 and 4.

Krista has a telling pattern of delayed fullness. Look at the noon column on the Week 1 chart. She had lunch at noon and was still hungry at 1 p.m. She had dinner at 7 p.m, still felt empty at 8 p.m, and kept eating. Her stomach finally got the message at 9 p.m., by which time she was stuffed.

EXAMPLE 9

Krista, Week 1

## Body Signals Chart, Week 1

| CATEGORY | DESCRIPTIONS | BASELINE DATA—NO CHANGES | | | | | | | | | | | | | | | | |
|---|---|---|---|---|---|---|---|---|---|---|---|---|---|---|---|---|---|---|
| Timeline | Circle Wake-up | 6AM | 7 | 8 | 9 | 10 | 11 | 12PM | 1 | 2 | 3 | 4 | 5 | 6 | 7 | 8 | 9 | 10 | 11 |
| **Food** <br> *Numbers go in this section* | Proteins | | 3 | | | | | 4 | | | | | | | 4 | | | | |
| | Complex carbs | | | | | | | | | | | | | | | | | | |
| | Simple carbs | | 6 | | | | | 4 | | | | | | | 4 | 5 | | | |
| | Fats | | 1 | | | | | 2 | | | | | | | 2 | 5 | | | |
| Check | **Equal/NutraSweet** | | | | | | | | | | | | | | | | | | |
| **Drink** <br> *Dots go in this section* | Water | | | | | | | | | | | | | | | | | | |
| | Pop | | | | | | | | | | | | | | | | | | |
| | Diet pop | | | | | | | • | | | | | | | | • | | | |
| | Coffee | | • | | | | | | | | | | | | • | | | | |
| | Herbal drink | | | | | | | | | | | | | | | | | | |
| | Milk | | • | | | | | | | | | | | | | | | | |
| | Juice | | | | | | | | | | | | | | | | | | |
| | Alcohol | | | | | | | | | | | | | | | | | | |
| | Tea | | | | | | | | | | | | | | | | | | |
| Check | **Caffeine** | | ✔ | | | | | ✔ | | | | | | | | | | | |
| Timeline | | 6AM | 7 | 8 | 9 | 10 | 11 | 12PM | 1 | 2 | 3 | 4 | 5 | 6 | 7 | 8 | 9 | 10 | 11 |
| **Fullness** | Stuffed | | | | | | | | | | | | | | | | | | |
| | Comfortable | | | | | | | | | | | | | | | | | | |
| | Empty | | | | | | | | | | | | | | | | | | |
| **Hunger** | Starving | | | | | | | | | | | | | | | | | | |
| | Really hungry | | | | | | | | | | | | | | | | | | |
| | Mildly hungry | | | | | | | | | | | | | | | | | | |
| | Not hungry | | | | | | | | | | | | | | | | | | |
| **Appetite** | Craving food | | | | | | | | | | | | | | | | | | |
| | Food focused | | | | | | | | | | | | | | | | | | |
| | Quiet | | | | | | | | | | | | | | | | | | |
| **Satiety** | Satiated | | | | | | | | | | | | | | | | | | |
| | Not | | | | | | | | | | | | | | | | | | |
| **Energy** | High | | | | | | | | | | | | | | | | | | |
| | Medium | | | | | | | | | | | | | | | | | | |
| | Low | | | | | | | | | | | | | | | | | | |

Now look at Krista's hunger indicators. She started eating at 7 p.m. and still felt starved at 8 p.m. Hunger, or lack of comfortable fullness after an hour of eating, is a classic sign of serotonin insufficiency.

Krista's appetite follows a similar pattern. Even though she ate at noon, she still wanted more food at 1 p.m. Not until 2 p.m. did her appetite quiet down. Then in the evening, she was still craving food at 8 p.m., even though she'd been eating for an hour.

We can differentiate a serotonin deficiency from an NPY/PYY problem in several ways. First, although Krista had a long gap between lunch and dinner, she did eat a breakfast that included protein. Her appetite began to increase *before* lunch and dinner. She awakened hungry and wanting to eat. Her satiety was delayed after her lunch and dinner, but she did become satiated.

Now look at Krista's chart from Week 4, shown on the next page. Notice that, now that Krista is eating turkey, she is reaching fullness and satiety during her meals. Boosting her serotonin levels has normalized her eating.

EXAMPLE 10

## Krista, Week 4

## Body Signals Chart, Week 4

| CATEGORY | DESCRIPTIONS | CHANGE: ADD TRYPTOPHAN ONCE A DAY | | | | | | | | | | | | | | | | |
|---|---|---|---|---|---|---|---|---|---|---|---|---|---|---|---|---|---|---|
| Timeline | Circle Wake-up | (6AM) | 7 | 8 | 9 | 10 | 11 | 12PM | 1 | 2 | 3 | 4 | 5 | 6 | 7 | 8 | 9 | 10 | 11 |
| **Food** Numbers go in this section | Proteins | | 4 | | | 5 | | 4 | | | 5 | | | 4 | | 5 | | | |
| | Complex carbs | | 3 | | | 5 | | | | | 5 | | 7 | 3 | | 5 | | | |
| | Simple carbs | | 1 | | | | | 4 | | | | | 3 | 2 | | | | | |
| | Fats | | 2 | | | | | 2 | | | | | | 1 | | | | | |
| Check | **Tryptophan** | | | | | | | | | | | | | ✔ | | | | | |
| Check | **Equal/NutraSweet** | | | | | | | | | | | | | | | | | | |
| **Drink** Dots go in this section | Water | | | | | • | | • | | | • | | | • | | | | | |
| | Pop | | | | | | | | | | | | | | | | | | |
| | Diet pop | | | | | | | | | | | | | | | | | | |
| | Coffee | • | | | | | | | | | | | | | | • | | | |
| | Herbal drink | | | | | | | | | | | | | | | | | | |
| | Milk | | | | | | | | | | | | | | | | | | |
| | Juice | | | | | • | | • | | | • | | | • | | | | | |
| | Alcohol | | | | | | | | | | | | | | | | | | |
| | Tea | | | | | | | | | | | | | | | • | | | |
| Check | **Caffeine** | | | | | | | | | | | | | | | | | | |
| Timeline | | 6AM | 7 | 8 | 9 | 10 | 11 | 12PM | 1 | 2 | 3 | 4 | 5 | 6 | 7 | 8 | 9 | 10 | 11 |
| **Fullness** | Stuffed | | | | | | | | | | | | | | | | | | |
| | Comfortable | | | | | | | | | | | | | | | | | | |
| | Empty | | | | | | | | | | | | | | | | | | |
| **Hunger** | Starving | | | | | | | | | | | | | | | | | | |
| | Really hungry | | | | | | | | | | | | | | | | | | |
| | Mildly hungry | | | | | | | | | | | | | | | | | | |
| | Not hungry | | | | | | | | | | | | | | | | | | |
| **Appetite** | Craving food | | | | | | | | | | | | | | | | | | |
| | Food focused | | | | | | | | | | | | | | | | | | |
| | Quiet | | | | | | | | | | | | | | | | | | |
| **Satiety** | Satiated | | | | | | | | | | | | | | | | | | |
| | Not | | | | | | | | | | | | | | | | | | |
| **Energy** | High | | | | | | | | | | | | | | | | | | |
| | Medium | | | | | | | | | | | | | | | | | | |
| | Low | | | | | | | | | | | | | | | | | | |

Below is Fania's Week 4 chart:

EXAMPLE 11

Fania, Week 4

**Body Signals Chart, Week 4**

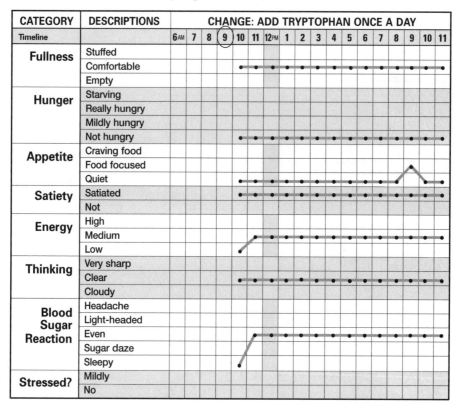

By Week 4, Fania's levels are remarkably even. Her tummy is comfortable throughout the day, and she isn't craving food. Her energy level is even and her thinking is consistently clear. The daily headaches that were bothering her at the beginning are still gone.

Now, don't worry if you don't have levels this even by Week 4. It is natural to have an increase in hunger and appetite before a regular mealtime.

**Focus: Fullness and Satiety Rows**

Problems:

- Delayed fullness after a meal
- Delayed satiety after a meal
- Continued eating after a meal

*Signs of Progress:*

- Comfortable fullness after meals
- Hunger that is stopped by meals
- Appetite that is stopped by meals
- Satiety that is reached sooner after meals
- Hunger soon after waking
- Breakfast soon after waking
- Lower hunger and appetite spikes
- Improved thinking, mood, and energy levels
- More even blood sugar and energy levels
- Reduced stress
- Increased consciousness of what's going on in your body
- More easily soothed
- Increased sense of well-being
- Decreased vulnerability

What you're looking for this week is the degree to which serotonin has improved your response to eating. Since you began eating turkey (and tryptophan), what has happened to your fullness and satiety indicators? How is your feeling of hunger affected after you start eating? How soon after you start eating are you reaching fullness or satiety? How does this compare to your body's responses during Week 1?

Sometimes, when people start getting enough serotonin, they suddenly feel clearer, as if their minds have abruptly shifted into greater sanity. What changes do you notice?

Also, notice what has happened to your feelings of stress. Compare the stress line of your Week 1 and Week 4 Body Signals Charts.

### Changes Due to Increased Tryptophan

Once again, examine your charts from Week 4. Highlight peaks and valleys, circle successes, and pick a new color marker for highlighting improved serotonin delivery. Compare your Week 4 charts with charts from Week 3. In the chart below, put slashes in the boxes to indicate positive changes. Put a slash for each instance of change. Remember that any box may contain multiple slashes.

### Changes Due to Increased Tryptophan

| Indicator | Achieved Sooner | Stopped w/Meal | Improved | Decreased | |
|---|---|---|---|---|---|
| Fullness | | | | | |
| Hunger | | | | | |
| Appetite | | | | | |
| Satiety | | | | | |
| Thinking | | | | | |
| Mood | | | | | |
| Stress | | | | | |
| Consciousness | | | | | |
| Comfort-seeking through food | | | | | |
| Vulnerability | | | | | |
| Other serotonin successes | | | | | Grand Total |
| **Total Progress** | | | | | |

Finally, count the slashes in each column and put the totals in the last line. Then add the totals and put that sum in the Grand Total box.

## Super-Big Pat on the Back

If you've made it to this point, you've done a lot of work and paid really significant attention to yourself. You now have summary worksheets that shout the successes you've made from following this program for four weeks.

Any improvement in your appetite, satiety, hunger, and fullness levels means that each change contributed toward repair of your disordered appetite. The question now is this: Have you done all you need to do, or is a big dragon still scratching at your door?

We're going to look for one more pattern on your charts. I'll give you a hint.

Here's another one of Berthe's charts. What do you notice about her indicators after 6 p.m.? Look at the circled areas.

### Body Signals Chart, Week 1

| CATEGORY | DESCRIPTIONS | BASELINE DATA—NO CHANGES | | | | | | | | | | | | | | | | |
|---|---|---|---|---|---|---|---|---|---|---|---|---|---|---|---|---|---|---|
| Timeline | Circle Wake-up | 6AM | 7 | 8 | 9 | 10 | 11 | 12PM | 1 | 2 | 3 | 4 | 5 | 6 | 7 | 8 | 9 | 10 | 11 |
| **Food** <br> *Numbers go in this section* | Proteins | | | | | | 2 | | | | | | | 5 | | | | | |
| | Complex carbs | | | | | | 3 | | | | | | | 2 | | | | | |
| | Simple carbs | | | | | | 5 | | | | | | | 1 | 5 | 5 | 5 | | |
| | Fats | | | | | | | | | | | | | 2 | 5 | 5 | 5 | | |
| Timeline | | 6AM | 7 | 8 | 9 | 10 | 11 | 12PM | 1 | 2 | 3 | 4 | 5 | 6 | 7 | 8 | 9 | 10 | 11 |
| **Fullness** | Stuffed | | | | | | | | | | | | | | | | | | |
| | Comfortable | | | | | | | | | | | | | | | | | | |
| | Empty | | | | | | | | | | | | | | | | | | |
| **Hunger** | Starving | | | | | | | | | | | | | | | | | | |
| | Really hungry | | | | | | | | | | | | | | | | | | |
| | Mildly hungry | | | | | | | | | | | | | | | | | | |
| | Not hungry | | | | | | | | | | | | | | | | | | |
| **Appetite** | Craving food | | | | | | | | | | | | | | | | | | |
| | Food focused | | | | | | | | | | | | | | | | | | |
| | Quiet | | | | | | | | | | | | | | | | | | |
| **Satiety** | Satiated | | | | | | | | | | | | | | | | | | |
| | Not | | | | | | | | | | | | | | | | | | |

By 8 p.m. Berthe is stuffed and has no hunger. Yet she keeps craving food and continues eating for hours after her dinner at 6 p.m. Granted, she skipped breakfast and waited too long for dinner, but even accounting for a rise in NPY after she started her evening meal, what kept her appetite going?

Here are two more charts. What do you notice about them? Hint: Look toward the end of the day.

EXAMPLE 13

Fania

## Body Signals Chart, Week 3

| CATEGORY | DESCRIPTIONS | CHANGE: EAT 50/50 SNACKS | | | | | | | | | | | | | | | | |
|---|---|---|---|---|---|---|---|---|---|---|---|---|---|---|---|---|---|---|
| Timeline | Circle Wake-up | 6AM | 7 | 8 | 9 | 10 | 11 | 12PM | 1 | 2 | 3 | 4 | 5 | 6 | 7 | 8 | 9 | 10 | 11 |
| **Food** Numbers go in this section | Proteins | | | | 5 | | 5 | | | | | 5 | | | 3 | | | | |
| | Complex carbs | | | | 5 | | 4 | | | | | 5 | | | 2 | | | | |
| | Simple carbs | | | | | | 1 | | | | | | | | 2 | | | 5 | |
| | Fats | | | | | | | | | | | | | | 3 | | | 5 | |
| Check | Equal/NutraSweet | | | | | | | | | | | | | | | | | | |
| **Drink** Dots go in this section | Water | | | | • | • | • | • | • | • | | | • | | • | | | | |
| | Pop | | | | | | | | | | | | | | | | | | |
| | Diet pop | | | | | | | | | | | | | | | | | | |
| | Coffee | | | | | | | | | | | | | | | | | | |
| | Herbal drink | | | | | | | | | | | | | | | | | | |
| | Milk | | | | | | | | | | | | | | | | | | |
| | Juice | | | | | | | | | | | | | | | | | | |
| | Alcohol | | | | | | | | | | | | | | | | | | |
| | Tea | | | | | | | | | | | | | | | | | | |
| Check | Caffeine | | | | | | | | | | | | | | | | | | |
| Timeline | | 6AM | 7 | 8 | 9 | 10 | 11 | 12PM | 1 | 2 | 3 | 4 | 5 | 6 | 7 | 8 | 9 | 10 | 11 |
| **Fullness** | Stuffed | | | | | | | | | | | | | | | | | | |
| | Comfortable | | | | | | | | | | | | | | | | | | |
| | Empty | | | | | | | | | | | | | | | | | | |
| **Hunger** | Starving | | | | | | | | | | | | | | | | | | |
| | Really hungry | | | | | | | | | | | | | | | | | | |
| | Mildly hungry | | | | | | | | | | | | | | | | | | |
| | Not hungry | | | | | | | | | | | | | | | | | | |
| **Appetite** | Craving food | | | | | | | | | | | | | | | | | | |
| | Food focused | | | | | | | | | | | | | | | | | | |
| | Quiet | | | | | | | | | | | | | | | | | | |
| **Satiety** | Satiated | | | | | | | | | | | | | | | | | | |
| | Not | | | | | | | | | | | | | | | | | | |
| **Energy** | High | | | | | | | | | | | | | | | | | | |
| | Medium | | | | | | | | | | | | | | | | | | |
| | Low | | | | | | | | | | | | | | | | | | |

In Example 13, Fania did almost everything right. Skipping lunch wasn't ideal, but she still had two meals and two healthy snacks. She had a bit of an NPY rebound when she snacked after missing lunch, but her levels recovered fairly quickly. She wasn't hungry at 10 p.m., so what accounts for the rise in appetite and the high-carb/high-fat snack? Let's look at one more chart:

EXAMPLE 14

**Maddie**

### Body Signals Chart, Week 1

| CATEGORY | DESCRIPTIONS | BASELINE DATA—NO CHANGES | | | | | | | | | | | | | | | | |
|---|---|---|---|---|---|---|---|---|---|---|---|---|---|---|---|---|---|---|
| **Timeline** | Circle Wake-up | 6AM | 7 | 8 | 9 | 10 | 11 | 12PM | 1 | 2 | 3 | 4 | 5 | 6 | 7 | 8 | 9 | 10 | 11 |
| **Food** | Proteins | | 5 | | | | | 6 | | | | | | | | | | | |
| | Complex carbs | | 5 | | | | | 3 | | | | | | | | | | | |
| *Numbers go in this section* | Simple carbs | | | | | | | | 10 | 10 | 10 | | | | | | | | |
| | Fats | | | | | | | 1 | | | | | | | | | | | |
| *Check* | **Equal/NutraSweet** | | | | | | | | | | | | | | | | | | |
| **Drink** | Water | | | | | | | | | | | | | | | | | | |
| | Pop | | | | | | | | | | | | | | | | | | |
| *Dots go in this section* | Diet pop | | | | | | | • | | | | | | | | | | | |
| | Coffee | | • | | | | | | | | | | | | | | | | |
| | Herbal drink | | | | | | | | | | | | | | | | | | |
| | Milk | | | | | | | | | | | | | | | | | | |
| | Juice | | | | | | | | | | | | | | | | | | |
| | Alcohol | | | | | | | | | | | | | | | | | | |
| | Tea | | | | | | | | | | | | | | | | | | |
| *Check* | **Caffeine** | | | | | | | | | | | | | | | | | | |
| **Timeline** | | 6AM | 7 | 8 | 9 | 10 | 11 | 12PM | 1 | 2 | 3 | 4 | 5 | 6 | 7 | 8 | 9 | 10 | 11 |
| **Fullness** | Stuffed | | | | | | | | | | | | | | | | | | |
| | Comfortable | | | | | | | | | | | | | | | | | | |
| | Empty | | | | | | | | | | | | | | | | | | |
| **Hunger** | Starving | | | | | | | | | | | | | | | | | | |
| | Really hungry | | | | | | | | | | | | | | | | | | |
| | Mildly hungry | | | | | | | | | | | | | | | | | | |
| | Not hungry | | | | | | | | | | | | | | | | | | |
| **Appetite** | Craving food | | | | | | | | | | | | | | | | | | |
| | Food focused | | | | | | | | | | | | | | | | | | |
| | Quiet | | | | | | | | | | | | | | | | | | |
| **Satiety** | Satiated | | | | | | | | | | | | | | | | | | |
| | Not | | | | | | | | | | | | | | | | | | |
| **Energy** | High | | | | | | | | | | | | | | | | | | |
| | Medium | | | | | | | | | | | | | | | | | | |
| | Low | | | | | | | | | | | | | | | | | | |

In Example 14, Maddie forgot her midmorning snack, but she had breakfast and lunch, both in good proportions. At 1 p.m., she was comfortably full and her hunger was fading. She even had satiety. But she wanted to eat and from 1 to 4 p.m., she had a string of simple-carb foods. Simple carbs and/or fatty foods three hours in a row qualifies as a binge.

Now look at Iona's chart.

EXAMPLE 15

Iona

## Body Signals Chart, Week 1

| CATEGORY | DESCRIPTIONS | BASELINE DATA—NO CHANGES | | | | | | | | | | | | | | | | |
|----------|--------------|------|---|---|---|----|----|------|---|---|---|---|---|---|---|---|----|----|
| Timeline | Circle Wake-up | 6AM | 7 | 8 | 9 | 10 | 11 | 12PM | 1 | 2 | 3 | 4 | 5 | 6 | 7 | 8 | 9 | 10 | 11 |
| **Food** Numbers go in this section | Proteins | | | 5 | | | 5 | | 5 | | | | 5 | | | | | |
| | Complex carbs | | | 3 | | | 4 | 10 | 2 | | | | | | | | | |
| | Simple carbs | | | 2 | | | 1 | | 2 | | 10 | 5 | | | | | | |
| | Fats | | | | | | | | 1 | | | 5 | 5 | | | | | |
| Check | Equal/NutraSweet | | | | | | | | | | | | | | | | | |
| **Drink** Dots go in this section | Water | | • | | | • | | | | | | | | | | | | |
| | Pop | | | | | | | | | | | | | | | | | |
| | Diet pop | | | | | | | | | | • | | | | | | | |
| | Coffee | | | | | | | | | | | | | | | | | |
| | Herbal drink | | | | | | | | | | | | | | | | | |
| | Milk | | | | | | | | | • | | | | | | | | |
| | Juice | | • | | | | | | | | | | | | | | | |
| | Alcohol | | | | | | | | | | | | | | | | | |
| | Tea | | | | | | | | | | | | | | | | | |
| Check | Caffeine | | | ✔ | | | | | | ✔ | | | | | | | | |
| Timeline | | 6AM | 7 | 8 | 9 | 10 | 11 | 12PM | 1 | 2 | 3 | 4 | 5 | 6 | 7 | 8 | 9 | 10 | 11 |
| **Fullness** | Stuffed | | | | | | | | | | | | | | | | | |
| | Comfortable | | | | | | | | | | | | | | | | | |
| | Empty | | | | | | | | | | | | | | | | | |
| **Hunger** | Starving | | | | | | | | | | | | | | | | | |
| | Really hungry | | | | | | | | | | | | | | | | | |
| | Mildly hungry | | | | | | | | | | | | | | | | | |
| | Not hungry | | | | | | | | | | | | | | | | | |
| **Appetite** | Craving food | | | | | | | | | | | | | | | | | |
| | Food focused | | | | | | | | | | | | | | | | | |
| | Quiet | | | | | | | | | | | | | | | | | |
| **Satiety** | Satiated | | | | | | | | | | | | | | | | | |
| | Not | | | | | | | | | | | | | | | | | |
| **Energy** | High | | | | | | | | | | | | | | | | | |
| | Medium | | | | | | | | | | | | | | | | | |
| | Low | | | | | | | | | | | | | | | | | |

Iona had breakfast even though she awakened satiated. Good for her. The fact that she was satiated and had no hunger upon awakening tells us she was probably eating late the night before. She had either a snack or an early lunch at 11 a.m. and a meal at 1 p.m. At noon she had a snack consisting entirely of carbs. What's going on here?

It looks like Iona was craving food until she had that snack. Then, after the snack, she had hunger that wouldn't quit. Her appetite became quiet, but she wasn't satiated.

At 3 and 4 p.m., we see what looks like a binge profile: simple carb and fat eating for two hours. If you look at Berthe's chart on page 117, her eating from 7 p.m. on also qualifies as a binge.

What we are seeing in all four women's cases is eating that is outside of any misalignment of alimentary or gustatory biochemicals. This eating is not about nutrition.

In all four cases, the eating is similar: a combination of fat or simple carbs following soon after a well-balanced meal, usually at the end of the day.

But although the behavior is similar, the stimuli are different. Here we see a mix of fullness, emptiness, hunger, no hunger, appetite, no appetite, satiety, and no satiety. This eating is occurring even when the person has been faithfully following the four-week regimen. Something else is going on. Another powerful factor is still at work.

What kind of eating is this? Addictive eating—eating in order to affect feelings or mood. In a couple of chapters, we'll look for a similar pattern in your charts.

If you have followed the four-week eating maps, and deep inside you a motor is humming, restlessly awaiting your return to comfort eating, then we can't stop here. A diet or weight-loss program can only be successful for you if we tackle the next major cause of appetite disorder: food addiction.

• • •

*Opening*

*Today's Agenda*

1. Help each other

   • Highlight charts

   • Read and interpret charts

   • Find successes

2. Discussion topics (pick any or all):

   • What you discovered

   • How you feel about what you learned

   • What the successes mean to you

*Closing*

# 16

# Tracks

❧ FROM NOW on, you will follow your own track through this book, based on the appetite changes that occur as you implement each step and food change.

The goal is to rebuild your natural satiety, to manage the stimuli—both chemical and emotional—that boost your appetite, and to normalize your hunger, so that it rises before a meal and disappears after a meal.

Notice your moments of satiety. You may experience this as a feeling of peace around food, as the disappearance of food thoughts and driven eating, or as a lack of interest in eating. Once your satiety starts building, guard it. Don't risk losing it by being haphazard with the changes that restored it.

Satiety is your most precious guardian against disordered appetite. Each step you've taken thus far and the steps you will take in coming weeks are all for the purpose of restoring satiety and reducing appetite stimulation.

Remember that satiety and appetite are always in fluctuation, responding to the conditions that you create through your choices and actions. The balance is delicate and can be easily tipped if you become lax with your program, especially in the early days of your recovery, when the changes are only starting to be programmed into your neural networks.

**STEP 9**

Determine which track to follow.

Be wary of a seduction that is the longing of most disordered eaters—a deep longing to just be normal. Those of us who've been controlled by food yearn to have a simple, normal relationship with it. We want to be able to take it or leave it, to have a meal and then leave it with no further concern about food until the next regular mealtime.

The irony is this: You can have that carefree relationship with eating, as long as you take care to protect your satiety. Protect your satiety by following your personal eating map, the one you are designing based on the appropriate track for you. Thus, you *can* have what you want, *as long as* you follow your daily practice, which you will now define. Below is a description of the first two tracks. If you do not fit the criteria for either of these tracks, continue with the next chapter and Step 10.

## Track A Criteria

Check each item that is true for you.

☐ With eating changes one and two, your appetite operates normally.

☐ You achieve satiety after meals and snacks.

☐ Your portions are getting smaller as you get used to eating five or six meals or snacks each day.

☐ You are comfortable with the routine of replenishing snacks and ensuring they are stashed where you need them.

☐ You don't have to fight yourself to replace or eat snacks. You don't feel an internal stubbornness that makes you resist the planning and shopping required to keep snacks going.

☐ You are not bingeing *at all.*

☐ You have no desire to binge.

☐ You are not turning to food for soothing or comfort.

☐ When you are done with a meal or snack, you don't give food another thought until it's time for the next snack or meal.

If you answered yes to *every one* of the above criteria, follow **Track A.**

> **Track A Eating Map:**
> - Eat every two to three hours, for as long as you are awake.
> - Eat snacks that are 50/50 protein/complex carbs.
> - Do not eat snacks made from flour, wheat, sugar, or simple carbs.
> - Take 50/50 snacks with you wherever you go.

*Jump to Chapter 20.*

**Track B Criteria**

Check each item that is true for you.

☐ With eating changes one, two, and three, your appetite operates normally.

☐ You achieve satiety after meals and snacks.

☐ Your portions are getting smaller as you get used to eating five or six meals or snacks each day.

☐ You are comfortable with the routine of replenishing snacks and ensuring they are stashed where you need them.

☐ You don't have to fight yourself to replace or eat snacks. You do not feel an internal stubbornness that makes you resist the planning and shopping required to keep snacks going.

☐ You are not bingeing *at all.*

☐ You have no desire to binge.

☐ You are not turning to food for soothing or comfort.

☐ When you are done with a meal or snack, you don't give food another thought until it's time for the next snack or meal.

If you answered yes to *every one* of the above criteria, follow **Track B**.

**Track B Eating Map:**

- Eat every two to three hours, for as long as you are awake.

- Eat snacks that are 50/50 protein/complex carbs.

- Do not eat snacks that are made from flour, wheat, sugar, or simple carbs.

- Take 50/50 snacks with you wherever you go.

- Eat at least four ounces of turkey two or three times a week, depending on which amount maintains your satiety. You may substitute turkey with another source of tryptophan such as milk, sesame seeds, or tahini. Make sure your food intake gives you the equivalent of about 380 mg of tryptophan.

- If your stress level goes up, increase your intake of tryptophan.

*Now jump to Chapter 20.*

Not fitting these criteria? Not to worry, you are on Track C and the plan just continues. Proceed with the next chapter and Step 10.

**Stepping Forward**

Here's a quick look at what you can expect in upcoming chapters.

Step 10: Understand the addictive cycle.

Step 11: Consider powerlessness.

Step 12: Assess the likelihood that you are a food addict.

Step 13: Solidify your satiety.

Step 14: Switch best friends.

Step 15: Strengthen your support.

Step 16: Identify your trigger foods.

Step 17: Define your abstinence.

Step 18: Prepare for abstinence.

Step 19: Begin your first abstinence.

Step 20: Solidify your abstinence.

Step 21: Expand your support.

Step 22: Reduce the stress in your life.

Step 23: Keep priorities clear. Put recovery first.

• • •

# 17

# The Addictive Cycle

❧ DEEP INSIDE your head, in your midbrain at the top of the brain stem, practically at the center, is the ventral tegmental area (VTA). Frankly, this area is pretty primitive. It wants what it wants, when it wants it.

FIGURE 10

**The Brain**

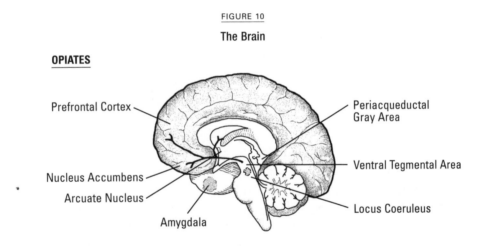

Neurons here manufacture the neurotransmitter dopamine, and then deliver it to the nucleus accumbens, which is a bit forward and a part of the basal ganglia. The nucleus accumbens is your euphoria center. When this part of your brain is activated, you experience satisfaction and pleasure.

Although differing addictive substances act on various other parts of the brain, all addiction involves the VTA and the nucleus accumbens, acting through the neurotransmitter dopamine. Almost every substance abused by humans has been shown to increase dopamine levels in the nucleus accumbens.

Endorphins also act on the VTA. The VTA has endorphin receptors that can be stimulated both by intake of opiate drugs, such as morphine or heroin, and by internal opioids, such as dynorphin, beta-endorphin, and enkephalin.

Even if you aren't a food addict, you may have noticed that eating food can give you pleasure. Eating is essential to survival, and you are wired to enjoy the activities that promote survival. Thus, eating naturally stimulates your pleasure center (see the box below).

Certain foods stimulate an especially rapid or intense pleasure response. For example, foods high in sugar, chocolate, or alcohol content are particularly adept at promoting endorphin release. For many people, when these internal opiates hit the nucleus accumbens, it's as good as a drug.

**STEP 10**

Understand the addictive cycle.

So what is it that causes some of us to respond dramatically to sugary foods, while other folks leave half of their pie uneaten? (Food addicts will universally say, "Leave dessert on the plate? I don't get that.")

---

**HOW WE KNOW WHAT WE KNOW—TWO TOOLS**

**Tool 1:**

Much of the basis for understanding brain function originates in animal research. Certain animals have body parts that are structurally similar to ours. Studies done on these animals illumine the likelihood of how those same parts work in humans.

For example, the rat brain has certain similarities to the human brain. (This is not a political statement.) By studying reactions in rat brains, we can build experiments for understanding the human brain.

**Tool 2:**

Each single piece of research is built on thousands of studies that went before it. For example, through years of patient observation and experimentation, scientists have discovered chemicals that either stimulate or block specific neurons. By applying a stimulus, we can see what a certain part does. By applying a block, we can see what happens when a certain part isn't working. Much of food addiction research follows this method—of either stimulating or blocking specific neurons in certain parts of the brain, and then noticing what happens to appetite.

---

Two theoretical possibilities and one pretty sure bet are emerging from the latest research. These include (1) sensitivity to reward, (2) opioid-induced consumatory behavior, and (3) stress-induced feeding.

### Sensitivity to Reward[1]

According to researchers Davis, Strachan, and Berkson, "Sensitivity to reward (STR)—a personality trait firmly rooted in the neurobiology of the mesolimbic dopamine system—has been strongly implicated in the risk for addiction."[2] Here we have an explanation for the development of food addiction.

Some of us are sensitive to reward. In other words, when presented with a substance that activates our pleasure and reward center (our VTA and nucleus accumbens), we have a particularly strong reaction to it. We are more reactive than, say, someone not vulnerable to addiction. If we are sensitive to reward, a pleasurable stimulus has quite an impact on us. It registers big time.

Now here's an interesting aspect to this research. An unexpected finding was that obese women were more anhedonic than overweight women. *Anhedonic* means, literally, "no pleasure"—that is, having a threshold resistant to the experience of pleasure. Doesn't it make incredible sense that if someone just naturally experiences less pleasure than others, she will sit up and take notice if something finally works to give her some?

As a person's capacity for pleasure decreases, her need for something that will provide pleasure increases. This theory may explain the critical difference between those who find pleasure before they've crossed the line into obesity and those who have to eat past that point to finally relieve their pleasure deficiency.

Obesity, in this case, is a side effect.

These studies about sensitivity to reward give us a clue to two risk factors that lead to overeating and overweight:

- A reduced ability to obtain pleasure from ordinary things
- A constitutional sensitivity to the rewards provided by food

### Opioid-Induced Feeding

Several studies demonstrate that intermittent, excessive sugar intake causes opioid dependence.[3] Eating an excess of sugar on a regular basis actually changes the way genes express themselves in the brain, causing physical alteration. The brain's pleasure receptors in the nucleus accumbens increase in a profile similar to morphine dependence.[4]

## Stress-Induced Feeding

We're almost certain that stress makes people more reactive to stimulation of the nucleus accumbens. Stress and trauma, especially when prolonged, wear down the brain. Both relief and effort neurotransmitters (serotonin and norepinephrine) get used up, as our entire system focuses on warding off threat. When stress becomes our usual state, our brain looks for something to intervene.

Certain chemicals are capable of turning off this overworked brain. These include the following:

- External opiates (drugs such as opium, heroin, and morphine)
- Internal opioids (in the form of neurochemicals such as dopamine, endorphins, and dynorphin)
- Alcohol
- Benzodiazepines (drugs such as Valium and Librium)
- Tranquilizers
- Serotonin

Unfortunately, everything on this list is addictive except serotonin. (Interestingly, serotonin is not a big player in the nucleus accumbens, but all the other chemicals on this list can build a pathway to this part of the brain. Perhaps something can only become addictive if it creates a pathway to the nucleus accumbens.)

## A Tale of Three Theories

These three constructs go well together.

1. What if stress and trauma, gobbling up the brain's resources, cause a person to experience less pleasure, and therefore to be particularly responsive to sources of relief such as the internal opioids stimulated by eating sugar?

2. Obviously, a person will return to a dependable source of relief, and, over time, this *habit* of using sugar for relief induces the physical changes that result in full-blown sugar addiction.

3. We have other studies that show that injecting opioids can lead to a 300 percent increase in fat and sugar intake,[5] and that eating sugar can cause a 33 percent increase in meal size.[6] The increased fat intake observed in the first study occurred after fullness had been achieved. Thus, this eating had nothing to do with hunger. Thinking back to those charts two chapters ago, we found a similar pattern: binge eating after fullness had been achieved.

Here's what the process looks like:

FIGURE 11

**Pleasure and Pain Sequences**

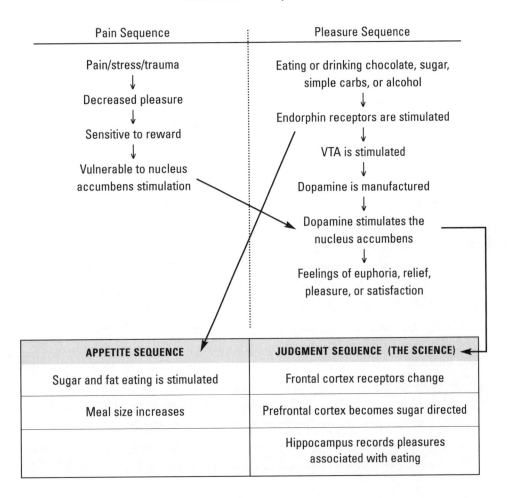

| Pain Sequence | Pleasure Sequence |
|---|---|
| Pain/stress/trauma<br>↓<br>Decreased pleasure<br>↓<br>Sensitive to reward<br>↓<br>Vulnerable to nucleus accumbens stimulation | Eating or drinking chocolate, sugar, simple carbs, or alcohol<br>↓<br>Endorphin receptors are stimulated<br>↓<br>VTA is stimulated<br>↓<br>Dopamine is manufactured<br>↓<br>Dopamine stimulates the nucleus accumbens<br>↓<br>Feelings of euphoria, relief, pleasure, or satisfaction |

| APPETITE SEQUENCE | JUDGMENT SEQUENCE (THE SCIENCE) |
|---|---|
| Sugar and fat eating is stimulated | Frontal cortex receptors change |
| Meal size increases | Prefrontal cortex becomes sugar directed |
|  | Hippocampus records pleasures associated with eating |

*To bring all this down to earth, imagine*
*how a plate of brownies captures your mind.*

### The Experience

You're at a party and a good friend is telling you about seeing her ex in the diaper section at Food Mart. The two of you are deep in speculation about the meaning of this when the hostess strolls by with a tray of brownies.

Even though you are looking at your friend and the brownies are only sighted out of the corner of your eye, you track their progress across the room and to the buffet without moving your head. Your eyes are still on your friend, but your attention is glued to the brownies.

Your behavior hasn't changed. You are nodding your head and "uh-huhing" as if you were still listening. Meanwhile, a plan is forming about how you will disengage from your friend and meander across the room, arriving at the buffet table ostensibly by accident.

You tune back into her conversation sufficiently to interrupt with a comment. "Oh, my leg has a cramp. I need to walk it off. I'll be right back." This is a lie. Your leg is not cramping.

You are an upright woman who, ordinarily, wouldn't dream of lying. You aren't even good at lying. However, this lie flows silkily from your lips without a qualm of conscience. In fact, it doesn't even register that you are lying. Your attention is so focused on your plan to get next to the brownies that you are minimally aware of anything else.

By the way, this plan isn't all that conscious. You are barely aware of what you are doing. Your focus on the brownies has even eclipsed your awareness of yourself. You're almost in a trance. Later, you'll remember very little of what transpired between the entrance of the brownies and your first bite.

### The Science

What went on here?

Dopamine neurons that lead from the VTA and nucleus accumbens to the frontal cortex, particularly the prefrontal cortex, fired when your addictive substance entered the room. The frontal cortex overvalued your drug (the brownies) as a pleasure source, and it undervalued alternative pleasure sources, such as your conversation with your friend.[7] If you were in a state of sugar withdrawal, this discrepancy in assigning value would have been even greater.

The prefrontal cortex fixated your attention on the brownies and activated your motivation toward getting them. It made the plan for you. The brain's locus coeruleus allowed you to lie because it thinks it's okay for you to do whatever you need to do in order to get your drug.

It's also possible that a decrease in D2 dopamine receptors in the prefrontal cortex, caused by eating sugar,[8] impaired your judgment and created temporary amnesia. This process could have caused you to forget anything not associated with snatching the brownies—including your pre-party commitment to abstain from sugar. It could be the reason that your judgment was impaired as you reached for your third brownie and made plans to sneak a couple more brownies later.

FIGURE 12

| JUDGMENT SEQUENCE (THE EXPERIENCE) |
| --- |
| Sugar (or fat) overvalued |
| Other pleasure sources undervalued |
| Attention selectively directed toward sugar (or fat) |
| Motivation centered on obtaining sugar or fat |
| Plans constructed and carried out |
| Higher values take back seat (lying is okay) |
| Satisfaction or pleasure |
| Temporary amnesia |
| Associated pleasures get recorded |

This last point on the judgment sequence has to do with the pleasure pyramids that get constructed around addictive use. The hippocampus preserves agreeable memories and details associated with using the addictive substance, to the point where subsequent exposure to the association will trigger the desire to use. (For example, addicts in recovery from cocaine use can be triggered by seeing a mound of flour or by having money in their pockets.)

Food addicts have scads of pleasure associations with eating: eating and reading; movies and popcorn; taking a risk and getting a special dessert; seeing the dentist and getting a food reward afterward; Saturday night pizza, videos, and beer; the state fair and BBQ, cotton candy, and elephant ears. Associative eating thus seems justified, and an addict will often defend her eating if a friend is sharing the experience: "Normally I don't eat this, but I had a hard decade."

### The Addictive Cycle

Although I've combined the above three constructs as a single unified theory, each can stand alone. I've used trauma or stress as the entry and first phase of the addictive cycle, but any point can serve as the funnel that sucks a person into food addiction.

FIGURE 13

**The Cycle of Addiction**

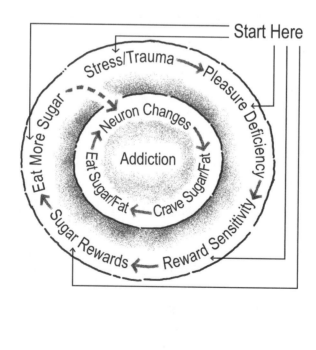

The addiction cycle is found in the inner part of the circle. It explains why addictions get progressively worse over time if there is no intervention. Once neurons and receptors are altered as a result of using, they perpetuate further use. The altered receptors are the point of craving. They have multiplied, or they have become more or less sensitive as a result of the sustained chemical flood. When the flood ebbs, they empty and want to be filled. The receptors stimulate a craving for the substance, whether it be alcohol, heroin, fat, or sugar, and that craving leads to seeking, obtaining, and ingesting more of the substance. The excessive use promotes even more neuron changes, and once this cycle starts, it keeps going: Neuron changes promote use and use promotes changes.

Recovery that includes abstinence from the addictive substance eventually takes these neurons off-line, but they never go away. They can fade out of the picture when they aren't used, but they are only dormant, not gone. This explains why some people can be abstinent from smoking or alcohol for umpteen years, smoke one cigarette or sip one martini, and within the week, be using at the same level as or worse than when they stopped. It's as if no time has passed in the brain's chronology.

I'm reminded of a demonstration at the fair by a vendor selling those little vacuums that suck the air out of storage bags so that marshmallows end up like little desiccated sponges. Those marshmallow dots can sit in your cabinet for twenty years, but if you pull the bag open, they'll pop right up. Reusing your substance after a period of abstinence is like giving your addictive neurons air. They'll pop right up, absorb the pined-for substance, and go straight back into operation.

### Will Pretzels Do?

Throughout this chapter, I've referred exclusively to sugar as the gateway substance that carries a person from overuse into addiction. Do carbs lead to the same consequence?

So far, most studies involve sugar. However, the body reacts similarly to simple carbs, particularly in large quantities. Simple carbs are broken down and metabolized quickly. Saltine crackers, for example, are converted to sugar, which is partially absorbed even while still in your mouth.

The threshold for triggering an addictive response may be slightly higher with carbs than sugar. You may need to eat slightly more carbs than sugar to get the satisfaction you're after, but for many people, they do create that addictive response. In fact, for some, it's bread, rather than sugar, that rings their chimes.

Even complex carbs, if eaten in sufficient quantity, can trigger addictive relief. Contentment may come more slowly, but it will eventually arrive.

### Pass the Butter

Once neuron changes occur, a craving for fatty foods may enter the picture. A yen for fat typically starts to accompany sugar and carb cravings. You may remember a time when hard candy (pure sugar) spun your wheel, but nowadays chips and dip lead to nirvana.

The aristocrats of food addiction are the foods that combine sugar, carbs, and fat (and salt, for some folks). Add chocolate and you're really done for. Not only is chocolate usually mixed with salt, fat, and sugar, but it also contains a chemical similar to that found in coffee and tea. Chocolate contains theobromine, which is a methylxanthine, like caffeine (in coffee) and theophylline (in tea).

By adding a caffeine-like substance to the mix—chocolate + sugar + fat—you give yourself a one-two punch. Caffeine sparks insulin release, which gets serotonin going. Then the triple combination carries on to get the endorphin-dopamine system fired up. Serotonin bestows relief until the addictive response takes over.

### Crossover from Sister Addictions

Recovering alcoholics are vulnerable to becoming starch addicts because the addiction cycles are so similar. You may remember from Chapter 14 that serotonin deficiency is a risk factor for sugar or carb addiction.

---

**AMERICA'S MOST WANTED: CARB-FAT COMBINATIONS**

- Ice cream
- Brownies
- Cookies
- Chips and dip
- Pancakes or waffles (with butter and syrup) and bacon or sausage
- Hash browns
- French fries
- Fudge
- Pizza
- Pasta, sauce, and garlic bread

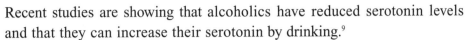

Recent studies are showing that alcoholics have reduced serotonin levels and that they can increase their serotonin by drinking.[9]

When they become abstinent from alcohol, they can easily and unconsciously revive their serotonin levels by eating carbs. This slides them smoothly back into the addictive cycle with carbs as the abused substance.

For years it was not uncommon to find a bowl of candy at AA meetings, and monthly sobriety birthdays are still sometimes celebrated with cake. Members may routinely bring doughnuts or cookies, mechanically using food-stimulated, addictive biochemicals as a soother while talking sobriety.

I'm not suggesting that carb addiction is inevitable for alcoholics in recovery. And, certainly, I'm not advising anyone to solve a serotonin deficiency by drinking or eating addictively. There are healthy solutions to serotonin problems such as eating change three. What I'm simply saying is that science has now found a clear link between the two addictions.

### Why Isn't Serotonin Stopping Your Appetite When You Eat Addictively?

Back in Chapter 14, you learned that serotonin enhances satiety. So you may be wondering, *Why doesn't eating lots of sugar or carbs trigger the production of serotonin and lead to satiety?*

This is a good question. Now here's the answer. If you have sufficient supplies of tryptophan, serotonin will be readily released after eating starch, decreasing your appetite.

*Addiction trumps satiety.*

Here's the catch: As dopamine in the nucleus accumbens rises, serotonin simultaneously declines. Thus your supply of a natural appetite regulator dwindles, and you are prevented from achieving satiety. The addictive process overpowers the body's natural mechanisms that would otherwise halt eating.

### Congratulations!

This was a big chapter, and possibly the hardest in the book. The good news is that you are done with the technical part of this book. I know this chunk was complicated, but big guns are needed to blast false beliefs out of the minds of binge eaters. Nearly all binge eaters are convinced that they are weak-willed and lacking in self-discipline, and that just isn't true. Body chemicals are the real culprits.

By now, I hope you have been persuaded that overeating is not even in the same country as discipline or self-control. It's comparing apples to scissors.

If you overeat, it's because you have an appetite disorder. And if all other factors have been accounted for by the first four weeks of this program, what's left is food addiction. Digesting and understanding this chapter is Step 10. If you need to sleep on it and read it again, please do.

It's not necessary to remember the names of the brain parts or the chemicals discussed in this chapter. There won't be a quiz. What is important is that you understand the following realities:

- Addictive eating is a chemically motivated chain of events.
- Once the addictive process is triggered, it will continue until it is satisfied by the eating of addictive foods.
- Because food addiction operates under the radar of your conscious thought, you can be seeking food without any real awareness.
- It's not possible to interrupt the addictive process with a strong and fervent statement, such as, "I will not overeat today!"
- Promises, threats, rewards, or punishments have no impact on this cycle.
- Intelligence and education don't interrupt the chain reaction that results in eating.

• • •

## Support Meeting 4

*Opening*

*Today's Agenda*

Pick one or more of the following as discussion topics.

1. How this chapter impacts my belief that I'm undisciplined

2. How this chapter illuminates some of the things I do in order to eat

3. Examples from my own experience of

- Valuing food over other pleasures

- Going into a trance on the way to food or eating

- Telling a lie even though I am a principled and/or spiritual person

- Getting amnesia and eating, even though I made a promise to myself that I wouldn't eat a certain way

- Threats or promises that made no difference in my eating choices

- Sensitivity to reward

- Noticing that others seem to derive more pleasure than I do in certain situations

- Powerful food associations like movies and popcorn

- My individual entry point on the addictive cycle

*Closing*

# 18

# I Am Powerless
# over Eating

WHEN ADDICTS go to Twelve Step recovery meetings, one of the first things they hear is, "I am powerless over _____ (alcohol, gambling, food, nicotine, etc.)."

After reading the last chapter, perhaps you can see where this declaration comes from. Once the addictive cycle is stimulated, we are powerless to stop it.

That's not to say nothing can be done.

Oh, yes, something can be done. You are already halfway toward doing it.

Let's toss around this issue of powerlessness, because you are about to make two important assessments: (1) whether the addictive cycle is causing what's left of your appetite disorder and (2) what your level of abstinence needs to be. Both matters are connected to the issue of powerlessness.

Many of us have an aversion to admitting powerlessness. Both women and men with appetite disorders have suffered far too much powerlessness already. We may have been abused because we had no power in our families. We may have been powerless over people who hurt or threatened us. Perhaps we've even made life choices from our own need to gain power over what happens to us. Thus, to say flat out, "I'm powerless," can go against our innermost instincts.

**STEP 11**

Consider powerlessness.

And for those of us who use affirmations to improve our lives, such a statement can seem like a negative affirmation.

Fair enough. Yet there is another, more important side to all of this.

In the last chapter you read that the hippocampus records pleasurable associations, such as movies and popcorn, and that having one can stimulate the desire for the other. The hippocampus and the amygdala also archive traumatic associations, like a glowering look and being yelled at. If your amygdala makes this association, then a glowering look can produce as much fear as being yelled at.

In the "It's not fair!" category is the reality that some of the positive things we have to do in order to recover are associated *negatively* with past trauma. For example, most typical addicts would limp a mile with a twisted ankle rather than ask for help. Many of us were betrayed or hurt if we asked for help, so we have an aversion to doing it. *But to recover we need to overcome this aversion because recovery day after day isn't possible without help.*

Let me share an example from my life. While I helped build a house that was designed to support and nurture my writing, I had to find temporary quarters. The only dwelling that met both my logistical needs and my budget was a small trailer. The last time I lived in a trailer I was abused. So as I was driving to the trailer for the first time, I was filled with dread and horror. But I made myself open the door to that trailer, walk in, and begin a temporary life there because it had to be done in order to reach my dreams. The situation was hard, but now my negative association with trailers is broken because it became a completely sufficient little place where I found contentment. (And now I'm in my dream house, watching the birds through a window as I write.)

When we have a powerful negative association with something, we tend to view it as a dead end. We perceive the situation as if life or progress stops there, as if there's no road leading beyond this thing. *This is an illusion.* Almost always there's a road out, if we will let ourselves use the vehicles that will take us beyond the edge of our vision.

### Positive Actions—Negative Associations

Some of the negatively associated but positive actions that can get food addicts stuck on the shadow side of recovery are

- Sitting at a table to eat
- Calling a friend when you're hurting
- Structuring food or meals

- Eating real meals
- Eating healthy foods
- Eating in front of others
- Restricting certain foods
- Preparing meals
- Planning meals
- Declaring a certain food off-limits
- Telling people about your feelings
- Telling people about your mistakes
- Telling people about your rebellion
- Expressing anger
- Expressing grief
- Really crying
- Stepping out of the compliant/defiant dance (more on this shortly)
- Asking for help
- Admitting powerlessness

Many people deal with these negatively associated actions by avoiding them, but some we absolutely, positively need to do in order to move forward with recovery. *If we want our lives to change, we have to grit our teeth and break the association.*

Let's look at a handful of these negatively associated actions.

### Sitting at a Table to Eat

If your childhood supper table was a torture chamber, you'll naturally have a negative association with sitting at a table for meals. You may compensate by eating out of the skillet, eating while standing at the counter, eating while reading or watching TV, or eating while driving.

The hitch is that it is important for a food addict to know she has eaten. It's also helpful for her to break any associations she has with eating. For example, if you separate the act of eating from the act of watching TV, then TV has less power to trigger you to eat.

Sitting at a table to eat doesn't need to be a rule, but it is one way to give yourself an environment of recovery from an addiction that finds temptation in every direction.

### Calling a Friend When You're Hurting

This action is an imperative for recovery. We have to have a solid way to prevent pain and find relief so we can stop depending on food to make us feel better.

### Preparing Food and Structuring or Planning Meals

These actions get spoiled for women if, as little girls, they were forced to prepare or deal with food in painful circumstances. Perhaps a sergeant major mother made meal preparation monstrous, or a perfectionist parent tormented you if you set the table wrong. Perhaps you served the men of the family while taking a backseat. Maybe some family members got the good stuff while you got the dregs. Do any of these food situations ring a bell?

If you were the family Cinderella, it may be difficult to be a servant to yourself. Yet structuring meals and preparing food are essential for success as a recovering food addict. When we don't plan, we are vulnerable to impulsive decisions, unavoidable food smells, and getting too hungry. We need to always have our snack food available and, since we are consuming it, we need to commit to a system for replacing it.

### Not Eating Certain Foods

Soon we'll talk about abstinence. You'll identify your trigger foods and determine which foods must be eliminated from your plate. Even though the scope of your first abstinence will be your choice, what if you have an aversion to designating a food as off-limits?

This is an important issue to handle because if certain foods always trigger your appetite and you don't take them off of your list, you'll be plagued by your appetite disorder no matter what diet you choose. This issue is so important that I'll use it as an example later in this chapter, when I demonstrate how to convert a negative association into a positive one.

### Expressing Feelings

Being able to express feelings is a cornerstone of recovery. Children learn to hide feelings if they are shamed, punished, or threatened for having them. ("I'll give you something to cry about!") Yet, we must allow ourselves to feel

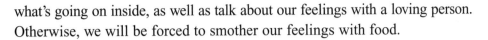

what's going on inside, as well as talk about our feelings with a loving person. Otherwise, we will be forced to smother our feelings with food.

### The Compliant/Defiant Dance

We each do our own set of steps in the dance of compliance or defiance. Some of us present a compliant appearance while behaving defiantly as soon as we're out of sight. Some of us react with automatic defiance. And others comply even when it's not good for them.

Which is your inclination? If you are an automatic complier, you'll tend to follow every directive in whatever diet you choose, even though I've shown you that you must discriminate. If you are a defier, you'll be in a "yes, but" relationship with the principles in this book. If you comply on the surface and defy behind closed doors, you'll be torn when you make good choices and be vulnerable to rebelling for no apparent reason. Getting conscious about your particular dance will help you.

### Powerlessness

Yes, we're back to this. There are factual, biochemical, and spiritual reasons for allowing yourself to admit you are powerless over the addictive chain reaction in your body.

Fact: We are all powerless in this way—once the levers trip, we'll end up eating addictively, unless we use our tools in time.

Now the biochemistry angle: By trying hard to defeat our addiction, we activate our effort neurotransmitter, norepinephrine, which fires up the binge center of the hypothalamus and stimulates our appetite. This is the catch-22 of food addiction recovery. *Trying hard will always lead to bingeing if it is sustained for a long enough period.*

And finally, let's listen to what our Spirit says.

*I'm not crazy about admitting that I make mistakes or that I'm less of a person than I want to be. I don't like noticing that I fall short of the goals I set for myself. Yet, accepting the reality of this, accepting that my canoe is in the human river, helps me.*

*It helps me stop trying to make superhuman efforts to do what can't be done (reducing my norepinephrine levels). It helps me remember that I, like everyone, need others.*

*If I were the superwoman I'd like to be, I wouldn't need anybody. But I do need people. I need my friends. I need them the way I need oxygen.*

We were constructed to need others, and recovery forces us to overcome our pathological isolation and independence so that we can open the door to connection. Connection saves us. It is what enables us to step into the unknown world that addiction has blocked.

This passage from isolation to connection has a sacred nature. It opens us to our grander selves, to the kernel inside us that is perfect and good, that is our strand to all other life.

Once in my early recovery, I cried, "I am unraveled," and it was soon after that that I began weaving myself into the strands of others. The paradox of recovery is that it both unravels and knits us.

. . .

Remember to use an opening and closing each meeting so that the meeting has transitions into and out of the group. The suggested meeting formats for openings and closings are in Appendix A.

## Opening

### Today's Agenda

OPTION 1: *Discussion Questions*

1. What items on the positive action list (pages 142–143) can you imagine doing?

2. Talk about a positive action that has a negative association for you.

3. What does the word *powerless* mean to you?

4. What other word could you substitute for the idea of powerlessness? Why would that word work better for you?

5. In what way are you able to see that you are powerless over food and eating?

6. When you think about how your own body operates when it is stalking sugar, fat, starch, or chocolate, do you see it as a conscious process or one that is hidden from you?

7. What names do you call yourself when you overeat? Are these accurate considering the automatic nature of the addition cycle?

8. What is the difference between being powerless and being weak-willed or lacking discipline?

9. Can you identify other processes in your body that you are powerless over? (Examples: breathing, seeing, menstruating, aging.) Do you have the same feeling of being undisciplined (or weak-willed, etc.) when these processes are operating?

Support Meeting 5 *continued*

OPTION 2: *Exercise: Converting a Negative Association*
*(see example on pages 149–150)*

1. Look at the list of positive actions that have negative associations on pages 142–143. Check the ones that apply to you.

2. Pick the one that feels easiest to change.

3. Talk about the childhood events that gave this action a negative association. As you talk, share your feelings.

4. Notice that this is in your past rather than in your present.

5. Notice that in the present, your recovery partner is joining you in your experience. You are not alone.

6. Bring yourself into the present moment. Express how your present life is different from the situation you've been describing.

7. Start building new, positive associations. Do one or more of the following:

   a. With your recovery partner, role-play taking that positive action.
   b. Visualize taking that positive action while being surrounded by the light of your spiritual source. Visualize a positive outcome.
   c. State an affirmation that includes doing the positive action and enjoying a positive outcome.
   d. Make a plan to do the positive action with your recovery partner sometime soon.

8. Thank your recovery partner.

**Closing**

> *Here's one example of how the conversion exercise in Option 2 might work.*

1. I've checked six items on the list.

2. I'm picking the one about declaring a food off-limits.

3. In my heart, I know I'm addicted to sugar. But when I think of saying that sugary foods are off-limits, I feel this wall come up. My mother was always telling me I couldn't eat this or I couldn't eat that. She was always trying to control my eating and when I feel that control slipping over my shoulders, I feel like a boxer. I just want to kick and scream and fight till my last breath. I want to scream, "You can't control me. You can't tell me what to do!"

   I'm feeling my rebellion now. It is really strong. I feel so angry. I am enraged that she tried to control me when she had no control at all. She couldn't control my father, she couldn't protect us, she couldn't leave. She was a wimp. How dare she constrict me when she couldn't even manage herself.

   I just want to scream at her: "Get away. Leave me alone."

   I think I need to feel this for a while. I just need to let myself be angry for a while. I'm so mad and so angry. Grrrrr.

4. Okay, I'm ready to continue the exercise. I'm aware that this was in the past. No one is telling me I have to stop eating sugar. I can see for myself that sugar is keeping me trapped in this addiction. If I decide to abstain, it is my choice.

5. You are listening to me. You are not telling me what to do. I'm not alone now.

6. I can make choices now. I'm in charge of my life now. I choose my meals, my mealtimes, my food. I can have what I want. And I can choose to have what is healthy for me.

7. Affirmation: I choose to eat healthy food, and I enjoy choosing foods that protect me from the addiction cycle.

   Now I'm visualizing making healthy food choices while I surround myself with spiritual energy. I'm picturing a table with fresh vegetables and luscious fruit, and I can have whatever I want on that table. The table is surrounded with light. I can feel the energy of my Source all around me. I take a bite of some really crisp celery. I love the crunch. The flavor is like spring. I feel the nutrients entering my body and my body responds with a feeling of lightness. I feel healthy and strong. I am good to myself.

8. I want to suggest that we have a healthy meal together this week. I'd like to experience eating and abstaining in a light-hearted situation. Thank you for listening to me and supporting me.

*End exercise example.*

### The Recovery Partner's Role

- Listen with compassion. (For details, see "Effective Listening Skills" on pages 171–176.)

- Attune to your partner.

- Affirm any similarities and commonalities, while keeping your focus on your recovery partner.

- To the extent you are willing and able, build new, positive associations along with your partner.

# 19

# Curious?

✂ HAVE YOU figured out if you're an addictive eater yet? If you're not sure, take the following quiz.

### Quiz: Am I a Food Addict?

*Check all the statements that sometimes apply to you.*

☐ I eat to make the stresses of the day go away.

☐ I have this motor running deep inside that starts planning what I'll eat way before I get done with work. I can't say this plan starts out consciously, but a picture of a restaurant will begin as a fuzzy image and then become clear, and I'll know that's where I'm going. If pressed, I could even say what I will eat there, even though that choice is not conscious at first either.

☐ If I'm alone, once I start eating potato chips, I don't stop until the bag is empty. Add dip and they're sure to disappear.

☐ A meal is just something to get out of the way so I can eat dessert. Sometimes I eat dessert for another hour or two.*

☐ If I'm alone, once I start eating in the evening, I can eat nonstop for a couple of hours or more.*

☐ I eat from the time I get home until the time I go to bed unless I distract myself by playing computer games or doing some other activity over and over.*

☐ If I feel scared or threatened, I just bide my time until I can get to some food.

☐ I know that I'm eating to push away feelings of loneliness.

☐ I wouldn't consider leaving half a piece of pie. In fact, give me the whole pie and walk away.

☐ If there is leftover dessert, the thought of it haunts me until I go back to the kitchen and finish it off. Sometimes I'll sliver it to death, one small serving at a time, hoping no one will notice.

☐ When I feel really let down or disappointed, I need to eat something soothing, like ice cream or pudding.

☐ Occasionally, I don't turn to food and it surprises me. For example, after my grandfather died, I couldn't eat much for weeks. But then once I started eating, I couldn't stop. Soon I was eating the way I usually do.

☐ I can make healthy food choices for lunch and dinner, and then in the evening, pow!, I'm out of the gate and diving into all sorts of food.

☐ I crave sweets.

☐ When I accomplish something, I want to celebrate with ice cream or some special dessert.

☐ When I was on a certain diet, I was free of cravings. I thought, *Now I'm changed. Now I know I'll be able to control my eating. I'll be able to have one doughnut and stop with that.* I really believed it. And I did stop with the first doughnut. But the next day, the second doughnut grabbed me and after that, I couldn't stop with one anymore.

☐ Sometimes I secretly look at someone with a terrible disease and think, *At least they aren't tormented by food.* And just for a moment, it seems better to have a disease that stops the torment than to suffer this miserable captivity every day.

☐ I crave fried foods.

☐ Have a potato without the butter and sour cream? What's the point?

☐ I want so much to stop eating the way I do. But I'm terrified when I think of not being able to have the foods I love.

- ☐ Sometimes I think, *If I got diabetes or had a heart attack, then I could stop eating the way I do.* But I know people who have had serious health problems and are still trapped by eating.

- ☐ People say to me, "How can you still eat like that when you are at such risk for a serious problem?" I react defensively or shrug it off when I hear this, but inside I feel helpless. I can't stop.

- ☐ I've actually burned my mouth because I couldn't wait for food to cool before I ate it.

- ☐ I hide evidence that I've been eating.

- ☐ Just reading this list upsets me so much that I want to eat.

- ☐ The only time I lie is when it has to do with food and eating.

- ☐ I make up excuses so that no one knows I'm late because I hit a drive-through restaurant.

- ☐ I justify why I can eat this or that.

- ☐ I've actually finished the dessert on someone else's plate when I was in the kitchen and no one could see.

- ☐ Every once in a while, I'll feel peace around food and think, *Oh, this has finally changed.* I feel lighter and joyous, thinking I'm out from under this mantle. But then the fixation with eating always comes back, pulling me under again.

- ☐ I believe that if I were just spiritual enough, my problems with food would go away.

All of the above statements are common to food addicts. If you checked more than ten statements, you are thinking and behaving like an addict. Three of the statements near the beginning of the list are marked with an asterisk. These statements signify binge eating thoughts and behaviors. If you checked one or more of these statements, please estimate, on the average, how many times in a week that statement is true. If you have two or more episodes a week of such eating, you meet one of the qualifications of binge eating disorder, which you now know is actually an appetite disorder.

## Are You Eating Like an Addict?

In Step 8, you identified eating caused by NPY surges and serotonin deficiency. By changing how frequently you eat and adding two or three snacks a day, you've already improved and calmed your appetite-stimulated eating. Now, pull out your Body Signals Charts. Let's take a look at them and find out if you're eating like an addict. This time you're going to look for eating that isn't accounted for by NPY, serotonin, or energy needs. (Doing this analysis is another good time to meet with your recovery partner.)

The following charts demonstrate what addictive eating looks like. Each chart reveals a different aspect.

EXAMPLE 1

Berthe

### Body Signals Chart, Week 1

| CATEGORY | DESCRIPTIONS | BASELINE DATA—NO CHANGES | | | | | | | | | | | | | | | | |
|---|---|---|---|---|---|---|---|---|---|---|---|---|---|---|---|---|---|---|
| Timeline | Circle Wake-up | 6AM | 7 | 8 | 9 | 10 | 11 | 12PM | 1 | 2 | 3 | 4 | 5 | 6 | 7 | 8 | 9 | 10 | 11 |
| **Food** <br> *Numbers go in this section* | Proteins | | | | | | 2 | | | | | | | 5 | | | | | |
| | Complex carbs | | | | | | 3 | | | | | | | 2 | | | | | |
| | Simple carbs | | | | | | 5 | | | | | | | 1 | 5 | 5 | 5 | | |
| | Fats | | | | | | | | | | | | | 2 | 5 | 5 | 5 | | |
| Timeline | | 6AM | 7 | 8 | 9 | 10 | 11 | 12PM | 1 | 2 | 3 | 4 | 5 | 6 | 7 | 8 | 9 | 10 | 11 |
| **Fullness** | Stuffed | | | | | | | | | | | | | | | | | | |
| | Comfortable | | | | | | | | | | | | | | | | | | |
| | Empty | | | | | | | | | | | | | | | | | | |
| **Hunger** | Starving | | | | | | | | | | | | | | | | | | |
| | Really hungry | | | | | | | | | | | | | | | | | | |
| | Mildly hungry | | | | | | | | | | | | | | | | | | |
| | Not hungry | | | | | | | | | | | | | | | | | | |
| **Appetite** | Craving food | | | | | | | | | | | | | | | | | | |
| | Food focused | | | | | | | | | | | | | | | | | | |
| | Quiet | | | | | | | | | | | | | | | | | | |
| **Satiety** | Satiated | | | | | | | | | | | | | | | | | | |
| | Not | | | | | | | | | | | | | | | | | | |

Berthe's hunger was satisfied by lunch (serotonin was working), and she was comfortably full until the dinner hour approached (dotted circle). She did have an NPY surge in appetite after lunch because she skipped breakfast, but eventually PYY kicked in and she achieved satiety (dashed circle).

So what happened after supper? The first jump in appetite could be caused by NPY. After all, it had been a long time since lunch—seven hours. Still, her appetite stayed ferocious for the rest of the night (square). And look at the food choices—she ate mixed carbs and fats three hours in a row (solid circle).

Appetite that doesn't quit and prolonged eating of carbs and fats despite being stuffed is a giveaway. Berthe is experiencing addictive eating that shows involvement of the ventral tegmental area.

**Focus:**

- Sugar, flour, and fat rows
- Appetite rows

**Problems:**

- Eating that continues after a meal or snack
- Choosing foods that are composed mainly of sugar, flour, and/or fat
- Appetite that continues after a meal or snack
- Extreme appetite
- Food cravings

Look at your own charts and identify evidence of this type of eating. Circle times of appetite or lack of satiety that last long after meals or snacks that are composed primarily of simple carbs and/or fats. Label this VTA, to indicate involvement of the ventral tegmental area.

Now let's look at a second example, shown on the next page.

Iona is hungry despite regular eating (dotted oval). She's not satiated despite having a quiet appetite (dashed oval). This could indicate a problem with serotonin. Still, at 3 and 4 p.m., she shows a telltale pattern (solid circle). She has a 100 percent simple carb snack, followed by a mix of fats and simple carbs. Iona may have a serotonin issue, but she is also being triggered to eat.

Something else is happening here too. Do you notice that she didn't fill out her chart after 7 p.m.? It is possible that she went to bed quite early, but the other possibility is that she didn't want to record what she was eating or felt defiance or rebellion about keeping her chart.

EXAMPLE 2

Iona

## Body Signals Chart, Week 2

| CATEGORY | DESCRIPTIONS | CHANGE: EAT EVERY 2–3 HOURS | | | | | | | | | | | | | | | | |
|---|---|---|---|---|---|---|---|---|---|---|---|---|---|---|---|---|---|---|
| Timeline | Circle Wake-up | 6AM | 7 | 8 | 9 | 10 | 11 | 12PM | 1 | 2 | 3 | 4 | 5 | 6 | 7 | 8 | 9 | 10 | 11 |
| **Food** | Proteins | | | 5 | | | 5 | | 5 | | | | | 5 | | | | | |
| | Complex carbs | | | 3 | | | 5 | 10 | 2 | | | | | | | | | | |
| *Numbers go in this section* | Simple carbs | | | 2 | | | | | 2 | | 10 | 5 | | | | | | | |
| | Fats | | | | | | | | 1 | | | 5 | | 5 | | | | | |
| *Check* | **Equal/NutraSweet** | | | | | | | | | | | | | | | | | | |
| **Drink** | Water | | • | | | • | | | | | | | | | | | | | |
| | Pop | | | | | | | | | | | | | | | | | | |
| *Dots go in this section* | Diet pop | | | | | | | | | | | • | | | | | | | |
| | Coffee | | | | | | | | | | | | | | | | | | |
| | Herbal drink | | | | | | | | | | | | | | | | | | |
| | Milk | | | | | | | | | | • | | | | | | | | |
| | Juice | | | • | | | | | | | | | | | | | | | |
| | Alcohol | | | | | | | | | | | | | | | | | | |
| | Tea | | | | | | | | | | | | | | | | | | |
| *Check* | **Caffeine** | | ✔ | | | | | | | | ✔ | | | | | | | | |
| Timeline | | 6AM | 7 | 8 | 9 | 10 | 11 | 12PM | 1 | 2 | 3 | 4 | 5 | 6 | 7 | 8 | 9 | 10 | 11 |
| **Fullness** | Stuffed | | | | | | | | | | | | | | | | | | |
| | Comfortable | | | | | | | | | | | | | | | | | | |
| | Empty | | | | | | | | | | | | | | | | | | |
| **Hunger** | Starving | | | | | | | | | | | | | | | | | | |
| | Really hungry | | | | | | | | | | | | | | | | | | |
| | Mildly hungry | | | | | | | | | | | | | | | | | | |
| | Not hungry | | | | | | | | | | | | | | | | | | |
| **Appetite** | Craving food | | | | | | | | | | | | | | | | | | |
| | Food focused | | | | | | | | | | | | | | | | | | |
| | Quiet | | | | | | | | | | | | | | | | | | |
| **Satiety** | Satiated | | | | | | | | | | | | | | | | | | |
| | Not | | | | | | | | | | | | | | | | | | |

Let's look at yet another example.

EXAMPLE 3

## Maddie

### Body Signals Chart, Week 1

| CATEGORY | DESCRIPTIONS | BASELINE DATA—NO CHANGES | | | | | | | | | | | | | | | | | |
|---|---|---|---|---|---|---|---|---|---|---|---|---|---|---|---|---|---|---|---|
| Timeline | Circle Wake-up | 6AM | 7 | 8 | 9 | 10 | 11 | 12PM | 1 | 2 | 3 | 4 | 5 | 6 | 7 | 8 | 9 | 10 | 11 |
| **Food** | Proteins | | 5 | | | | | 6 | | | | | | | | | | | |
| | Complex carbs | | 5 | | | | | 3 | | | | | | | | | | | |
| Numbers go in this section | Simple carbs | | | | | | | | 10 | 10 | 10 | | | | | | | | |
| | Fats | | | | | | | 1 | | | | | | | | | | | |
| Check | Equal/NutraSweet | | | | | | | | | | | | | | | | | | |
| **Drink** | Water | | | | | | | | | | | | | | | | | | |
| | Pop | | | | | | | | | | | | | | | | | | |
| Dots go in this section | Diet pop | | | | | | | • | | | | | | | | | | | |
| | Coffee | • | | | | | | | | | | | | | | | | | |
| | Herbal drink | | | | | | | | | | | | | | | | | | |
| | Milk | | | | | | | | | | | | | | | | | | |
| | Juice | | | | | | | | | | | | | | | | | | |
| | Alcohol | | | | | | | | | | | | | | | | | | |
| | Tea | | | | | | | | | | | | | | | | | | |
| Check | Caffeine | | | | | | | | | | | | | | | | | | |
| Timeline | | 6AM | 7 | 8 | 9 | 10 | 11 | 12PM | 1 | 2 | 3 | 4 | 5 | 6 | 7 | 8 | 9 | 10 | 11 |
| **Fullness** | Stuffed | | | | | | | | | | | | | | | | | | |
| | Comfortable | | | | | | | | | | | | | | | | | | |
| | Empty | | | | | | | | | | | | | | | | | | |
| **Hunger** | Starving | | | | | | | | | | | | | | | | | | |
| | Really hungry | | | | | | | | | | | | | | | | | | |
| | Mildly hungry | | | | | | | | | | | | | | | | | | |
| | Not hungry | | | | | | | | | | | | | | | | | | |
| **Appetite** | Craving food | | | | | | | | | | | | | | | | | | |
| | Food focused | | | | | | | | | | | | | | | | | | |
| | Quiet | | | | | | | | | | | | | | | | | | |
| **Satiety** | Satiated | | | | | | | | | | | | | | | | | | |
| | Not | | | | | | | | | | | | | | | | | | |

Maddie's meals satisfied her hunger (dotted ovals), and her serotonin is working. Her appetite was satisfied by breakfast and rose before lunch, which shows normal NPY performance (dashed circle). Because she shows normal NPY, PYY, and serotonin functioning, why did she still have an appetite for three hours after lunch (square)?

Her food choices reveal the answer. Three hours of eating simple carbs shows that an addictive cycle is in operation; the food she is eating is causing her to eat.

**Focus:**

- Sugar, flour, and fat rows

**Problem:**

- Eating that is triggered by consuming sugar or flour

Now look at your charts. Circle any strings of carb and/or fat eating that follow ingestion of simple carbs. Label these DP/NA for dopamine involvement of the nucleus accumbens.

Now look back at Maddie's chart for a moment. What else do you notice about it? That's right. She stopped filling it out at 5 p.m. She went underground.

I see so many charts like this: careful records until late afternoon or evening when suddenly they appear empty for the rest of the day. Either I work with a population that goes to bed extraordinarily early, or these folks don't want anyone (including themselves) to know how they are spending the rest of the evening.

Let's analyze this. They chose to be in a recovery program and know that chart-keeping helps them in the long run. Despite that, they stopped dotting their charts. In addition, they are breaking the commitment they made to themselves when they agreed to chart.

Something affected their judgment, which can only mean involvement of the frontal cortex. Dopamine pathways to the cortex are being affected by the nucleus accumbens. The eating itself is causing the change in perspective.

The locus coeruleus says it's okay to break a commitment if a food fix is needed. And temporary amnesia (forgetting the commitment to chart) shows that the hippocampus is being affected.

This tells us that the whole brain is now involved in the addiction. It's a serious condition and, if ignored, it will only get worse.

At about this time, many people become angry and start resenting the charting. Can you guess why?

All of this attention on their eating is upsetting the addictive cycle. Addicts get angry when you come between them and their drug, and this program does just that. Even though we aren't abstaining from food yet, the comfort the addiction provides is being interrupted. These flying sparks are further evidence of the addiction.

**Focus:**

- Columns that aren't filled out, even though you were awake

**Problem:**

- No record of eating, appetite, or other body signals

Count the number of charts that you haven't filled out or finished. Mark each of these unfinished spots FC/WB for frontal cortex/whole brain.

EXAMPLE 4

## Vonna

### Body Signals Chart, Week 4

| CATEGORY | DESCRIPTIONS | CHANGE: ADD TRYPTOPHAN ONCE A DAY | | | | | | | | | | | | | | | | |
|---|---|---|---|---|---|---|---|---|---|---|---|---|---|---|---|---|---|---|
| Timeline | Circle Wake-up | 6AM | ⑦ | 8 | 9 | 10 | 11 | 12PM | 1 | 2 | 3 | 4 | 5 | 6 | 7 | 8 | 9 | 10 | 11 |
| **Food** | Proteins | | | 7 | | 5 | | 3 | | | 5 | | | 5 | | | | | |
| | Complex carbs | | | 3 | | 5 | | 5 | | | 5 | | | 4 | | | | | |
| *Numbers go in this section* | Flour | | | | | | | | | | | | | | 5 | | | | |
| | Sugar | | | | | | | | | | | | | | | | 5 | 5 | 5 |
| | Fats | | | | | | | 2 | | | | | | 1 | 5 | 5 | 5 | 5 | |
| Check | **Tryptophan** | | | | | | | | | | | | | ✔ | | | | | |
| Check | **Equal/NutraSweet** | | | | | | | | | | | | | | | | | | |
| Timeline | | 6AM | 7 | 8 | 9 | 10 | 11 | 12PM | 1 | 2 | 3 | 4 | 5 | 6 | 7 | 8 | 9 | 10 | 11 |
| **Fullness** | Stuffed | | | | | | | | | | | | | | | | | | |
| | Comfortable | | | | | | | | | | | | | | | | | | |
| | Empty | | | | | | | | | | | | | | | | | | |
| **Hunger** | Starving | | | | | | | | | | | | | | | | | | |
| | Really hungry | | | | | | | | | | | | | | | | | | |
| | Mildly hungry | | | | | | | | | | | | | | | | | | |
| | Not hungry | | | | | | | | | | | | | | | | | | |
| **Appetite** | Craving food | | | | | | | | | | | | | | | | | | |
| | Food focused | | | | | | | | | | | | | | | | | | |
| | Quiet | | | | | | | | | | | | | | | | | | |
| **Satiety** | Satiated | | | | | | | | | | | | | | | | | | |
| | Not | | | | | | | | | | | | | | | | | | |
| **Stressed?** | Highly | | | | | | | | | | | | | | | | | | |
| | Mildly | | | | | | | | | | | | | | | | | | |
| | No | | | | | | | | | | | | | | | | | | |

After four weeks on the program, Vonna's hunger and appetite levels are managed. Her serotonin and NPY/PYY levels are in good balance, as evidenced by hunger and appetite levels that are stopped by meals (dotted ovals).

Then look what happens at 2 p.m. Vonna experiences stress (bottom rectangle). Soon after, her appetite increases (upper rectangle). This increase could be the normal appetite that should occur before the evening meal—and, in fact, the meal does stop Vonna's hunger and restores comfortable fullness.

However, the meal has no impact on Vonna's appetite. She remains driven toward food, as her eating shows. At 7 p.m., she has flour and fat, followed by three hours of fat and sugar eating.

What was the trigger? What started the binge? The simple answer is stress. Norepinephrine built up in her system for six hours. Eating finally stopped the stress at 9 p.m. (arrows). But we already know that serotonin isn't what fixed it. Her rise in hunger at 8 p.m. tells us that (dashed rectangle). At 8 p.m. serotonin stopped helping her, even though it had been working at 6 p.m.

Four indicators prove that the addictive cycle took over:

1. Vonna's serotonin level plummeted. We know that was caused by a rise in dopamine in the nucleus accumbens.

2. Her stress was soothed. Because serotonin didn't fix it, endorphins must have done the job.

3. Her eating continued. The endorphins that relieved the stress also promoted addictive eating.

4. She chose the type of foods encouraged by the addiction: fats and simple carbs.

**Focus:**

- Stress and eating rows

**Problems:**

- Increased stress
- Addictive eating

Now look at your own charts. Where do you find eating that follows an increase in stress? Circle this eating and label it NE, for norepinephrine.

**STEP 12**

Assess the likelihood that you are a food addict.

Pull together all the indicators of addiction-stimulated eating. Count the number of labels for each category and fill in the totals. What do you think? Is your appetite influenced, in part, by the addictive cycle?

| Indicator: | VTA | DP/NA | FC/WB | NE |
|---|---|---|---|---|
| TOTALS: | | | | |

---

**BRAIN ALTERATIONS COMMENSURATE WITH ADDICTION**

**VTA**—Ventral tegmental area
- Appetite stimulated by the opioids released from eating sugar, starch, and/or chocolate

**DP/NA**—Dopamine/Nucleus accumbens
- Eating triggered by consumption of sugar, flour, and/or fat, leading to alteration of receptors on the nucleus accumbens and involving dopamine transmission

**FC/WB**—Frontal and prefrontal cortex and whole brain involvement
- Judgment, memory, priorities, and ethical behavior being influenced by the addictive response

**NE**—Norepinephrine
- Eating to find comfort from norepinephrine-stimulated appetite caused by stress

*Opening*

*Today's Agenda*

1. Help each other mark and label charts, and compile sums.

2. Discuss one or more of the following:

   • Do I have a food (sugar/carb/fat) addiction?

   • How do I feel about what I see in my charts?

   • How does it feel to say any of the following statements out loud?

     — I am powerless over food/eating.

     — I am powerless over my appetite once it is triggered.

     — This evidence proves my eating is a result of my biochemicals. Therefore it has nothing to do with willpower.

*(Feel free to substitute your own phrase for "powerless."*
*For example, "I can't help myself in the face of food.")*

*Closing*

# 20

# Current Eating Map

᪥ CONGRATULATIONS! You've made enormous progress.

Can you feel that you're honing in on why you eat what you eat? Can you sense that you're almost ready to remove the final barriers to losing weight?

You have a few more decisions to make before you design your final eating map. Until then, here's the structure for your eating, day by day:

- Eat every two to three hours so that you have five or six meals or snacks per day.
- Eat snacks that are 50/50—50 percent protein and 50 percent complex carbs.
- Make sure your snacks are free of flour, wheat, sugar, or simple carbs.
- Take snacks with you wherever you go.
- Eat at least four ounces of turkey (or the tryptophan equivalent in milk, etc.) three times each week.
- When your stress goes up, increase your intake of tryptophan.

## Body Signals Chart

You can decide whether or not to continue keeping your Body Signals Chart daily. A more compact one is provided for you now that you've gathered your basic data.

**STEP 13**

Solidify your satiety.

Nearly every nutrition authority will tell you that you will improve your eating by keeping a daily record of everything you eat. While that's true, my experience with clients has been that they'll keep a food diary for a short while and then abandon it. And it's easy to see why; when we get busy or stressed, it's easy to ditch something that is complex and takes time.

The point of a food diary is to stay conscious of what you are putting in your mouth. By keeping a daily Body Signals Chart, you can stay just as conscious with half the time and effort, especially since you now have four weeks of experience using one.

Of course you can manipulate these charts, just as you can manipulate a food diary, or even an eating report to your recovery partner. By now, you can reckon what *that* means—manipulation is the addictive brain at work.

Some people use the Body Signals Chart as a red flag of unwillingness. If they start to develop a bad attitude about the chart, they know they are straying into addict-land and they have something to talk about with their recovery partner.

## Current Chart

This chart is different from the previous ones. If you eat turkey (or an equivalent tryptophan source), you'll put the proportion in the proteins box and also check the turkey/tryptophan row.

Fluids are now separated according to sweetener. Any drink that is not sweetened in any way gets a dot for each eight ounces in the "no sugar added" box. A drink that is 100 percent natural fruit juice is counted as juice. However, if a drink is sweetened with *any* sugar, corn syrup, or fructose, it gets a dot in the "contains sugar" box. Splenda, NutraSweet, Equal, saccharin, and Sweet 'N Low drinks are counted as artificially sweet. Drinks sweetened only by the herb stevia can be counted as sugar-free. If a drink also has caffeine in it, add a check to the caffeine box. Milk is considered sugar-free, and it also gets a tryptophan credit. As before, three and a half eight-ounce glasses of milk get a check in the turkey/tryptophan box.

# Body Signals Chart, Ongoing

Date: _____

| CATEGORY | DESCRIPTIONS | TRYPTOPHAN 3 TIMES A WEEK | | | | | | | | | | | | | | | | | | | | | | |
|---|---|---|---|---|---|---|---|---|---|---|---|---|---|---|---|---|---|---|---|---|---|---|---|---|---|
| Timeline | Circle Wake-up | 6AM | 7 | 8 | 9 | 10 | 11 | 12PM | 1 | 2 | 3 | 4 | 5 | 6 | 7 | 8 | 9 | 10 | 11 | 12AM | 1 | 2 | 3 | 4 | 5 |
| **Food** Numbers go in this section | Proteins | | | | | | | | | | | | | | | | | | | | | | | | |
| | Complex carbs | | | | | | | | | | | | | | | | | | | | | | | | |
| | Flour | | | | | | | | | | | | | | | | | | | | | | | | |
| | Sugar | | | | | | | | | | | | | | | | | | | | | | | | |
| | Fats | | | | | | | | | | | | | | | | | | | | | | | | |
| Check | **Tryptophan** | | | | | | | | | | | | | | | | | | | | | | | | |
| Check | **Equal/NutraSweet** | | | | | | | | | | | | | | | | | | | | | | | | |
| **Fluids** Dots go in this section | Juice | | | | | | | | | | | | | | | | | | | | | | | | |
| | No sugar added | | | | | | | | | | | | | | | | | | | | | | | | |
| | Contains sugar | | | | | | | | | | | | | | | | | | | | | | | | |
| | Artificially sweet | | | | | | | | | | | | | | | | | | | | | | | | |
| Check | **Caffeine** | | | | | | | | | | | | | | | | | | | | | | | | |
| Timeline | | 6AM | 7 | 8 | 9 | 10 | 11 | 12PM | 1 | 2 | 3 | 4 | 5 | 6 | 7 | 8 | 9 | 10 | 11 | 12AM | 1 | 2 | 3 | 4 | 5 |
| **Hunger** | Starving | | | | | | | | | | | | | | | | | | | | | | | | |
| | Really hungry | | | | | | | | | | | | | | | | | | | | | | | | |
| | Mildly hungry | | | | | | | | | | | | | | | | | | | | | | | | |
| | Not hungry | | | | | | | | | | | | | | | | | | | | | | | | |
| **Appetite** | Craving food | | | | | | | | | | | | | | | | | | | | | | | | |
| | Food focused | | | | | | | | | | | | | | | | | | | | | | | | |
| | Quiet | | | | | | | | | | | | | | | | | | | | | | | | |
| **Satiety** | Satiated | | | | | | | | | | | | | | | | | | | | | | | | |
| | Not | | | | | | | | | | | | | | | | | | | | | | | | |
| **Stressed?** | Highly | | | | | | | | | | | | | | | | | | | | | | | | |
| | Mildly | | | | | | | | | | | | | | | | | | | | | | | | |
| | No | | | | | | | | | | | | | | | | | | | | | | | | |
| **Seeking Comfort?** | | | | | | | | | | | | | | | | | | | | | | | | | |
| Timeline | | 6AM | 7 | 8 | 9 | 10 | 11 | 12PM | 1 | 2 | 3 | 4 | 5 | 6 | 7 | 8 | 9 | 10 | 11 | 12AM | 1 | 2 | 3 | 4 | 5 |

Duplicating this page for personal use is permissible.

## Opening

## Today's Agenda

Discuss one or more of the following topics, or pick your own:

- Keeping my Body Signals Chart as an indicator of my willingness
- My decision to keep (or not keep) using the chart
- My willingness to follow the ongoing eating map
- Venting my rebellious feelings
- Converting another item on the positive action with negative association list (see the exercise on page 148)
- Reminding myself of my reasons for choosing to confront my eating
- Reinspiring myself and thinking about the life I want to lead

## Track Update

If you are on Tracks A or B, jump to the "Friendship Skills" section of the next chapter on pages 168–169.

If you are on Track C, continue with the start of the next chapter.

## Closing

# 21

# Switching Best Friends

MANY FOOD addicts testify that food is their most dependable friend, and that they'll turn to eating sooner than call a friend or ask for a hug.

By now you know the biochemical reason for this: The prefrontal cortex is assigning a higher value to the pleasure derived from food than to pleasurable contact with humans.

To change this dynamic, you'll have to deliberately defy your frontal cortex because you can only make the intricate changes that make a lasting difference on your appetite by building new neuron pathways.

You already know you can white-knuckle it through a diet for a little while, but that it won't last. The good news is you're about to make a very powerful change, and you'll have white knuckles for only about a week.

Bear in mind how powerful an addiction can be. It can lure you back like a Greek siren. To prevent this, you can either stay tied to a mast, like Odysseus—making it hard to drive or sit at a computer—or you can make your way through a transition that will be hard at first, but will get easier.

You are about to wallop your appetite disorder by making a decision and then acting on it. After a few weeks of discomfort, you will begin to feel you are on an astonishing island of peace when it comes to eating. You'll be surprised by other things too.

Perhaps your thinking will seem sharper than you knew it could be. Perhaps your vision will be clearer. Once you get the imbalanced, addictive chemicals out of your body, the changes will be your bonus.

But first, you'll need backup. When you confront your addiction, you'll be in for a wrestling match. Also, I'm sorry to say, your addiction is bigger than you are. It's sneakier. It has hidden resources. And it doesn't play fair.

You just can't go it alone. My proof? You've already tried that, haven't you? Think about how many times you have tried to fix this problem by yourself.

With this step, we are going to improve your skills at calling for backup. If you are a cop or a firefighter, a rescue worker or a soldier, you already know how powerful a team can be. You already know how to call for backup.

**STEP 14**

Switch best friends.

Granted, this will be harder because you will be learning to ask for help for yourself, rather than somebody else.

But get this: You aren't alone in thinking this is hard. Thousands of other people reading this book think it's hard to ask for help too. Imagine, thousands of other people reading this book are all thinking it's hard to ask for help. So, check out www.annekatherine.org. At my Web site, you'll find ways to contact those other folks. Meeting people online gives you twenty-four-hour backup.

But it's important that you build support with actual warm, materialized people too. An addiction thrives on isolation, and it can entice you back by keeping you from social contact.

You really can change your brain. The neuron pathways involved in addiction will go off-line as you build new pathways around support and abstinence.

Plus, the more we practice the tools of recovery, the stronger our new neural networks will become. As we create new positive associations, we reinforce those new connections inside our heads. In this way, we get our brains on our side, metaphorically speaking. Recovery gets easier the longer we practice it because the brain is now on board to help us.

So you see, the next few changes will only be hard at first. This gives you a good reason to keep going. Your appetite disorder will soon begin to leave you alone, freeing you from addictive captivity. With the goo cleaned out of your brain, you will improve your life in ways that today you can't even imagine.

### Friendship Skills (Tracks A and B join us here)

Call a meeting with your recovery partner because you'll be doing the following skill building together. You'll need a timer and each of you will need your book.

Being a good friend and building a new friendship are like riding a bicycle. They involve skills that can be learned.

The most important skills involved in being a friend have to do with the capacity to be honest, trustworthy, and honorable. You and your recovery partner have already agreed to behave in these ways by not revealing confidences or gossiping about each other. You also know not to take any sensitive information your friend has shared with you and use it against her.

The other important friendship skills have to do with being present, showing up, and listening. These skills are not just about being a good friend to someone else; they reveal your genuine self, something food addicts tend to hide. After all, how can your partner be there for you if you aren't there for yourself?

Giving and receiving have to go both ways. Otherwise, the boundaries fray and the relationship becomes less healthy.

Every once in a while, we may discover we're with a recovery partner who's a compulsive taker. This trait may show up as someone taking an hour to your five minutes, or, after asking how you are, interrupting you frequently to tell about how she is. If this happens, you can give your partner a couple of chances by pointing out the discrepancy and asking her to delay sharing until you have finished. If this works, you've both gained something. If this doesn't work, look for a new recovery partner.

Naturally, any friendship has to be built. Sometimes we just click with a person, and we can go straight to revealing our deepest feelings. More often, though, we build safety with each other by taking a small risk and seeing what happens.

Friendship skills include effective listening and authentic talking. The skills required for a successful recovery partnership are even more refined. Listening has to be of sufficient quality to help your partner move forward. Talking has to be honest and focused so that it offers authentic expression.

## Skill Building

Effective listening and focused talking are two skills most of us can always improve. Even those of us who make a living at listening—therapists, counselors, health care professionals, spiritual leaders, and so on—can benefit from a refresher.

Trimming the fat from what we say can also radically improve the quality of a conversation. We all add little side comments to protect ourselves from looking foolish or taking too much risk, but these comments act like static and impact an interchange.

Watch out for redundancy and vagueness, which are boring and sedating. Redundancy is saying the same thing more than once. My observation is that people who are redundant aren't used to being listened to. They say the same thing multiple times until they get some indication that they've been heard. Watch your own tendency to do this, and train yourself to say things once. If you're worried that you haven't been heard, ask your friend what she heard you say.

Also watch for a tendency toward vagueness—communication that is cloudy or inexact. Your recovery partner will have trouble acting as a true friend if she can't see who you are.

Some indicators of vagueness are

*I don't know.*

*She was . . . you know.*

*It was okay.*

*I'm fine.*

*I'm not sure.*

*Whatever.*

*That's different. (Doesn't explain how or in what way.)*

*I can't explain/describe it.*

*He's special/unique. (Doesn't explain how or in what way.)*

*Maybe.*

If you don't make the effort to see and explain what's really going on inside you, your partner won't have any material to work with. It's not reasonable to make her spend more effort to connect with you than you are willing to put into connecting with yourself.

**Skill Practice**

Do this exercise with your recovery partner. It will help each of you build both your talking and listening skills.

1. Pick one of the following topics or choose your own.

2. Decide who will talk and who will listen first.

3. The talker will use the focused talking protocol (beginning on page 176).

4. The listener will practice the listening skills described below. It's fine to either work with all of the listening skills at once or to focus on a different one each time the two of you have a mindful conversation. You choose.

*Possible topics*

• What I went through today just getting here.

• My frustration with work is . . .

• When I think about confronting my addiction, I feel . . .

• When I think about turning to you for support with my recovery, I feel . . .

• When I think about giving support to you, I feel . . .

• As we practice these support-building skills, I feel . . .

• My concern about building this friendship is . . .

*Effective Listening Skills*

■ **REFLECTIVE LISTENING**

Reflect back to the talker the gist or essence of what you heard her say. In the examples on the next page, notice that the response doesn't have to be exact or long. A little bit goes a long way in showing that you are paying attention.

| Speaker | Listener |
|---|---|
| "I'm furious." | "Really mad." |
| "I'm exhausted." | "Spent." |
| "I graded papers for two hours, went to a boring, endless faculty meeting, and then had parent-teacher conferences." | "You did a lot." |
| "I told Tom I'd have to meet with you at least once a week, and probably would call you every day, and he clammed up. I get so manipulated by that. He won't talk, then I feel responsible for making him feel better." | "You were trying to take care of yourself, and you ended up feeling responsible for him." |

## ■ LISTENING FOR FEELINGS, ATTUNING

Reflect the feelings the talker is revealing either through her words, metaphors, delivery, or body language. (Metaphors are actually even more effective than feeling words.) Examples:

| Speaker | Listener |
|---|---|
| "I could stomp and scream." | "Pound the ground." |
| "I've tried so hard and nothing makes any difference to her." | "You sound discouraged." |
| "I graded papers for two hours, went to a boring, endless faculty meeting, and then had parent-teacher conferences." | "You sound tired." |
| "It's like a knot in my belly." | "Tied tight." |
| "It's like there's a brick wall between us." | "Yeah, hard and immovable." |

■ **MATCHING INTENSITY**

Modulate your response so that it has a similar energy and intensity as the speaker's. Examples:

| Speaker | Listener |
| --- | --- |
| "I COULD STOMP AND SCREAM." | "REALLY MAD." |
| "I've tried so hard and nothing makes any difference to her." (whispering) | "You sound discouraged." (very quietly) |
| "I graded papers for two hours, went to a boring, endless faculty meeting, and then had parent-teacher conferences." (with a sigh) | "Phew." (letting out a breath) |

■ **ASKING OPEN-ENDED QUESTIONS**

Invite the speaker to explore more of her experience. Examples:

• Tell me more.

• What did you notice?

• How did that feel?

• Where do you feel that inside of your body?

■ **JOINING***

Join with some part of her experience, add a bit of your own experience, and toss the ball back to her. With this technique, you build a common picture together. It's almost like making a film of your common experience that includes the uniqueness and complexity that each of you contributes. In the example shown on the next page, the arrows and highlighted words show how each partner joined the other; the remaining words show how each blended in her own experience.

---

* Used with permission. This technique comes from the work of Yvonne Agazarian and Systems-Centered Training® and is part of a more comprehensive skill that allows for the growth and transformation of human systems including individuals, families, groups, and organizations. See Appendix C.

| Speaker | Listener |
|---|---|
| "I'm mad at the hundreds of diets I tried and failed. I'm mad that I thought something was wrong with me." | "I feel mad too. I'm realizing just how many years I've struggled with this." |
| "Yes, I've felt bad about myself for so many years and so many hours, and I've put up with snide comments or smiled when someone teased me in a mean way." | "Yeah, I've pretended to laugh when someone was really ripping my guts out. 'Just put the potatoes in front of Sally, then she won't have to strain her arm.' Ooh, I am so mad at that." |
| "Me too. I am furious. I'd like to lock my family in a room and read this book to them." | "Okay. That works for me." |
| Genuine laughter ←———————→ Genuine laughter | |

## Avoiding Common Listening Errors

■ **PROBLEM SOLVING**

A common mistake is to snatch and hold the conversational ball by offering solutions. The listener's intent is usually to help the talker feel better. However, this has the opposite effect. The talker ends up being cut off before she's completed her process, which can leave her feeling stuck or worse. Most women and some men would rather be understood than have the problem solved for them.

■ **PREMATURE COMFORTING**

Comfort feels great *at the end* of talking something out. But it can be interruptive if it occurs in the middle of someone's sharing. Giving comfort early in a conversation usually makes the listener feel better, but the person speaking and being comforted usually feels cut off.

■ **JUDGING**

Judgmental or critical comments will dry up the stream of talk in a jiffy. Plus, the critical person loses the other person's trust. She won't feel safe enough to reveal herself.

■ **COMPARING**

Negative comparisons come in two versions. The first is putting down the talker: "Sally had that happen too, but she had the guts to stop the creep in his tracks." The second is putting down yourself: "You do that so much better than I do. I'm clumsy at it." Both cause harm for someone.

When you're mindfully listening, limit positive comparisons as well. These snatch your partner's attention from her inner self and force her to compare herself with others. For example, if your recovery partner says, "I knew I'd feel better if I waited a day or two," and you respond with "Honey, you understand that better than anyone else I know," you're actually changing the subject from what the talker felt and did to what a savvy person she is.

■ **EXPLAINING**

This is yet another form of snatching the conversational ball. Remember, you're the listener, not the talker.

Beware of asking why she did or felt something. This is always a stopper. When we pause to figure out our motivation or stimulus, we interrupt our flow toward self-discovery.

Sometimes a why question from the listener is a hidden criticism. The speaker will be invited to defend herself, and she will abandon the edge she was exploring.

In the following example, a why question diverts the speaker from exploring her anger:

> "When he asked for my engagement ring, I just threw it at him and ran to my car."

> "Why didn't you keep it?"

> "I didn't want it. It's a symbol of betrayal."

> "It was valuable. You could have sold it."

■ **TAKING HER AWAY FROM HER POINT**

More ball snatching. Catch yourself and refocus on the speaker.

■ **INTERRUPTING**

If you're a compulsive talker, or simply very chatty, it's usually better to say very little and just listen, rather than risk getting triggered into talking when it's your partner's turn.

Your skill level as a listener will improve as you practice. While you are listening to your recovery partner, don't think about what skills to use; just pay attention to her, saying very little unless you are joining. Remember, the most important thing you can do is listen compassionately, attuning yourself to her and staying receptive.

## Focused Talking Protocol—SHARP

Our ability to receive help depends in part upon what we communicate. If I'm heartbroken, but covering it up by chatting cheerily, how can I expect my recovery partner to empathize and be present for me? You must give your partner enough to work with.

The more you focus inside yourself, on your own feelings, the more you can achieve through talking.

A sequence of talking skills called SHARP can help you do this. SHARP stands for Settle, Here and now, Attend, Reveal, and Process. (See next page.)

These listening and speaking skills are immensely valuable, but you needn't use them 100 percent of the time. In the next chapter, for example, you'll find scripts that you and your recovery partner can use to support each other through the critical moments of recovery.

As the two of you work together, you'll sense when your friend has dropped down into herself and needs quality listening. And you'll start to recognize when *you* need to pause and use the focused talking protocol so that you can get at what's eating you (or making you want to eat).

Consistently practicing both focused talking and effective listening will not only make you a better communicator and friend, but it will also begin to make a noticeable difference in your need to use food as a soother.*

---

* Canadians, replace the word *soother* with *pain reliever.*

## FOCUSED TALKING PROTOCOL—SHARP

1. **S**ettle
    a. Sit down.
    b. Align your body, feet on the floor, with your spine erect.
    c. Become still.
    d. Settle, like motes of earth settle to the bottom of a pond.

2. **H**ere and now
    a. Bring yourself into the present moment.
    b. Breathe in, all the way down to your belly button.
    c. Slowly release the breath.

3. **A**ttend
    a. Feel the center of your being.
    b. Turn your attention inward, toward your own physical and emotional sensations.

4. **R**eveal
    a. As you focus on your inner self, describe what you see or feel.
    b. Express feelings, metaphors, anything that is going on in you.
    c. Be as clear and specific as you can. "My heart feels empty; I'm angry and a little scared" is more powerful than "I'm upset" or "I'm frustrated."
    d. Remember, no matter how hard it is to feel what you encounter inside yourself, if you will express it, you will move through it and past it.

5. **P**rocess
    a. Peel away the layers, one by one, expressing what you feel with each layer.
    b. Perceive and stay attuned to your inner flow.
    c. Put every aspect of your experience into words or word pictures.

If at all possible, meet with your recovery partner once a week. We humans seem to be able to keep on track with whatever program we're on for about a week. After that, somehow our focus starts to fade away. Regular support meetings will bolster you as you continue to fix your appetite disorder.

And now some more good news: You're already two-thirds of the way through the process of mending your appetite disorder. You just have a little further to go.

. . .

*Opening*

*Today's Agenda*

**Skill Practice**

Taking turns, each of you use the focused talking protocol and effective listening skills to explore a topic that matters to you. You can choose from the topic list on page 171, from the following list, or from your own concerns.

- Converting another negative association into a positive action (see the exercise on page 148)

- How it feels to be really listened to

- How it feels to practice focused talking

- Which of your family members and friends really listen, and whether these are the ones you talk with the most

- Which of your family members and friends don't listen well, and whether you're more protective about what you reveal to them

- Your willingness to give this recovery friendship a chance to be as soothing as food

- Your willingness to meet once a week with your recovery partner to support each other face to face

*Closing*

# 22

# Support Dialogues

WHEN YOU first added two or three snacks a day, it went against the grain, didn't it? Adding regular repasts was quite an adjustment, especially if you used to dump most of your eating into one bulky evening meal.

By now, you've had four weeks to get used to this way of eating. You've become accustomed to shopping for snacks, getting snack bags ready, and stashing them wherever you spend time.

The next step is similar, and at first, it may feel awkward. But if you persist with it, it will become one of the best presents you've ever given yourself.

You're about to change the way you get support from others. Right now, your relationship to support is similar to your old relationship to meals when you'd skip them. Here was something you wanted and needed, yet you deprived yourself of it.

Likewise, very few food addicts walk around with a sufficient amount of daily comfort. Most of the women I've worked with are starved for comfort and have endured lifetimes of deficiency.

**STEP 15**

Strengthen your support.

Given that, you'd think these same women would leap at the chance to receive support. But they don't. For most, the old pattern of handling matters privately feels safest.

How about you? Have you rushed to embrace the process of building a recovery relationship, or have you dragged your feet?

If you've held back, was this because you don't need any more comfort and support? Does your cup of support run over, day after day?

Most of you are probably answering, "No."

So what makes it so hard to turn to your recovery partner for help? The following are possible reasons for resisting support *(and my response to each one).*

1. You don't know how to ask. *I'm going to teach you.*

2. You don't know what will help. *What will help is more support, so you can get used to having it. When there are big gaps in support, you have to overcome your resistance every time you receive it. With regular support, it gets easier to accept it.*

3. You're afraid of appearing needy. *Or you're afraid that if you get a little, you'll want too much. Or you fear that the neediness that's been asleep inside you will wake up and make you miserable. You'll be surprised at how far a little bit of help will go. Notice that when you are really understood, you turn the corner toward feeling better.*

4. You're afraid of being seen as weak or foolish, or you're afraid of being ridiculed, hurt, or rejected. Or, you're just not used to having support; you've always handled everything by yourself.

   *These are all reasons based on past experience and—I'm guessing—young experience. Since we're born with the natural ability to receive help, we have to be trained to turn away from it. If our training is harsh and hurtful, we carry a painful lesson deep inside us. We learn not to ask for or accept help, and we learn to rely on ourselves—and on food.*

I want you to consider something. When you let the past rule you in this way, you are acting as if today were still the past. You are acting as if the whole world is operating the way your family did when you were young.

**Now Protocol**

Try something with me now. Yes, right now.

Sit comfortably with your spine in alignment and both feet on the floor. Breathe deeply and slowly, taking in air all the way down to your knees. Do this a couple of times.

Bring yourself fully into this present moment, into right now.

Reflect on these thoughts:

- *The past is past.*
- *The present is present.*
- *You are here, right now.*
- *You are safe, right now.*
- *You know how to survive.*
- *Not only did you survive, but you are also strong and adult now.*
- *You will never let anyone hurt you the way you were hurt in the past.*
- *You can handle things.*
- *You have skills.*
- *You have choices.*
- *You can let yourself be supported.*
- *You deserve support.*
- *You are in this moment.*
- *You are here, right now.*

Whenever debris from the past arises and threatens to keep you from making good choices, use this exercise to center yourself in the present. You may also want to read Thich Nhat Hanh's wonderful book on being present in the here and now, *The Miracle of Mindfulness*.

## Using Support

You are on a ramp toward the most significant change you can make to quiet your appetite disorder. This chapter and the next are your final preparation for this change. Trust me when I say that you'll catapult your odds of being successful if you surrender to the advice presented in this chapter.

Suggestion 1:  Talk to your recovery partner every morning.

Suggestion 2:  Talk to your recovery partner soon after you get home from work every day.

I'm going to give you a precise structure to use for these phone calls. Please follow it. Sometimes people think they ought to be creative and embroider the structure with social niceties, but I want you to resist this tendency. For one thing, that would muddy the intent of the phone conversation. For another, it would lengthen the calls.

*Dialogue Structures*

In each case, I'll give the instructions and the rationale, an example of the dialogue in use, practice tips, and, lastly, the structure itself. Meet with your recovery partner and practice each one.

## Daily Vitamin Call

Start your day by connecting with a loving human. It makes a world of difference; plus it will remind you that you aren't alone.

You can use this call to affirm your vision for the day, to describe how you've set yourself up for success, or to clear feelings. You can pinpoint the challenging events of the day and arrange support for those times. You can share your eating plan. You can recite the first three steps of Twelve Step recovery programs (pages 239–240). You can also end with a brief prayer.

I have a warning, which I'll repeat again and again. *Do not turn this call into a social chat.* Most people have very little time in the morning. Keep this call to three minutes max. If you disrespect this time boundary, one or both of you will start dreading the call, eventually stop doing it, and lose this vital tool.

*Sample Dialogue*

Answerer: "Hello?"

Caller: "Hi, it's _____ (name)."

A: "Hi."

C: "I'm picturing myself enjoying an abstinent day. I see myself making healthy food choices and following the plan. My snacks are packed and ready to go, and backup snacks are at work and in my car."

A: "Good job. And I'm holding the same picture for you."

C: "My challenge today is meeting my sister after work to shop for Mom's birthday present. The mall is full of food triggers, and my sister will want to get food at one of my trigger places."

A: "What is your prevention plan?"

C: "We could decide before we drive what we want to get her. We could park right outside that store and stay out of the rest of the mall. When we're done, I could eat my snack in the car and she could join me when she's through eating."

A: "Great plan. Also, take your phone. Call me before, during, or after you shop if you want to, or all three."

C: "Thanks. Your turn."

A: "I see myself leaving early for work so that I'm not rushed getting there. I have my snacks in the car already. I enjoy my snacks and feel good about soothing my appetite.

"My challenge today is the departmental lunch meeting. I see myself choosing the salad option and enjoying it. I've already arranged to sit next to Sandy, who is a wise eater and doesn't choose bread or dessert. I'm having turkey for my snack midmorning so that I'm fortified for lunch. I plan to call you after lunch so that if I get triggered by someone else's choices, I have a way to get my consciousness back. In fact, I've already programmed my phone to ring and remind me to call."

C: "Wow! Superior planning."

A: "Share prayer?"

C: "Sure."

C&A: "God, grant us the serenity to accept the things we can't change, to change the things we can, and the wisdom to know the difference. Amen."

C&A: "Bye."

*Principles:*

1. Get in. Get out. Notice that these women had no social chat, no caretaking, and no conversational fat. They did the job and closed the call. The entire call took two minutes.

2. The caller goes first. Food addicts have a tendency to start support calls by asking about the other person. Don't. If it's your quarter, you go first. Plunge right into the vitamin call agenda.

3. C was encouraged by A to do her own problem solving around her sister's likely action of hovering near trigger foods. A asked, "What is your prevention plan?" rather than offering solutions. This kept the

responsibility for handling the situation with C. (We food addicts have to avoid our tendency toward codependence.) Offer solutions only if your partner specifically asks.

4. Making a call for help was encouraged by both women. A reminded C that she could call as much as needed to get through the mall unscathed. And C responded positively to A's commitment to calling her after the lunch meeting.

Since many of us dread rejection, it helps us to receive frequent reminders that it's more than okay to call when needed.

*How to Practice*

At your meeting, practice the daily vitamin call. Each of you take a turn being the caller. (*Note: You'll need a timer.*)

1. Sit back to back, each with the dialogue agenda in front of you. The taller person is C.

2. Both of you:

   a. Pretend it is tomorrow morning. Think about what part of the day you'd like to improve. Decide what you'll do to improve it. Affirm, visualize, or make a plan for that improvement.

   b. Think about what your greatest challenge will be tomorrow, either to your eating or to your stress level. Decide what would help you.

3. Set the timer for three minutes.

4. C says, "Ring." A answers, and you begin the dialogue.

*Dialogue Agenda*

1. Greeting

2. C expresses one or more of the following:

   a. Vision for the day

   b. Affirmations for the day

   c. Commitment to healthy eating for the day

   d. Steps 1, 2, and 3 (from a Twelve Step recovery program, pages 239–240).

   e. Food plan—specifically what you will eat at each meal and snack today

    f. Positive setups—how you will set yourself up for success

    g. Challenges you foresee either to staying on your food plan or to handling stress

    h. Your plan for handling these challenges

3. A offers supportive comments and cheers, and she champions problem solving

4. A and C switch roles and repeat steps two and three

5. Both exchange encouragement to call for help

6. Close and adieu

### Evening Relief Call

For most food addicts, evening is their most vulnerable time. They've used up their energy and resiliency at work and come home with diminished resources. When they are clobbered with difficult feelings, food is their primary defense. This is why an evening relief call is so very important.

It's astonishing what a difference a brief phone call can make to bolster us. One of the myths many of us hold is that our need is bottomless. We believe that we need tons and tons of care.

We fear that the emptiness inside is infinite. We conjure up a scenario where, if someone started filling us, we'd turn into a leech and suck that person dry. We have trained ourselves to take and ask for very little, always guarding against imagined abandonment caused by asking too much.

The exercises in this chapter are, in part, to train you out of this thinking, and, in part, to let you research your myths.

Pay attention to what actually happens when you get a little help. Notice how you feel after a smidgeon of connection.

As with the vitamin call, making a human connection is more important than what you actually say. The dialogue is to help you learn how to keep the conversation on point, but the most important thing about the call is that you reached out and someone answered.

*Sample Dialogue*

    A: "Hello?"

    C: "It's _____ (name)."

A: "Hi."

C: "What's your time boundary?"

A: "I've got ten minutes. What's yours?"

C: "I've got all evening, but ten is good." (C sets the timer for five minutes.)

A: "Go."

C: "I could report successes with my plan and eating, but the main thing is that I'm just spent. When I walked in the house, it seemed so quiet and empty. I felt the loneliness well up . . ." (C sounds choked up.)

A: "Hmm. You sound sad."

C: "I am." (Pauses with a sound of soft crying.)

A: (With presence and caring.) "Let the tears just flow."

C: "I am so sad." (Pause.)

A: "Take your time. I'm here. What are you noticing inside your body?"

C: "I'm feeling completely alone in the world. It's like there's a hole inside of me."

A: "Like a big, empty hole?"

C: "Yeah." (Crying.)

A: (Acts fully present without words, using an occasional comforting sound so that C can tell she's listening and waiting patiently as C moves through this feeling.)

C: (More crying.) "Phew. That took me by surprise. I didn't know that was in there."

A: "It caught you off guard. Very important work."

C: "How about you?"

A: "I join you in feeling sad and alone. I had such a great day at work. I was brilliant and solved six crises in a single bound. And then as I was driving home, I realized, I could never share this with Tom and get the response I want. He'd either minimize my success, explain it, or top it. And then I felt alone. (Pause.) I'm feeling sad."

C: "Hmm (comforting, inviting sound). I hear your sadness. Take your time."

A: "Now I'm pissed. Damn it. I'm so angry that my husband can't see me."

C: "Yeah. Angry that he can't show up for you."

A: "Yeah. Man, I'm so mad. Grrrrrrrr."

C: "Grrrrr." (Supportive grring.)

A: "I want to throw something."

C: "What do you want to throw?"

A: "Tom."

C: "Okay. I support you in that."

A: (Starts laughing.) "Okay, I'm through it."

C: "Well done."

A: "You too. Thanks."

C: "Thanks. By the way, congratulations on being a hero at work."

A: "Hey, thanks, that's just what I wanted someone to recognize. I'm going to bask in that a moment."

C: "Hero, hero."

A: "You want to plan for the evening?"

C: "I'll sit down and eat dinner. Then I'll get up from the table and stretch out on the couch and read my new magazine. Then I'll decide whether to do housework for no more than thirty minutes or read for the rest of the evening."

A: "Good plan. I'm going to sit down and eat dinner. Then I'll get up, make my snacks for tomorrow, put them in my car, start a load of laundry, and then watch TV and knit."

C: "Good plan. Thanks for being there."

A: "Thanks for being there."

C: "Bye."

A: "Bye."

If you want to, read the example again, and identify the listening skills the partners used. Notice they did not distract themselves with "he said's" or "she said's." They did not search for reasons but went straight into their present experience. Notice also that they guided each other into focused talking.

This call took about nine minutes. With but a short call, they tuned in, cleared themselves of their difficult feelings, shifted past them, and were able to envision a manageable and restorative evening. Their connection decreased their isolation and freed energy for using the evening well.

It might seem unrealistic that two people could zero in on deep feelings so quickly, and then move through them that fast. Although real dialogues are bound to last a bit longer, this shortened sample dialogue illustrates the important highlights of the evening relief call. With practice and a safe partner, it does become possible to move quickly into the depth of awareness that lets us move out of difficult places.

Of course, your evening relief calls may not always be about tough feelings. You'll have successes or joys or just ordinary aspects of living to share with your partner too. However, since we have a tendency to put on a good face even when things are bad, we will gain more if we search for anything that might be wrong as we make this call. Being perpetually upbeat will prevent the honest dialogue that can open up your creativity for using your evening for something besides eating.

### How to Practice

In a face-to-face meeting with your recovery partner, practice an evening relief call:

1. Sit back to back, each with the dialogue agenda in front of you. The shorter person will be C.
2. C: Begin the focused talking protocol—SHARP—by taking yourself through the quiet preparatory steps.
3. A: Prepare to be an effective listener.
4. C: Say, "Ring." When A answers, you begin the dialogue.

### Dialogue Agenda

1. Greet each other.
2. Negotiate the time boundary. (If C has eight minutes and A has ten minutes, the call should last no more than eight minutes.) In any case, the call should not last more than ten minutes.
3. Divide this time in half and set the timer for half the minutes available. *It is very important that you each take an equal amount of time to talk.* If one of you has a difficult issue and needs more time one night, then the other is to take an equivalent amount of extra time the next night. If the timer goes off before C is done talking, she finishes up quickly.
4. C: Begin focused talking (SHARP).

5. A: Listen effectively.

6. Switch roles and repeat steps three to five.

7. Make a plan for the evening (optional).

8. Say thanks and good-bye. If you haven't used up the time, say good-bye anyway.

(Remember, you must guard against turning this into a social chat. If you forget this discipline, the call will lose its power. One of you will grow to dread it, and these support calls will soon disappear.)

## Help Call

This is the call you make to your recovery partner when you notice any sign that your appetite has been activated. These signs include:

- Thoughts of food
- Food pictures
- Plans for going to a dangerous restaurant (such as a bakery, fast food joint, or buffet)
- Skipping your snack or (horrors) a meal
- Daydreaming about sugar, chocolate, fat, or starchy food
- Taking a bite of a food that contains sugar, chocolate, fat, or starch
- Feeling stubborn
- Feeling defensive
- Feeling pressured
- Feeling stressed
- Feeling afraid or alarmed
- Feeling discouraged
- Feeling sad
- Feeling alone
- Feeling overwhelmed
- Plummeting into despair
- Feeling like a little kid
- Feeling numb

- Making a plan to do something compulsively (e.g., shop, gamble, spend money, have sex, work, play computer games, or eat)
- Being or feeling rejected
- Being or feeling disappointed
- Feeling defiant or rebellious
- Becoming fixated on weight
- Comparing yourself to others
- Receiving very bad news
- Being treated meanly, rudely, or unkindly
- Being treated thoughtlessly
- Being criticized or judged
- Feeling left out of something that matters to you
- Being traumatized or harmed

*Sample Dialogue*

C: "Help!"

A: "I have twenty minutes max." (She sets the timer.) "What happened?"

C: "My mom cancelled again."

A: "I'm so sorry."

C: "I noticed I plummeted into feeling little and unimportant and then I remembered that was a sign I was in trouble."

A: "Good for you. Now, breathe. Settle."

C: (Takes a deep breath.)

A: "Align your body and center yourself. Tune into the here and now."

C: "Okay."

A: "Pay close attention to your insides. Then talk to me."

C: (Breathes.) "Okay... I'm feeling so small. I have this feeling that I don't matter to anyone."

A: "Yeah, you feel like you don't matter."

C: "Yeah." (C pauses.) "It's almost a drowning feeling, like I'm disappearing under water, and moving farther away from the surface. I'm reaching my hand out, but no one is there to pull me up."

A: "No one to reach for you."

C: "Yeah. I'm sinking."
A: "Going down."

C: "The loneliness is pressing me down."
A: "It's heavy."

C: "More like oppressive."
A: "Oppressive."

C: "Yeah, that's it. Like it's gonna squeeze the air out of me. But now I feel myself getting mad. I'm thinking, I won't let you. I won't let you do this to me. I feel myself pushing back. I'm coming back and I'm getting stronger. I'm bigger now, an adult."
A: "You're returning."

C: "Yes, I am. I'm returning to the present. I'm here. I'm an adult. And I'm royally ticked off at my mom."
A: "You gotta right to be."

C: "Man, that was a bad one. I can't believe I could go down so fast. And then that I could come back just as fast. Before, I never would have believed that I could recover from an emotional blow so quickly."
A: "You did the right thing. You remembered to connect, to call me. That made all the difference."

C: "Yes, it did. Thanks so much for being there."
A: "Welcome."

C: "I'm done."
A: "Good job."

C: "I can go now."
A: "Actually, listening to you helped me tune into something going on for me. Do you have five minutes?"

C: "Yes, I do. Go ahead."
A: "Okay, I'll settle in and use the SHARP protocol like the book taught us."

or

C: "I hate to say this, but I actually don't right now. However, I will have time in an hour."
A: "Thanks, I'll call you in an hour. Bye."

A help dialogue always starts immediately by the caller saying, "Help!" as soon as the phone is answered. This cuts to the chase, saves time, and prevents both partners from being distracted. (Presumably, neither one of you has many people who would call and say, "Help!" right off the bat. So you can safely assume that it is your recovery partner on the line when you answer and hear "Help!")

Notice that C started the call with no embroidery or chit-chat and no misleading opening like, "How are you?" which may have sidetracked the caller from her purpose. C was too upset to remember to check A's time boundaries, so A took care of that. The first thing she did was set a limit for the length of the conversation.

As you saw, A guided C into using the SHARP focused talking protocol. When we're severely agitated, we may not remember the SHARP guidelines. A, being in a calmer state, had the resources to apply the tool.

The word *help* signaled A to go into gear as an effective listener. A shifted quickly into using her listening skills, which was efficient in supporting C's exploration of her body's sensations and feelings.

Most of the time, A hit right on the nose with her responses. She didn't need to be fancy. If she couldn't think of a good listening response quickly, she just repeated an important word that C used.

Remember,

> Forget the social conventions. You're in deep water.
>
> You see a lifeboat.
>
> Call for a line.
>
> Get right to the point.
>
> Get support
>
> and hang up.

At one point in the conversation, A used a descriptive word (heavy) that didn't quite fit for C. The response still helped C clarify her feelings because she paused and reached for a better-fitting word. A accepted that clarification (rather than going back to her word and trying to push for it), and C moved quickly forward.

The most challenging part about handling a help call is ending it. A may be tempted to act as a caretaker. C may be tempted to "pay" for the call by giving something back to A.

But a help call is the only type of support call that doesn't require taking turns. It's important for all of us to be free to ask for help without fearing we'll get tangled up in a time-consuming interchange.

If A has an issue that surfaces because of C's call, it's fine for her to mention it. However, it's critical for C to be honest about her own time boundaries. Neither person must make a sacrifice to help the other, or else a partner's availability—or even the entire partner relationship—will soon peter out.

Both recovery partners must always be honest about time boundaries, and both must always respect the other's limits. Then, when A calls back, C can be open and A can feel safe.

Since we food addicts tend to sacrifice ourselves, I say again: *Always set and respect time boundaries.* A helpful idea is to place a timer next to your phone so that you can always set it easily. (And since you already know not to turn this into a social call, I won't even mention it.)

### How to Practice

In a face-to-face meeting with your recovery partner, practice a help call:

1. Sit back to back, each with the dialogue agenda in front of you. The person with the darker hair will be C.
2. This first time through, end the call as soon as C has completed her work or time is up, whichever comes first.
3. C says, "Ring." A answers, and you begin the dialogue.

### Dialogue

C: "Help!"

A: "I've got fifteen minutes. What's going on?" (A sets the timer.)

C: Relates the problem.

A: Guides C into using the SHARP protocol and uses effective listening skills.

C: Follows A's guidance and begins to use focused talking.

When C is finished or time is up, whichever comes first, end the call using one of the following alternate endings.

If you like, practice either or both of these endings.

### Alternate ending 1.  *A requests time. C has time.*

A: "Listening to you has helped me see that I have an issue too. Do you have time?"

C: "I have ten minutes." (C sets the timer.)

A: States her issue, using SHARP.

C: Guides A in using SHARP, while switching to effective listening.

### Alternate ending 2.  *A requests time. C doesn't have time right now.*

A: "Listening to you has helped me see that I have an issue too. Do you have time?"

C: "I don't now. I will at 10 o'clock."

A: "I'll call you then. Bye."

C: "I'll look forward to it. Thank you so much. Bye."

### Using Voice Mail

Many times, just *making* a help call can make a difference, even if voice mail answers instead of your partner. Here are some tips for using voice mail for support calls.

Get your own private mailbox, if possible. If that's not possible, let your recovery partner know who else has access to it—and make sure that person will keep messages from your recovery partner confidential.

Let your partner know the length of a message that is okay to leave. Let your partner know if it is all right to leave a message in two or three parts, over two or three voice mails in a row. And if you find yourself *purposely* making your support call when you know your partner won't be there, that is a sign that a help call (in which you actually talk to your partner) is in order.

### Using E-mail

Another good way to reach out to each other is through e-mail. If you have limits around e-mail—how often you check it, when you're able (and not able) to access it, time constraints, and so on—make these clearly known to your partner. Of course you should let her know if anyone else has access to your e-mail.

Remember, neither e-mail nor voice mail is a substitute for the real-time connection that's possible with a phone call.

• • •

## Support Meeting 9

### Opening

### Today's Agenda

1. Practice one of the three dialogues, the one that seems easiest. Discuss:

   a. How I felt when I was C

   b. How I felt when I was A

2. Discuss one or more of the following topics:
   - My willingness to follow the two suggestions from page 183.
   - My personal reasons for resisting support (you might want to list these and follow up with the optional exercise)

3. Decide whether or not you will accept the suggestions

4. Exchange phone numbers and e-mail addresses (optional) and explain your limits for using each method of connecting with each other. Discuss the best times to call each other. Respect each other's time boundaries for receiving calls. (How early or how late she accepts calls; whether it's okay to call her at work.) Plan to take turns being the caller for vitamin and relief calls.

### Optional Exercise: Convert your resistance

Of your reasons for resisting support, pick the easiest, and then practice the Now protocol, page 182.

### Track Update

If you are on Tracks A or B, jump to Chapter 29.
If you are on Track C, continue with the start of the next chapter.

### Closing

# 23

# Trigger Foods

❧ CERTAIN FOODS pull the trigger on your appetite. When you eat these foods, you are stimulated to eat. There are two types of trigger foods, which could be likened to the difference between a pistol and a shotgun.

A pistol trigger food stimulates you to eat more of that same food. Peanut butter is a pistol trigger food for some people. When some food addicts start eating peanut butter, they have difficulty stopping, and usually end up eating much more than they intended. However, for these people, eating peanut butter does not stimulate them to eat other foods or to eat other foods to excess.

A shotgun trigger food creates a wide pattern of eating, involving foods other than just the trigger food itself. Candy is a shotgun trigger food for most food addicts. Once we eat one type of candy, we want to eat more—not only of that particular type of candy, but also of other sweets as well. Shotgun trigger foods promote chain eating, grazing, bingeing, and foraging.

Most sugary and starchy foods are shotgun triggers for food addicts. Not only will they promote a higher intake of other sugars and starches, but also they'll boost appetite in general, causing us to eat bigger servings and bigger meals.

A food addict who routinely eats sweets or simple carbs also wants larger servings of meat and potatoes, more slices of pizza, or bigger helpings of lasagna. She'll be capable of eating two slices of pie plus ice cream for dessert, and then picking up a handful of chocolate mints after leaving the table. An hour later she could eat a pile of cookies and drink a soda.

**STEP 16**

Identify your trigger foods.

A food addict who eats doughnuts or pancakes for breakfast will be hungry for lunch before her nonaddicted companions are. She'll want to eat a large hamburger with all the trimmings, a full serving of fries, a couple of onion rings, and a large milk shake. And afterward, she'll still be interested in dessert.

While her nonaddicted friend chooses salad or soup, the food addict will crave meat, and she'll want it fried rather than baked. She'll prefer a starch over vegetables. Addictive foods shine in the spotlight; healthy foods become invisible.

Once food addicts are triggered, we have the capacity to consume a great quantity of food. Plus, other components of the addiction cycle are also triggered.

For instance, we notice what other people are eating. If they make healthy choices, we may feel inferior. If they eat smaller quantities, we may feel ashamed.

We become food-aware. We notice the portions on the plates around us. We are secretly envious or vexed if our sister's slice of pie or garlic bread is larger than ours. We may even make a plan to remedy the slight by eating later, when we're alone.

We become concerned about our next serving or portion. *How soon will no one notice if I go back for seconds? If I pretend to be fascinated in what he's saying while I casually slide that biscuit onto my plate, perhaps he won't pick up on it.*

When a normie (the nickname we use for people who don't have food addictions) eats a salad and half a sandwich and proclaims she's full, we can't relate. That does not seem to us like nearly enough food.

Do these fixations sound familiar? If so, I have good news. The more you stay with this program, the more satisfied you'll be with smaller portions. You'll start eating like a normie. In fact, a small amount of food will one day look like a lot. It will be plenty.

On the following page, I've listed some common trigger foods. You may already have a sense of what foods act as a trigger for you. Now decide which ones fire a pistol and which foods fire a shotgun of appetite.

*Pistol Trigger Foods*

On the following list, check the foods that you can't stop eating, but that don't trigger you to eat any other foods. If you proceed to *any* other eating after eating *one* of these foods, don't check it on this list. If you *add* any food to this one, don't check it on this list. For example, if you add butter to bread, check bread on the shotgun list instead of this one. If you go from one type of cookie to another type of cookie, check that cookie on the shotgun list.

☐ Dried fruit      ☐ Breads

☐ Peanut butter      ☐ Pasta

☐ Corn chips      ☐ Candy

☐ Nuts      ☐ Cookies

☐ Popcorn      ☐ Ice cream

☐ Potato chips      ☐ Sour cream

☐ Dip      ☐ Cream

☐ Trail mix      ☐ Butter

☐ Granola      ☐ White rice

☐ Cereal      ☐ _____

☐ Cream of wheat      ☐ _____

☐ Chocolate      ☐ _____

☐ Cheese spread      ☐ _____

☐ Herbed cream cheese      ☐ _____

☐ Cream cheese      ☐ _____

☐ Pizza      ☐ _____

☐ Pancakes

☐ Pretzels

*Shotgun Trigger Foods*

Check any of the following foods that trigger you to eat or that you eat in combination with other foods.

- ☐ Pretzels
- ☐ Pasta
- ☐ Pancakes and other breakfast starches eaten with syrup
- ☐ Pastries
- ☐ Pizza
- ☐ Breads, buns, biscuits
- ☐ Candy
- ☐ Chocolate
- ☐ Cookies
- ☐ Cake
- ☐ Pie
- ☐ Cereal
- ☐ Dip
- ☐ Ice cream
- ☐ Refined grains
- ☐ Chips
- ☐ Gravy
- ☐ Any dessert combining sugar, fat, and/or flour
- ☐ _____
- ☐ _____
- ☐ _____
- ☐ _____

If you are using the ongoing Body Signals Chart, you can look at it at the end of each day to discover ways in which your appetite may have been triggered. If you have eaten a pistol trigger food, your chart may look something like this:

| Timeline | Circle Wake-up | 6AM | 7 | 8 | 9 | 10 | 11 | 12PM | 1 | 2 | 3 | 4 | 5 | 6 | 7 | 8 | 9 | 10 | 11 |
|---|---|---|---|---|---|---|---|---|---|---|---|---|---|---|---|---|---|---|---|
| **Food** | Proteins | | | | | | | | | | | | | | | | | | |
| | Complex carbs | | | | | | | | | | | | | | | | | | |
| | Flour | | | | | | | | | | | | | | | | | | |
| | Sugar | | | | | | | | | | | | | | | | | | |
| | Fats | 10 | 10 | 10 | | | | | | | | | | | | | | | |

After eating a shotgun trigger food, you may see a pattern like the following:

| Timeline | Circle Wake-up | 6AM | 7 | 8 | 9 | 10 | 11 | 12PM | 1 | 2 | 3 | 4 | 5 | 6 | 7 | 8 | 9 | 10 | 11 |
|---|---|---|---|---|---|---|---|---|---|---|---|---|---|---|---|---|---|---|---|
| **Food** | Proteins | | | | | | | | | | | | | | | | | | |
| | Complex carbs | | | | | | | | | | | | | | | | | | |
| | Flour | 5 | | 3 | | | | | | | | | | | | | | | |
| | Sugar | | 5 | 2 | | | | | | | | | | | | | | | |
| | Fats | 5 | 5 | 5 | | | | | | | | | | | | | | | |

For the rest of this week, notice what foods cause a string of eating. Look at your Body Signals Chart at the end of each day, when you can still remember what you ate. If you see either a pistol or shotgun pattern, make a check by that food in the trigger foods lists. The blanks are for your personal trigger foods that aren't on the list.

. . .

## Support Meeting 10

*Opening*

*Today's Agenda*

1. Help each other figure out personal trigger foods and in which category they belong.

   Discuss one or more of the following:

   • How tempting it is to minimize the effect of a food on my appetite

   • My tendency to think of all food as either bad or good

   • My feelings about pinning down my trigger foods

   • Foods I want so badly to pretend aren't triggers for me

   • What it will be like to be free of the compulsion to eat

   • What I will do with my time when I'm not constantly thinking about food

2. Practice another dialogue from the chapter on support dialogues, pages 181–198. Remind yourselves of the two suggestions:

   a. Talk to your recovery partner every morning.

   b. Talk to your recovery partner soon after you get home from work each day.

*Closing*

# 24

# Abstinence

❧ THIS LITTLE DITTY is from the period in American history when alcohol was banned. People called the ban on alcohol temperance, but what they were really promoting was abstinence. Temperance is the moderate use of something; abstinence is refraining completely.

> Away, away with rum by gum,
> With rum, by gum,
> With rum, by gum.
> Away, away with rum by gum,
> It's the song of the Temperance Union.

In this chapter you will decide what foods you can eat temperately and which ones will require abstinence. You will also choose your first food to abstain from.

Achieving abstinence is a process. The abstinence you can manage today may be either more or less encompassing than the abstinence you will require in six months.

When I first got abstinent in the early '80s, I could manage to abstain from sugar one day at a time. Then as I got used to abstinence, and noticed that my life didn't end, I became more willing to refine it. At that point, I could expand my abstinence to include foods like ketchup and teriyaki, which contain sugar, but aren't technically sugar foods. For a while I even made my own sugar-free ketchup. (This was in the dark ages before more healthful condiments became available.) Over time, I lost my interest in ketchup and it moved into the non-trigger category.

I am not an alcoholic, but for years I abstained from all alcohol, reasoning that alcohol is made from sugar or starch, so it is a sugar food. However, I eventually added wine back to my list of nontrigger foods. I drink it rarely and don't want more than one glass of it at a time. And having some doesn't trigger me to eat.

Abstinence is a work in progress. As certain aspects of your life change, your abstinence profile will change as well.

**STEP 17**

Define your abstinence.

Some eating programs out there will tell you that *you absolutely must be abstinent of all the foods on our list*. If you feel safe with one of those programs and its list, feel free to adopt it.

My concern about programs that have long, encompassing lists is this: That kind of severe abstinence is hard to live with for an entire lifetime. My observation is that if people feel too restricted for too long—particularly from foods that are not their specific triggers—they will not only be unable to sustain that wide abstinence, but also when they blow, they'll blow big. (Think of the fasting mayor in the movie *Chocolat*, who loses control and binges on pounds of chocolate in the *chocolaterie* window.) These people will go back to eating everything on the list—and back to all their old eating patterns—and they'll have an aversion to ever returning to that list again.

Sometimes people will take a perfectly good program and become food Nazis. They'll actually reject or refuse to support people who do well with a more moderate abstinence.

My position is this: Everybody and every body is different. The foods that trigger the addiction cycle for one person are not necessarily the foods that trigger the cycle for someone else. When it comes to abstinence, one size does not fit all.

I see no point in staying away from food just to flex self-righteous muscles. What I mean by that is I don't agree with abstaining from food just for the sake of abstaining. Doing without is not a virtue in and of itself.

I'm not talking here about making the choice to be vegetarian or vegan or alcohol-free for health, planetary, religious, or spiritual purposes. Of course I support any people who avoid foods that pick at their conscience, cause an allergic reaction, or harm their health.

No, I'm referring to programs that insist on a wide abstinence just on the principle of the thing. People in such programs often fall into a class system. The wider abstainers are the aristocrats and the people who abstain on a more moderate basis are the underdogs, who are made to feel guilty and sneaky for eating a peanut.

Peanuts do trigger some people, but they don't trigger all people. For some, they are a pistol trigger but not a shotgun trigger. Furthermore, each pistol-triggered peanut picker is unique. Some will grab a handful of nuts and eat all ten nuts until they are gone. Others will go back, get the jar, and dump the whole thing in their laps.

There's a continuum. Your job is to pay attention to where you fall on the continuum of pistol-triggered peanut eating. If you can stop when you reach the sides of a finger bowl, don't have interest in more, and don't crave some other food afterward, how is this a problem?

Peanuts are not bad. They are not evil. They won't bring down the universe. We needn't get all bent out of shape over a peanut. Or a carrot or a banana.

Of course this makes a more delicate process out of defining abstinence. It takes careful observation, strict honesty, and a watchful eye toward the addictive brain.

Obviously, it would seem easier in the short run if I just told you what not to eat. However, in the long run, you will have more success if you create your own precise plan for abstinence. Plus, as you get better at watching your reaction to foods and correctly interpreting them as safe or dangerous for you, you'll be able to retool your abstinence as your body changes over time.

Still, we all know the addictive brain lies. For this reason, it's crucial to always work out abstinence boundaries with your recovery partner. Another food addict will be able to detect the wheedling, justifying patter of the addictive brain and help you stay honest with yourself.

### Determining Abstinence, Part 1

Now that you know which foods are your trigger foods and you have sorted them into pistol- and shotgun-trigger categories, you can decide how widely to define your first plan for abstinence.

My recommendation is to focus first on the shotgun triggers. You get more bang for your buck by eliminating shotgun triggers because they cause a wide pattern of eating.

Normally, I ask you to pick the easiest thing on a list to start with, but with abstinence, it's important to start with the most potent triggers. These are generally sugar, wheat, and/or flour—the Big Three.

Yes, there is some overlap in the last two categories. The wheat category includes all forms of wheat, including wheat flour; the flour category includes flour from all sources, including wheat. The lists are separate because, for some people, addictive eating is triggered by wheat in any form, including cream of wheat, bulgur, couscous made from wheat, and cracked wheat—but not from flour made from anything else, such as rice flour. In other people, however, addictive eating is triggered by any kind of flour, whether it's from rice, wheat, barley, or potatoes—yet these folks may do fine with nonflour forms of wheat, such as cream of wheat.

If only one of these three food categories is a shotgun trigger for you, use that food as your initial abstinence. If two or three of these are shotgun triggers for you, follow the instructions below.

If none of the Big Three are shotgun triggers for you, but certain other foods are, mentally replace the Big Three with those personal shotgun foods as you read on. And if you're fortunate enough to have no shotgun triggers, but have two or more pistol trigger foods, focus on these as you go through the abstinence selection process below.

Some people have more trouble with high-fat foods than Big Three foods. If that's the case for you, you can either skip to Chapter 35, page 339, and then come back to the chapter following this one, or you can think about this question: *What do you put your fatty food on?* (Do you eat a stick of butter or is a Big Three food the vehicle for it? Obviously, if you eliminate the vehicle, you'll also lose the passenger.)

The difficult decision you will be making now has to do with whether you are going to eliminate all of your Big Three shotgun triggers at once, or one at a time (assuming they are all shotgun triggers). Here are the pros and cons of each strategy.

By abstaining from the Big Three in unison, you:

| ADVANTAGES | DISADVANTAGES |
| --- | --- |
| Only go through withdrawal once, | but withdrawal is fierce. |
| Eliminate most food cravings, | but are more vulnerable to feeling deprived. |
| Become at peace with food and appetite. | |
| Find that abstinence boundaries are clear and easy to remember, | but if you slip or relapse, you generally start eating all three again. |

If you abstain from the Big Three one at a time:

| ADVANTAGES | DISADVANTAGES |
| --- | --- |
| Your withdrawal will be slightly less fierce, | but during withdrawal you will probably overeat any Big Three members you keep on your food plan. |
| You'll be less vulnerable to feeling deprived, | but the remaining culprits will continue to cause food cravings. |
| If you slip or relapse, you're more likely to confine the slip to that specific food group; | but you'll still be focused on food, and at times, you won't have peace with food or appetite. |

It helps to order the Big Three in terms of their personal potency for you. For many food addicts, sugar is the number one trigger. If that is true for you and you choose to become abstinent one Big Three food category at a time, then start with sugar abstinence.

Can I tell you whether abstaining from one Big Three food group at a time is better than abstaining from all three groups at once? No, I can't. For some people, it works best to get the whole withdrawal thing over with. The relief and clarity these folks experience when all the triggers are gone makes the bumpy transition worthwhile.

Others do better taking smaller steps. They understand that they won't lose all their food cravings until they get all the major shotgun triggers off their food plan. But they also need to prove to themselves that there's life after abstinence. As their use of support strengthens, they become more capable of adding to their abstinence.

Decide what will work for you in the long haul. The point is to sustain this program next year and the year after that. Whatever decision you make today can be refined as you see how it works for you.

You are now building your personal food plan. This is different from a diet. The word *diet* has come to mean food restriction—something you do only for a while and then stop doing. A food plan is your dietary code, your map for navigating kitchens, restaurants, parties, menus, and pantries.

Okay, are you ready? Fill in the following pledge to yourself, listing from one to three food categories.

---

**DECISION 1**

For now, I choose to abstain from the following food(s):

_____

_____

_____

_____

---

### Determining Abstinence, Part 2

Next you're going to decide where you'll draw the line regarding the foods that fall within your abstinent categories. For example, if you've chosen to abstain from the sugar category, are you going to eliminate every food that has any sugar in it?

Foods that have sugar include many sauces, ketchup, most frozen meals, canned peas and corn, even some salt. It's a long list. If you start reading labels, you'll be surprised to see how much sugar is out there.

Some people start with the big sugar items, such as most desserts, all candy, pies, cookies, cakes, ice cream, and so on. Some people eliminate any food that has sugar as the fifth or higher ingredient. (Be wary, if the item has more than one source of sugar—fructose, glucose, maltose, lactose,* honey, cane sugar, molasses, barley malt, maple syrup, or corn syrup solids—even if they are all below the fifth ingredient, that's a lot of sugar.)

Remember that you can always further refine your food plan. The first one doesn't have to be perfect. If something doesn't work, don't get mad at yourself or give up in frustration. Instead, change the plan, adding or removing foods as appropriate. Your food plan is a work in progress.

Aim for targeting the spot that lies between the seductive, come-hither messages sent by your addictive brain and tossing out items that don't trigger you.

| Come into my parlor, dearie! | Rejecting innocent foods |
|---|---|

▲

**Abstinence**

Just to complicate things, you'll need to take one more aspect into account: the threshold at which you are triggered. For some foods, your trigger threshold may be high. A cup of brown rice won't trigger you, but two cups will. For other foods, your threshold may be much more sensitive. A teaspoon of sugar in a gallon of soup won't trigger you, but a single cookie will.

---

* Any food that ends in *ose,* except cellulose and, possibly, sucralose.

So you need to decide how strict your abstinence from each food category will be. You decide where to draw the line. Below are gradation charts for each of the Big Three food categories. Draw a line at the point you will start your abstinence.

## Sugar Cube

Draw a line to represent your abstinence threshold. You will be choosing to eat the foods above the line. (If you are going to abstain from another Big Three category too, cross off any foods here that also fit in that other category.)

| |
|---|
| Savory soups, canned vegetables, processed meats, bacon |
| Ketchup, sauces, breads, breading |
| Molasses, maple syrup, honey, cactus syrup, date sugar, concentrated fruit syrup |
| Dried fruit, raisins, figs, dates |
| Sweet pickles, cranberry sauce, jelly, jam, relish, sweet soups, sweetened or candied vegetables, teriyaki |
| Desserts, pie, cookies, cake, ice cream, candy, doughnuts, syrup, sweet rolls, colas, soft drinks, sweeteners, sugar itself, artificial sweeteners (e.g., Splenda, Equal, NutraSweet) |

### Natural and Whole Sugars, Dried Fruit

Molasses, maple syrup, honey, cactus syrup, date sugar, and concentrated fruit syrups are all natural forms of sugar. Unlike white and brown sugar, they are not refined, so they have the more complex chemical structures that nature gave them. The more complex they are, the longer they take to metabolize. Therefore you may wonder if you should exclude them or include them.

Here we're presented with that old, annoying continuum again. It's entirely possible that once you've had a period of solid abstinence, you'll be able to have a teaspoon of a natural, unrefined, whole sweetener in tea or gelatin without being triggered. Quantity and context together make the difference. A small amount inside a larger, nontriggering food might not bother you.

The issue is whether you are better off eliminating them now and adding them back later, or keeping them on board.

Again, only you can decide. (And remember, there's no penalty for making a choice that doesn't work for you. If you realize that you need to redraw your line, by all means redraw it.)

If you continue eating natural sugars through your initial abstinence, the odds are that you'll overeat them. As a result, you won't get to experience that clean, awake feeling that a stricter abstinence soon gives you. You could well start substituting them as your new addictive substances and not be changing your life.

On the other hand, adding them back later carries risks too. Once you've settled peacefully into abstinence, toying with it can retrigger you.

My recommendation is that you eliminate the natural sugars for now. It's just too confusing to keep even natural sugars on your food plan at this point. Get your body cleaned out, and then revisit this question *in a couple of years*.

I make the same recommendation for dried and high-sugar fruits. Dried fruits are slightly less potent than natural sugars, but they are lower on the sugar cube because they come in larger servings. You can measure a teaspoon of honey, but few people eat just a slice of dried apricot.

The problem with dried fruit is that it's so easy to pop a handful without even realizing it. You've probably never eaten ten apricots or a whole pineapple in one sitting. However, it's not that hard to consume twenty dried apricot halves. They may be natural, but that kind of sugar load will set the addictive bells a-ringing. Dates and figs are the same—they are just too sweet.

Raisins might be okay. Need I say, they're small. You can select ten of them, put them in a baggie, and use them as part of a 50/50 snack. But keep an eye on yourself. Use the same criteria for raisins as for any food you eat.

*Criteria for Spotting Addictive Foods*

Just one yes answer to the following questions means particular foods should come off your list of approved foods.

- ☐ Do they trigger you?
- ☐ Do they make you want to eat more of them?
- ☐ Do you have difficulty stopping once you start eating them?

☐ Do you want to eat other things once you've eaten them?

☐ Do they haunt you the rest of the day?

☐ Do you want to go back to the container and get more?

☐ Do they trigger a binge?

Many of us find that once we're abstinent, we so prize that peaceful feeling of being set free from food tyranny that we don't want to risk being ensnared again. We notice when a food grabs us, and we back away fast. We don't want to return to the prison of food-on-the-brain.

Once you are peacefully abstinent, your addictive brain is a sleeping giant. But it's a light sleeper. It takes very little to wake it up, and once it stirs, it gets brawny fast.

### Artificial Sweeteners

The only alternative sweetener I trust is stevia. NutraSweet and Equal (which are both brands of aspartame) can be downright dangerous[1,2], so I hope you've already gotten rid of them. They are excitotoxins that overstimulate the brain and wear down its batteries.

Even if they weren't dangerous, they trigger appetite. Years ago, when Equal first blasted onto the market, folks who'd been abstinent for years were suddenly relapsing because they started drinking diet colas sweetened with aspartame. Drinking diet sodas may actually promote weight gain.[3]

Monosodium glutamate (MSG) causes most of the same problems in the body as aspartame. In animals, after doses of glutamate, lesions appear in the hypothalamus that lead to obesity. This obesity is not related to eating and can't be dieted away. Aspartame can produce the same lesions as glutamate.[4]

Splenda (sucralose) is just too new for us to know what its long-term effects may be. However, studies conducted before the sweetener was approved for consumption include a long list of adverse affects. Splenda is manufactured by adding three chlorine atoms to a sugar molecule, so I suspect that it may trigger many people to the same degree sugar does.

For these reasons, I've put Splenda, NutraSweet, and Equal in the lowest box of the sugar cube because of their triggering properties. To find peace from cravings, these have to go.

You may be crying out plaintively to me now, *What will I drink if I can't have pop?* My recommendation is water that you flavor with 100 percent fruit juice. Use a half cup of juice to every quart of water. If you want some fizz, use carbonated water. (Although carbonation may promote bone loss in postmenopausal women.)

One of my favorite beverages is four to eight ounces of unsweetened cranberry concentrate added to a quart of water, plus nine to twelve drops of stevia. I mix it up four quarts at a time and keep a steady supply on hand.

### Wheat Box

Draw a line that will be your abstinence threshold. You will be choosing to eat the foods above the line. You'll notice white rice appears here even though it isn't wheat. That's because it does trigger cravings and eating for some food addicts. If it doesn't trigger you, feel free to keep it on your approved foods list.

Remember that many foods with wheat also have added sugar. If you plan to be abstinent from sugar as well as wheat, then cross out any foods that have sugar in them.

| |
|---|
| Soufflés, meatloaf, hot dogs, frankfurters, sausage, lunch meat, bologna, sprouted wheat, crab cakes, malted milk, some brands of cottage cheese |
| Wheat-thickened soups, salad dressings |
| Beer, ale, root beer, instant chocolate drink mixes |
| Many sauces, creamed vegetables, gravies, creamed soup, most pudding, Yorkshire pudding, soups with noodles, scalloped potatoes, breaded vegetables, malt products, soy sauce, white rice |
| Yeast breads, rolls, croutons, biscuits, toast, dough, pizza crust, waffles, cakes, pancakes, noodles, pasta, macaroni, ravioli, dough-nuts, buns, stuffing, muffins, breadsticks, wheat couscous, crackers, wheat cereal, cream of wheat, pot pies, quiche, pita, piecrust, pasties, pirogies, phyllo dough, pastries, shortbreads, egg rolls, wontons, nachos, corn chips, tortilla chips, bread crumbs, bagels, shredded wheat, cornflakes and most packaged cereals, cornbread, graham crackers, pretzels, pies, breading, dumplings, popovers, blintzes, knishes, faro, ice cream cones, candy |

## Flour Box

Flour can be made out of a wide array of food products besides wheat. Draw a line that will be your abstinence threshold. You will be choosing to eat the foods above the line.

| |
|---|
| From legumes: soy, chickpea/garbanzo, dhokra, yellow pea, urad dal/black garam, carob |
| From vegetables: amaranth, quinoa |
| From roots: potato, tapioca, arrowroot, cassava |
| Nongluten: rice, wild rice, millet, sorghum, couscous (from millet), milo, rice cakes |
| From nonwheat grains or cereals: rye, barley, buckwheat, pumpernickel (coarsely ground rye), oats |
| From corn: cornstarch, corn flour, cornmeal, grits, polenta |
| From wheat grains: wheat, spelt, whole wheat, farina, couscous (from semolina), triticale, kamut, semolina |

## Whole Grains

Brown rice, oatmeal, popcorn, pearl barley, whole graham, wild rice, bulgur (whole wheat kernels that are steamed, dried, and crushed—not the same as cracked wheat), kasha, and tabouli (bulgur salad) are complete grains. If flour triggers addictive eating for you, then some of these foods may also trigger you. As with everything you eat, pay attention. If you catch yourself overeating any of these whole grains, gird yourself to discuss it with your recovery partner.

Grains, grasses, and cereals are all names for plants that yield a seed head that can be ground into flour. The bran and germ (such as wheat germ) are the nonfloury parts of the grain.

Generally, whole grains metabolize in the body more slowly than refined or enriched grains. Enriched flour is milled grain that has a bit of the original value put back. Enriched flour is like getting a dime in trade for a dollar.

Most wheat products and wheat flours, even those made from whole wheat, can cause an addictive response. Sometimes ancient organic grains and flours that haven't been bred for commercial purposes or genetically altered can be used sparingly as a thickener for soups and sugar-free desserts.

The items in the flour and wheat boxes are arranged according to their potency in stimulating an addictive response, which is based on my empirical (but not scientifically proven) observations. If your body requires that foods be put in a different order, adjust your chart accordingly.

Most people with food addictions need to draw their lines at least above the corn row in the flour box and the beer row in the wheat box in order to avoid being haunted by cravings. Many will need to draw their lines even higher.

The whole process of abstinence involves some trial and error. If, after three weeks of abstinence, you have no relief from food cravings, you have set the bar too low. Raise it to the next level and pay attention to your body, talking frequently with your recovery partner about how you are feeling.

**Other Foods**

Not much has been said yet about oil, butter, fats, or fatty foods. We'll get to those soon enough. One thing at a time. If you are choosing abstinence from the Big Three all at once, you have enough to do right now.

I'm not concerned about your portion sizes, either. You need to focus on one thing now—achieving abstinence. If you make too many changes at once, it will diffuse your attention. Stay focused—on abstinence.

Remember, this isn't the diet. This is your preparation for the diet you will choose later. You are treating your appetite disorder so that a diet can be successful.

## My First Abstinence—Eating Change Four

Summarize your abstinence here.

| I will abstain from: | Yes | No |
|---|---|---|
| Sugar | | |
| Wheat | | |
| Flour | | |

If you are abstaining from wheat or flour, please fill out this second chart as well:

| Whole-Grain Abstinence | Yes | No |
|---|---|---|
| Whole wheat | | |
| Brown/wild rice | | |
| Popcorn | | |
| Oatmeal | | |
| Pearl barley | | |
| Bulgur | | |

• • •

### *Opening*

### *Today's Agenda*

Work with your partner to define what you will abstain from. Be as forthright as possible in admitting what foods trigger you. Help each other to determine where to draw the line on the sugar, wheat, and/or flour boxes.

Make five copies of your first abstinence chart (page 220). Put one copy in your purse (or backpack or briefcase), one in your kitchen, one in your desk or at your workplace, and one in your car. Give the fifth one to your recovery partner.

### *Closing*

# 25

# Preparing for Abstinence

⚘ ARE YOU WILLING to set yourself up for success? Then you need to do some housecleaning before you start your abstinence. You need to clean all your trigger foods out of your house. This means all the foods that are below the lines you drew in the boxes of the last chapter.

**Cleanse the House**

You and your recovery partner might help each other with this task. Together, go through your kitchen, pantry, refrigerator, freezer, basement, garage—anywhere you store food—and put all the relevant sugar, flour, or wheat items into a box or bag. You can give these foods to a friend, take them to your church, or even throw them away. What you do with them doesn't matter, as long as you get them out of your house and out of your reach.

If you live with other people, have a meeting with them, explain what you are about to do, and find out how willing they are to support you. Ask them to honor your desire to keep your trigger foods out of your house, your reach, and your sight. Remind them that doing this will help you to be a healthier, happier, and lighter person. Also remind them that they are welcome to eat all of the banished foods themselves whenever they want, so long as they do it away from your home and away from you. (I have an entire book for people like the ones in your home, called *When Someone You Love Eats Too Much: What You Need to Know—and How to Help.* That book explains the chemistry of appetite disorders in a different way than in this book, and it gives the reader clear and practical suggestions for supporting you in your recovery.)

**STEP 18**

Prepare for abstinence.

Once your home is safe, get rid of all trigger foods in your car, desk, work area, purses, pockets, and backpack. Also throw away candy wrappers, empty chip bags, and junk food containers that are in your car or wastebaskets.

**Avoid Sight and Smell Triggers**

You will help yourself enormously by eliminating sight triggers. Sight triggers are pictures of foods that trigger you. Any magazines with food pictures on the cover should be stowed away. Don't leave an enticing picture with your trigger food staring at you from the coffee table while you're sitting on the couch. Go through your house and car and remove all such magazines. (If someone else in your home wants to read those magazines, ask that person to take them to work or keep them in the trunk of the car.)

If you have a subscription to a magazine that contains food pictures, either put the new issues aside during your first three months of abstinence, or have a friend rip out the pictures. When you're shopping for food, don't peruse the magazines by the checkout stand. Instead, read that little horoscope book or look at a puzzle.

The world will bombard you with food stimuli, so you have to take charge of toning them down. If you usually listen to a radio station that plays food ads, don't listen to that station, at least for now. Pop in a tape or CD instead. When you watch TV, mute the ads and don't watch them. Better yet, take a break from TV and read a book that doesn't have pictures.

Stay away from food as much as possible. Do hit-and-run shopping. Take a list, speed through the store, and get out. Smaller grocery stores are safer than gigantic supermarkets. And keep in mind this shopping tip: Most of the food you need is on the perimeter of the store, rather than in the aisles.

Need I say, don't read cookbooks or recipes—unless they're devoted totally to vegetables and salads.

**Here is a list of other things to avoid during your first abstinence. Do not**

1. Offer to bake cookies for the PTA or volunteer to provide any foods on your trigger list for any purpose or situation.
2. Buy your trigger foods for other people in the house. Let them get their stuff on their own—and make sure they keep it elsewhere, out of your sight.

3. Bake presents for people (including your family) at Christmas.

4. Go to or even walk past bakeries.

5. Linger in food courts.

6. Buy food as presents for others.

7. Carry trigger foods from one place to another. (For example, don't offer to deliver the leftover pie to a disabled neighbor.)

8. Cook one of your trigger foods for someone else.

9. Pretend you're strong enough to withstand the stimulation of any of the above. Remember, this isn't about willpower. It's about the chemical reactions in your body that can be initiated by the situations on this list, causing reactions that will result in cravings too powerful to resist.

Food smells are especially pernicious. Scent stimuli go straight to the animal part of your brain, not even filtering through your intelligent cortex, the thinking part of your brain. This is why scent is so evocative, conjuring up memories long forgotten. The aromas in bakeries and food courts, in kitchens and restaurants will go to work inside your body before you ever realize it. Therefore, you have to use good judgment about what you let your brain experience.

**Prepare for Confusion**

Remember, it's an addiction that you're fighting. Whenever people stop using their addictive substance, they go through withdrawal. So, as you get abstinent, your brain will be experiencing withdrawal from the chemicals it has grown to love. One of the symptoms of this withdrawal will probably be temporary confusion or a feeling of fogginess in the brain.

During this period, you'll be more at risk for pesky problems like locking your keys in the car, locking yourself out of the house, losing your keys, forgetting appointments, getting lost, and misplacing things. To minimize the impact of this problem, here's a "to-do" list.

*Pre-Abstinence "To-Do" List*

- Make a copy of all the keys on your key ring, plus two extra car keys and one extra house key.

- Hide the house key outside (and in a safe place), where you can find it.

- Put one spare car key in your purse.

- Hide the other spare car key in a little magnetic key case, or give it to a friend who is willing to rescue you if you get locked out.

- Make a copy of everything in your billfold—driver's license, insurance cards, credit cards—and keep those copies at home or at work (but not in your purse, briefcase, or backpack).

- If you will be traveling, make a copy of your passport and itinerary to keep inside your bag, and put your tickets and original itinerary in a bright folder.

- If you pay bridge, parking, or toll fees to get to work, fill a small manila envelope with the correct change and put it in the glove box in your car.

- Make copies of your calendar or date book for the next month, or print your schedule from your PDA and leave copies at work, at home, and in your car.

- Put Velcro on your cell phone and place receiving Velcro strips inside your car, in your purse or backpack, and on your desk.

- Make a copy of all your outgoing phone numbers on your cell phone or speed dial.

- Consider buying a locator—a gizmo that lets you locate your phone, wallet, car keys, PDA, and so on. You can usually find them at electronics stores for about twenty dollars.

- Consider joining AAA or another auto club. They'll rescue you if you get locked out of your car.

- Keep city and state road maps in your car.

- If possible, plan on making no big decisions for the first month of abstinence.

### Prepare for Nutritional Support

Remember to stay with the current eating map. Lay in supplies of turkey (or milk, or other sources of tryptophan) and grapefruit. For the first two weeks of your abstinence, you'll need to eat turkey, drink milk, or otherwise replenish tryptophan every day. As the addictive chemicals drain out of your body, serotonin will alleviate some of the discomfort. And serotonin will start working better for you, now that it isn't being shut off by dopamine.

I don't know why grapefruit helps with withdrawal, but it does. Eating grapefruit sections as part of a snack each day will help.

Designate a shelf in the fridge as your shelf by putting bright tape or ribbons on it. Tell the people in your household that anything on that shelf is off-limits. Because they can eat anything they want to, they are not allowed to gobble up your abstinent snacks.

Be sure to maintain a good supply of your snack ingredients, and mix up a couple of quarts of juice water.

### Prepare for People's Peccadilloes

Make a list of people in your immediate circle. Go down that list, one person at a time, and decide whether they are likely to support you or sabotage you. (Sabotage isn't always deliberate; it can also be the result of carelessness, selfishness, thoughtlessness, or immaturity.) A form is located on the next page.

Keep your plan for abstinence confidential from people on your sabotage list. Don't trust them to behave honorably now if they haven't in the past.

Take care about what you reveal to whom. Protect yourself by keeping thoughtful boundaries regarding your privacy. You'll be vulnerable while you're first in withdrawal, and the last thing you need is your jealous sister waving bonbons in your face.

You might think that since she's been harping about your weight for a decade, she'd applaud the effort you're making. Not necessarily. Previous comments about weight or size may have actually been weapons in a far subtler war.

As you learn to take care of yourself, the balance of power in your difficult relationships will shift. The people involved in them will be on you like brown on rice, if you let them—with questions, temptations, manipulations, insults, and invitations to eat.

| Person | Support | Sabotage |
|---|---|---|
| Spouse or partner | | |
| Kids (Add names below) _____ _____ _____ | | |
| Housemates/roommates (Add names below) _____ _____ _____ | | |
| Mom | | |
| Dad | | |
| Sister (Add names below) _____ _____ | | |
| Brother (Add names below) _____ _____ | | |
| Best friend | | |
| Good friends (Add names below) _____ _____ | | |
| Neighbor | | |
| Boss | | |
| Business partner | | |
| Co-workers | | |
| Staff | | |
| | | |
| | | |

For the people who will support you, decide the degree of support you'd like from each one, and ask them for it. Be as clear and detailed as possible, so they have a full understanding of what you need. If you can get the people inside your household on board, this will help a lot.

Here's a sample script for meeting with people you can trust to help and support you.

---

SAMPLE SCRIPT

### Setting Boundaries and Requesting Support

Thank you all for being here today.

I'm about to take a major step for my health and well-being, and I'm hoping you'll support me. I've realized I have an appetite disorder, and that's why I've had so much trouble trying to control the way I eat.

I've already taken important steps to recover from my appetite disorder, but the next one is the most challenging step of all, so I wanted to tell all of you how you can help me, if you're willing.

First, please don't offer me any foods that have lots of (add your trigger foods here) sugar, flour, or wheat.

Second, please don't eat desserts, candies, or breads (your trigger foods) in front of me.

Third, please don't bring these foods into the house (or office, etc.). You can eat them anywhere else you'd like, any time you want, so long as I'm not there. Please don't even bring them into the house while I'm gone; the aroma may linger and I may smell it when I come back. And scent is very powerful; it can make me crave the foods I shouldn't have.

Please don't eat the foods that I've prepared for my snacks or that I've packaged to take with me. Anything on the red-taped shelf in the fridge, and on the red-taped shelf in the second cupboard, should be considered off-limits to everyone but me.

And this might sound strange, but when we're having turkey, please save the last serving for me. The reason has to do with how the chemicals in turkey can help me to feel better.

---

Would you be willing to do these things for me, to help support my health and weight loss?

For the next three to five weeks, I'm going to be in withdrawal because part of my appetite disorder is caused by an addiction to certain foods. These foods are like drugs for my body, and the withdrawal is similar to the withdrawal people experience when they stop taking drugs. During this time, I need to experience as little stress as possible. Would you be willing to help me during this time?

Here are ways you can help:

- Be on standby if I lock my keys in the car or have other little problems that may occur because of the forgetfulness caused by withdrawal.

- Don't invite me to restaurants or offer to share snacks.

- Mute the TV every time a food commercial comes on.

- Field calls from my _____ (mother, father, sister, etc.). Please don't tell these people about my appetite disorder, or what I'm doing to recover from it. They'll only try to sabotage me, and maybe not even on purpose.

- Bear with me if I seem confused or disoriented at times.

- Help me to remember I'm in withdrawal and that it will pass—probably in three to five weeks.

And if you're willing to help me prepare for this journey, here are things we should cover.

Are there any big decisions we need to make this month? If so, let's make them today or soon, while I can think clearly.

If you want to be super helpful, you could

- Do the food shopping for the next month.

- Feed the kids for the next month.

- Do the cooking for the next month (following the guidelines of my eating program).

- Let me beg off going to (your mother's house for dinner, the extended family's Easter supper, etc.).

The upcoming challenges that concern me most are (the wedding, reunion, or holiday party; sabotage from _____ ; any food-centered event).

Could you help me with that?

Finally, I'd like to share with you that I've learned a lot recently about my body's chemistry and how it's the reason I've been overeating. What I'm doing now is changing the way my chemistry works. If you'd like to understand more about it too, I'd be happy to tell you more, or show you the book I'm reading.

Thank you. I appreciate your help so much. Your support can make a big difference for me.

. . .

## Support Meeting 12

*Opening*

*Today's Agenda*

- Discuss your plans for abstinence.

- Set specific times to help cleanse each other's houses.

- Decide whether it'll help you be more conscious if you go back to charting for the next three weeks. If so, use the chart on the next page.

- Help each other create your lists of potential supporters and saboteurs.
    — Work out who's trustworthy.
    — Decide what help you'd like from each person.
    — Make a plan for talking to your desired support people, either one by one or together.

- Reinforce your calling skills.
    — Practice the remaining dialogue from Chapter 22. (From the support dialogues—the daily vitamin call, the evening relief call, or the help call—practice the one you haven't rehearsed at previous meetings.)
    — Practice making a help call this week (see pages 191–197).

*Closing*

# Body Signals Chart, Withdrawal

Date: _____

| CATEGORY | DESCRIPTIONS | ADD TRYPTOPHAN ONCE A DAY | | | | | | | | | | | | | | | | | | | | | | |
|---|---|---|---|---|---|---|---|---|---|---|---|---|---|---|---|---|---|---|---|---|---|---|---|---|---|
| Timeline | Circle Wake-up | 6AM | 7 | 8 | 9 | 10 | 11 | 12PM | 1 | 2 | 3 | 4 | 5 | 6 | 7 | 8 | 9 | 10 | 11 | 12AM | 1 | 2 | 3 | 4 | 5 |
| **Food** *Numbers go in this section* | Proteins | | | | | | | | | | | | | | | | | | | | | | | | |
| | Complex carbs | | | | | | | | | | | | | | | | | | | | | | | | |
| | Flour | | | | | | | | | | | | | | | | | | | | | | | | |
| | Wheat | | | | | | | | | | | | | | | | | | | | | | | | |
| | Sugar | | | | | | | | | | | | | | | | | | | | | | | | |
| | Fats | | | | | | | | | | | | | | | | | | | | | | | | |
| *Check* | **Tryptophan** | | | | | | | | | | | | | | | | | | | | | | | | |
| *Check* | **Equal/NutraSweet** | | | | | | | | | | | | | | | | | | | | | | | | |
| **Fluids** *Dots go in this section* | No sugar added | | | | | | | | | | | | | | | | | | | | | | | | |
| | Contains sugar | | | | | | | | | | | | | | | | | | | | | | | | |
| | Artificially sweet | | | | | | | | | | | | | | | | | | | | | | | | |
| *Check* | **Caffeine** | | | | | | | | | | | | | | | | | | | | | | | | |
| Timeline | | 6AM | 7 | 8 | 9 | 10 | 11 | 12PM | 1 | 2 | 3 | 4 | 5 | 6 | 7 | 8 | 9 | 10 | 11 | 12AM | 1 | 2 | 3 | 4 | 5 |
| **Fullness** | Stuffed | | | | | | | | | | | | | | | | | | | | | | | | |
| | Comfortable | | | | | | | | | | | | | | | | | | | | | | | | |
| | Empty | | | | | | | | | | | | | | | | | | | | | | | | |
| **Hunger** | Starving | | | | | | | | | | | | | | | | | | | | | | | | |
| | Really hungry | | | | | | | | | | | | | | | | | | | | | | | | |
| | Mildly hungry | | | | | | | | | | | | | | | | | | | | | | | | |
| | Not hungry | | | | | | | | | | | | | | | | | | | | | | | | |
| **Appetite** | Craving food | | | | | | | | | | | | | | | | | | | | | | | | |
| | Food focused | | | | | | | | | | | | | | | | | | | | | | | | |
| | Quiet | | | | | | | | | | | | | | | | | | | | | | | | |
| **Satiety** | Satiated | | | | | | | | | | | | | | | | | | | | | | | | |
| | Not | | | | | | | | | | | | | | | | | | | | | | | | |
| **Energy** | High | | | | | | | | | | | | | | | | | | | | | | | | |
| | Medium | | | | | | | | | | | | | | | | | | | | | | | | |
| | Low | | | | | | | | | | | | | | | | | | | | | | | | |
| **Stressed?** | Highly | | | | | | | | | | | | | | | | | | | | | | | | |
| | Mildly | | | | | | | | | | | | | | | | | | | | | | | | |
| | No | | | | | | | | | | | | | | | | | | | | | | | | |
| Timeline | | 6AM | 7 | 8 | 9 | 10 | 11 | 12PM | 1 | 2 | 3 | 4 | 5 | 6 | 7 | 8 | 9 | 10 | 11 | 12AM | 1 | 2 | 3 | 4 | 5 |

Duplicating this page for personal use is permissible.

# 26

# First Abstinence

❧ HERE IT IS. We're at the top of the ramp. Everything you've done so far has prepared you for this moment. This isn't the last step, but it is the last big step. The changes you've already made will make this step manageable. It's steep, but it's not ten feet tall.

However much you've wanted your eating to change, a part of you has been in deep resistance to the idea. That's the part that knows that addictive chemicals were doing something for you. You probably won't appreciate just how much you've been counting on them until they drain from your body.

Withdrawal creates three chemical situations, two of which are temporary. The following paragraphs will explain.

## Neuron Firestorm

The neuron receptors involved in addiction require a dependable supply of neurotransmitters to keep them happy. When neurotransmitters become scarce, the receptors have a tantrum akin to a stubborn two-year-old in front of your boss's wife at the supermarket. They start screaming and yelling, "Feed me! Feed me!"

Sometimes they'll be loud. Sometimes they'll be sneaky. One minute you'll have an obvious, intense craving. The next minute you'll suddenly think it's a good idea to check out the new store at the mall—the one right next to the food court.

Symptoms of this firestorm include

- Strange, surprising cravings
- Sneaky, sabotaging ideas
- Subtle setups to get you to eat your trigger foods

**STEP 19**

Begin your first abstinence.

- Confusion
- Disorientation
- Forgetfulness

## Toppling Counterbalances

When a person uses a drug, the body counterbalances it. If you use a stimulant, the body will gear up its calming mechanisms. If you use a sedative, the body will reinforce alertness and reactivity. Take the drug away and the body's compensatory actions will suddenly be unopposed.

People who give up coffee can hardly stay awake. Alcoholics who stop drinking are, at first, jumpy and touchy. Thus, whatever way food affected your energy level, you'll temporarily have the opposite reaction.

Typically, people who abstain from sugar and starches experience
- Sleep difficulties
- Irritability
- Mood swings
- Grouchiness
- Touchiness
- A shortened fuse
- Anger
- Bursts of rage
- Increased sensitivity to pain

## Unsheathed Emotions

The addiction is doing something for you. When you stop using addictive foods, the addiction stops what it was doing. For many of us, eating cloaks feelings. Withdrawal takes the covers off. Any feelings we've been hiding from will come out into the open. These feelings will seem big, possibly overwhelming, because you aren't used to them. You may feel bombarded by them because they may all uncloak themselves at once. This doubtless sounds ugly, but remember: Withdrawal is temporary. I promise, it won't last forever.

*Withdrawal is temporary.*

### Why Withdrawal Passes

After a while, your receptors will accept the drought. They'll pout from time to time, and they'll keep a roving eye for triggers, but eventually they'll take a nap—that sleeping giant (light sleeper).

Because you will be continuing to follow your daily map, eating every two or three hours and having 50/50 snacks, your brain will begin major repair work once your addiction stops calling the shots. This may sound like a long time, but in about a year, you're going to feel a whole lot better.

Meanwhile, in a week, your body's counterbalancing will start to even out. Your body will figure out it's no longer being sedated, and the compensating neurons will calm down.

Your feelings will become manageable, if you are faithful about using your new skills to handle them. (These feelings, by the way, are real feelings. Their intensity may be augmented by the neuron firestorm, but this is the information you've kept yourself from knowing for a long time. This information is important. Your deep inner self has kept a record of your reactions to the world, and now it's delivering a pile of "While You Were Out" messages.)

In time, these feelings will become less intense, and you'll soon be able to sort them out. During this time, all the support skills you've practiced will very much be needed.

FIGURE 14

**Intensity of Withdrawal over Ten Days**

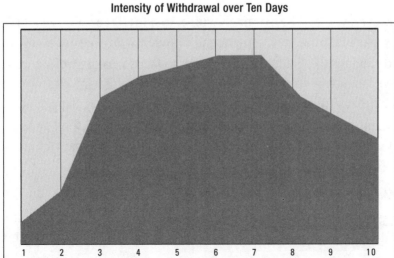

Your withdrawal may be less extreme, shorter, or more drawn out. It could resemble the following pattern.

Day 1: Hmm. Something's missing. I wonder what. I'm a little fuzzy.

Day 2: I seem to have forgotten something. I feel empty.

Day 3: Everyone is really irritating me. I want food.

Day 4: Snarl. Get out of my way.

Day 5: I'll just go eat everything at the mall. I'm sad and angry.

Day 6: Up. Down. High. Crash. Mad. Sad. Why am I doing this?

Day 7: It'll always be this way. I'll always be miserable.

Day 8: Hey, I feel better. My mind is clearer. I'm still mad and sad.

Day 9: Okay, I'm going to make it. But still, get out of my way.

Day 10: What was all the fuss about?

Again, your progression may be different. Every once in a while, someone has an easy withdrawal. My observation is that we only get one or two easy withdrawals in a lifetime. So, if you have smooth sailing, treasure it.

For most of us, withdrawal gets more intense by the third day, hits its peak somewhere between days five and seven, and then starts to diminish. It generally falls off fast, leaving you in pretty good shape by the end of the second week.

However, you will be extremely vulnerable to triggers throughout the first three weeks and must stay vigilant and in touch with your recovery partner.

The cravings of withdrawal are similar to the waves of grief we experience when we lose someone we love. These cravings will hit hard, rise, start to seem unbearable, and then disappear so quickly we forget they happened.

If, later on, you decide to reduce your intake of fried food and fat, withdrawal will hit much sooner—probably on the first day—and will continue to nag at you frequently for the first few days.

### First Aid Kit

To get you through withdrawal, you will need the equivalent of a first aid kit. The following pages discuss how to heal yourself during withdrawal.

*Your Recovery Partner*

She's your lifeline. If you followed the suggestions in Chapter 22, you've had lots of practice using the support dialogues every day. Now you'll see why these are so important. During the first weeks of abstinence, you'll need to be talking to each other throughout each day. Here is the recommended support schedule:

- Start each day with the daily vitamin call, page 184.
- Begin each evening with the evening relief call, page 187.
- Use the help call, page 191, as many times a day as needed.
- Use the SHARP protocol to handle your feelings, page 176, even when you can't reach your partner.

*The First Three Steps*

During withdrawal we get a chance to experience just how powerless we are over what goes on in our brains. We can support the brain with nutrition, hydration, and vitamins, and we can choose to get lots of support from others, but we can't govern the brain's course.

Recognizing powerlessness is one of those paradoxical experiences. It seems like we'd feel better if we could control everything, but when we can't, it can be such a relief to stop trying.

Let's review the first three steps of Twelve Step programs one more time. (Once we're abstinent, they start to make more sense than ever.)

1. *I am powerless over food.*

   There, it's out in the open. It's no longer a secret I'm keeping from myself. When it comes to addictive foods, all I can do is let go of them. I can't eat them in moderation. I can't be temperate. They have too much power over me. I can only stop eating them—with lots of help.

2. *I have come to believe a power greater than myself can restore me to sanity.*

   Well, if I can't do it, thank goodness something else is strong enough to make a difference. I can find all sorts of entities that are more powerful than I am—nature, my support group, the Creator, my God.

3. *I make a decision to turn my will and my life over to the care of this higher power.*

Okay, since my higher power is stronger than my addiction, I'm going to let Him/Her be in charge. My higher power has command over the universe, so my tiny little addiction ought to be a walk in the park. Here, Higher Power, you guide my life.

---

**The First Three Steps of Food Addicts Anonymous[1]**

1. We admitted that we were powerless over our food addiction—that our lives had become unmanageable.

2. Came to believe that a power greater than ourselves could restore us to sanity.

3. Made a decision to turn our will and our lives over to the care of God as we understood God.

---

Stating these three steps is a great way to start your day, and you can make them a part of your daily vitamin call.

### Gratitude Journal

When we've lost our perspective, counting our blessings is a way to remember just how lucky we really are. The more you look at what is working in your life, the more you'll notice other things that are going right.

On the next page is a simple gratitude journal you can keep. Make lots of copies and fill in a new page whenever you feel like it. If you make a routine of using the journal, you'll remember to turn to it when you're feeling lost or unhappy.

## Ten Things I Am Grateful For:

1. _____

2. _____

3. _____

4. _____

5. _____

6. _____

7. _____

8. _____

9. _____

10. _____

*Withdrawal Diary*

Keeping a journal of your experiences, thoughts, feelings, and cravings during the first week of withdrawal can be an enlightening experience.

After withdrawal is over, we tend to minimize what it was like, and we plain forget half of it, due to the erratic functioning of the mind. Reading about it a month or two later, you'll be amazed at all you went through. Your withdrawal diary is also a way to stay conscious of the fact that you are in the midst of a very active process and that you are doing it for a reason.

*One Day at a Time*

When I started my first abstinence, I was deeply concerned that I would never have a particular dessert* again my whole life. The weird thing about this is that I hardly ever had that dessert and didn't like it nearly as much as a lot of other sweets. Somehow, though, that dessert represented the pinnacle of eating, and I couldn't fathom a life without it.

Then I realized I could get through this one day without that sweet. And I did get through that day.

The next day, I thought, *I can get through this day without this sweet.*

Each day I made a new decision about getting through just that day, and before I knew it, I'd gone a month without any dessert. The months got easier after that, and soon a year, and then many years passed without my ever having that dessert.

Pull yourself back to this day, this hour, this moment. You just have to get through this one day, this next hour, this next minute.

Repeat these recovery mantras to yourself as often as you need:

For this one day, I choose to eat cleanly.

I can get through this hour without my drug food.

I can get through the next five minutes
without my drug food.

---

* Because you may, right now, be in withdrawal, I'm purposely not naming this dessert. I don't want to stimulate your appetite or your addiction with a food image.

**Being a Good Recovery Partner**

As you support each other through withdrawal, you'll need each other plenty. Here are some tips about how to help your friend.

- Be dependable. Show up and be available when you say you will.

- Remember to be an effective listener.

- Encourage your partner.

- Tell her "good job," "well done," "good plans," etc., often.

- Remind her that she's in withdrawal. She will actually forget at times why she's spacey, irritable, or having such strong feelings.

- Remind her that withdrawal is temporary, that right behind the opaque barrier, there's a path leading away from here to greater clarity and serenity.

- Remind her that she's building her health and her freedom to choose. When she gets free of the addictive chemicals, she's going to feel a lot better, and she'll have more choices. She's heading for a much more satisfying life.

- Remind her that she just has to get through the next minute without her drug food.

- Share your experiences and feelings with her.

• • •

## Track C (Achieving Abstinence Phase)

**Your Personalized Eating Map:**

☐ Eat every two to three hours, for as long as you are awake.

☐ Eat snacks that are 50/50, 50 percent protein/50 percent complex carbs.

☐ Do not eat snacks that contain flour, wheat, sugar, or simple carbs.

☐ Take 50/50 snacks with you wherever you go.

☐ Eat the equivalent of four ounces of turkey daily the first two weeks of abstinence and every other day for the rest of the month. You may substitute tryptophan from another source such as milk, sesame seeds, or tahini, making sure your daily intake is equivalent to about 380 food mg of tryptophan.

☐ Follow your plan for your first abstinence, according to the lines drawn in the sugar, wheat, and flour boxes (or the oil can, if you took the option offered on page 210).

**My First Abstinence**

Check one or more foods in the first column or Fats in the second column (from Chapter 35). You can work in either column but not both.

☐ Sugar

☐ Wheat     *or*     ☐ Fats and fatty foods

☐ Flour

• Start each day with a daily vitamin call.

• Make an evening relief call soon after work.

• Use the first aid kit (pages 238–242).

## Support Meeting 13

**Opening**

**Today's Agenda**

1. Decide what day you will each start your abstinence.

2. Discuss one or more of the following:

   • Which tools in the first aid kit I will use to get through withdrawal

   • The possible withdrawal symptoms that worry me most

   • How I can personalize the first three steps from Food Addicts Anonymous (FAA) so that they are meaningful to me

   • Whether or not I'll use the Body Signals Charts for the next one to three weeks

3. Read the first three steps from FAA and notice how it feels to say them aloud. Discuss this.

4. Set times for your daily vitamin calls, your evening relief calls, and the next meeting.

**Closing**

# 27

# Solidifying Abstinence

FOR THE NEXT three weeks, the most important thing you can do is strengthen your abstinence. The world may try to pull you off course, so here's what you can do to protect yourself.

- Stay in close touch with your recovery partner. Talk to her at least three times each day.

- Be very careful never to skip a meal or snack. Keep your satiety chemicals working for you.

- Put yourself first. If you're like a lot of food addicts, you tend to do more for others than for yourself. It's your turn now.

- Put abstinence first. As a part of the neuron firestorm, it sometimes seems like a good idea to stop everything else that's bad for you at the same time. My clients will say, "Oh, I'll stop smoking and quit caffeine while I'm at it." Please don't. This is the all-or-nothing thinking of an addict, and it's a setup. Attempting too much at once will create too much withdrawal.

- Drink a lot of water. Flush those impurities away.

- Take vitamins. If any part of your overeating has been from your body's efforts to get more nutrients, this will help. Plus, vitamins and antioxidants will help with cravings and cleansing your body.

**STEP 20**

Solidify your abstinence.

- Eat at least two or three whole fruits each day. The natural sugars will relieve some cravings. Remember the virtues of grapefruit.

- Have one of your fruits at the end of your dinner. It will help stop your appetite.

- Put a star on your Body Signals Chart each time you make it through another day of abstinence. (You'll now use the Withdrawal Chart on page 233.)
- Think about how much money you've saved by not buying your drug foods. What would you like to spend this money on instead?
- Do not cook two meals, one for you and one for your family. They can eat what you are eating. It's not like you're making them eat nothing but tofu and bean sprouts. If there's an uproar, perhaps they have addictions too and can benefit from this book.
- Consider expanding your support network (see Chapter 28).

### Put Yourself First

Are you thinking, *I don't want to be selfish?* I just wondered because I hear that a lot. Women I work with are concerned that they will be judged for taking care of themselves.

Have you really thought that through? What kind of person would judge you harshly for taking care of yourself?

Most of the time, we have fears like that because we were accused of being selfish as children. However, that was then; this is now.

You are an adult. The fact is that no one anywhere is more responsible than you for what happens to your body. You get to determine the course of your life, and that includes taking good care of yourself. (Still unconvinced? Okay, name one person whom you believe should not take good care of herself.)

People who would judge you for caring for yourself are probably being selfish themselves. They want you to take care of them. Remember, even nurses and rescue workers get time off. No job requires a person to work twenty-four hours a day, seven days a week, 365 days a year (although parenting comes close).

Here are some retorts to use if someone does accuse you of selfishness or otherwise gives you a hard time:

- Here's the crisis line number; they're waiting for your call.
- I'm not going to discuss this for one month. I've put it on my calendar to get back to you then.
- It *is* unusual for me to take care of myself. And I'm committed to learning

how. I hope you'll find it in your heart to support me.

- I'm angry that you keep asking that of me. I want you to stop.

- I'm angry that you aren't keeping your word. You said you would support me. Stop _____ and please _____ instead.

- Take that food right back outside. It's not okay to eat that in front of me.

- You're wondering where I put that dessert you bought? You violated our agreement when you brought it home. It's in the garbage can where I threw it.

- You say that like it's a bad thing. I take it as a compliment.

- I'm not participating in this argument. I'm taking a walk/making a call (to my recovery partner).

## Put Abstinence First

Keep it simple. Focus on just this one thing, abstinence. Believe me, it's a big enough project all by itself.

If you have abstinence, you have your life. You have choices. Your addictive brain rarely calls the shots anymore. Other things become easier too—things such as setting priorities, simplifying, sticking up for yourself, seeing through the hidden motives of others, and wisely managing your schedule and finances.

It's odd how life suddenly feels more orderly when our addiction is no longer running us. Suddenly, that first step, "We admitted that we were powerless over our food addiction and that our lives had become unmanageable," starts to make more sense.

I always thought, in the old days, that I ate because my life was unmanageable. I was shocked when I became abstinent and realized that it was the eating that *caused* the unmanageability. The longer I was abstinent, the more manageable my life became.

I didn't start doing anything significant with my life until I got abstinent and began working a recovery program. Until then, I was too busy treading water.

You can't begin to know the marvelous surprises that are waiting for you until you give your abstinence more time.

Something—maybe many things—will start getting better for you very soon.

## Sabotage City

Various people have agreed to support you in your abstinence and recovery, or at least to abide by certain principles. By the time you've gone through a week of abstinence, you'll know who kept their word and who didn't.

I want you to know something very important. If someone breaks his or her agreement with you, it's about that person, not about you. The number one cause of relapse in newly abstinent people is having their hearts broken by loved ones who let them down.

Some food addicts take this disappointment to mean that they aren't worthy of better treatment. They then think, *So what's the use? Might as well eat.*

Don't fall for this. This is sabotage, pure and simple. You're better off if someone says outright, "No, I won't do that for you." When someone makes a promise, we feel safe and let down our guard. If that person doesn't come through, that's sabotage.

So if, say, your spouse has promised to do something, like all the grocery shopping, or encouraging you to have breakfast, or not eating your trigger foods in front of you—and he has broken his promise, then he is the one with the problem. You don't even have to figure out what that problem is. Keep your attention on your own abstinence and set boundaries.

It's okay to remind him a couple of times about his promise. If he still doesn't respect your limits, then strengthen those limits.

For example, if your husband said he would do the grocery shopping, and he doesn't do it, find someone else. If family members bring home your trigger foods, start growling or yelling the moment you discover those foods and get rid of them. (Yelling or growling will give you something else to focus on while you are taking the contraband to the garbage can or throwing it at the tree.) If they walk into your presence eating your drug food, tell them to go right back out until they've finished it.

It's okay to give people appropriate, natural consequences. For example, if you have to shop after all, then you won't have time to run those errands they asked you to do. In the end, the shopping used up the time you'd allocated for errands. If you are busy decorating the tree with the drug foods they stuck in the fridge, of course you don't have time to cook dinner. They can heat some soup. Since someone ate your snack food supply, you had to replenish it rather than do the laundry. They'll have to do their own.

I hope you see the principle here. Don't turn yourself inside out and get too tired in order to make up for someone else's mistake. If someone makes life harder for you, take care of yourself first and let them take care of themselves. (Notice that other people's "punishment" involves things like doing their own laundry or cooking for themselves—none of which is painful or difficult.)

Treat these disappointments as research. You are in a rare position to find out what the people close to you are willing to bring to their relationship with you. This abstinence project will expose inequities in your relationships. It's an opportunity to see some truths you may have been blind to.

Be sure to keep calling your recovery partner regularly to let off steam.

*Don't let sabotage eat at you, or you will eat over it.*

. . .

## Support Meeting 14

*Opening*

*Today's Agenda*

Discuss one or more of the following:

- The hardest part of my first weeks of abstinence

- The positive changes I'm already noticing

- The changes showing up on my Withdrawal Body Signals Charts (page 233)

- How my family and friends are letting me down and how I feel about it

- How my family and friends are showing up for me and how I feel about it

- How I have/will set boundaries with the people who try to sabotage me

*Closing*

# 28

# More Support

❧ NOW IS THE TIME to consider expanding your support base. Many different kinds of groups are specifically devoted to recovery from addiction. Here are the pluses and minuses.

## Twelve Step Programs

All the different Twelve Step groups and programs have certain commonalities because they all spring from the granddaddy of recovery programs, Alcoholics Anonymous. The central program, principles, traditions, meetings, and structure are pretty much the same, though they are, of course, tailored to the appropriate addiction or compulsion.

Here we find the world experts on recovery. No other program or process in the world has as strong a success record with overcoming addiction as Twelve Step programs. For many decades, such programs have brought recovery to tens of millions of people. When you consider that no one profits from this, that there are no paid or professional leaders at meetings, that all the people directly involved in meetings are addicts in various stages of recovery, and that Twelve Step groups do no promotion, fund-raising, marketing, or advertising, this is an amazing record.

The offshoots alone are clear indicators of success. AA works so well that now there are Twelve Step programs for almost any compulsion or addiction. The Twelve Step structure is even being used for many physical and mental health issues. (Thank you, AA, for sharing your steps and traditions so freely.) Some professional addiction treatment programs follow the Twelve Step principles and processes,

**STEP 21**

Expand your support.

and many use Twelve Step programs as backup and expanded support.

Detractors of Twelve Step programs usually fall into two groups: addicts who haven't given them a chance, and family members who don't like it when their addict gets sober. I am amused when an addict says, "Oh, AA doesn't work." With a worldwide record of tens of millions of people in happy sobriety, AA doesn't have to defend itself.

The biggest reservation people have about Twelve Step programs sounds something like, "I don't agree with that Higher Power or God stuff." Frankly, this is usually the addictive brain talking. It has lots of thoughts designed to discourage you from getting help, and this is a pretty convincing one.

You don't have to believe in anyone else's interpretation of God to participate in a Twelve Step program. You don't have to believe in God at all. You can define your Higher Power any way you want. Whatever your choice, you will not be asked to identify or explain your Higher Power at any meeting.

Many people start out using their recovery meetings as their Higher Power. There's no question that a group is more powerful than an individual when it comes to confronting an addiction.

So any objection to "that religious stuff" doesn't hold water. (Anyway, if something works, big deal if you don't agree with the rationale behind it. If an Olympic skater attributes her gold medal to God rather than to her years of talent and training, so what? She still is graceful on the ice and a thrill to watch.)

The next biggest complaint about the Twelve Steps has to do with the admission of powerlessness. It is hard to admit something is getting the better of us. And yet, isn't that the truth? Why else would we continue doing something that makes us so miserable? Why else would we keep returning to diets even though they have never worked for us?

The Twelve Steps are a program of recovery. You start with the first step and, over time, you practice, study, or do exercises that help you advance through all twelve. Eventually it becomes apparent that these steps do more than treat your addiction. They become a model for living, a way to confront any stress or problem ethically, effectively, and with the support of other caring people.

Here's what you can expect if you go to a Twelve Step meeting. It will usually start and end on time, but if you get there late, it's not a big deal. Just enter quietly and find a seat. It's very likely someone will arrive later than you.

The meeting's leader will be from the members' ranks. Each week, the leader will probably change. The leader's job is to guide the meeting through a specific agenda that includes, usually, a reading of the Twelve Steps and Twelve Traditions, the reading of a short excerpt from recovery literature, people saying their first names and acknowledging their sobriety anniversaries. For example, "I'm Kyoto, and I've been in recovery for two years." (If you'd rather not use your real first name, it's fine to use a different one for meetings.)

The heart of the meeting occurs when it opens for anyone to talk. At this point, people can speak up, one at a time, and say what's on their minds. Each speaker gets to talk without interruption until finished. Questions, comments, advice, responses, and other forms of cross talk are discouraged. Questions can be asked and answered after the meeting.

Near the end is a brief closing that reminds everyone of the importance of anonymity—that is, protecting the privacy of others by not revealing their membership in the group to outsiders. Most meetings end with a group recitation of the Serenity Prayer.

All of these practices protect the safety of meetings, and they are why the Twelve Steps are so successful despite a lack of consistent or professional leadership. There are no dues, fees, application processes, membership lists, or records of who attends meetings. A basket is passed, and individuals can voluntarily toss in a buck or two.

You are not required to do anything at Twelve Step meetings. You may sit and listen or you may talk. Newcomers are enthusiastically welcomed (an unusual feature, since a well-bonded group usually has a resistance to new people).

Any level of recovery is honored, be it two hours or thirty years. In Twelve Step programs, sobriety is seen as more than just abstaining from your substance or compulsion. Sobriety encompasses an entire attitude of openness, honesty, and willingness. Recovering addicts know that a relapse occurs long before the substance is grabbed. It starts with a slip in sobriety and attitude.

Most people in Twelve Step programs do better if they find a sponsor, someone who has been sober longer and who is further along in working the Twelve Steps. Essentially, you and your recovery partner have been cosponsoring each other. Because you have achieved a level of trust with each other, I hope you'll keep that relationship going.

However, there's no such thing as too many resources. If you go to Twelve Step meetings and add a sponsor and other recovering friends to the list of people you call for support, great. Your odds of finding a warm body when you make a help call will improve.

As you can tell, I'm a big fan of Twelve Step programs. I've seen them work wonders for people I care about, no matter how far down in the pit they were when they started.

Before I started working my own Twelve Step program many years ago, I didn't think anything could stop my compulsive eating. It wasn't just the eating that was stealing my life; it was also the hours I thought about food, planned eating, and hid eating. I lost friends because I was too focused on food to respond in a timely fashion to invitations. My mind was too murky to accurately perceive social cues, and my thinking too limited to see that others were giving more than I was giving back. Eventually, I—or rather, my addiction— drove people away.

My food addiction cost me both wonderful people and important opportunities. I felt completely imprisoned by it, until I found—and kept going to—a Twelve Step program. The first few meetings I went to didn't suit me, but I kept trying different groups until one finally clicked.

Each Twelve Step group has a slightly different flavor. It can take a month of going to different meetings before you find a group that feels good. Shop around, trying a few different meetings a week. Give it a hearty try for one month. What have you got to lose?

Since there are Twelve Step recovery programs for overeaters, these are your best bet. However, if you live in an area that has no such meetings, then you can find a lot of help at AA.

Most AA meetings are open to anyone and everyone. A small percentage of AA meetings are "closed." This means that they are open only to alcoholics. Also, some Twelve Step meetings are specifically for men only or for women only. (For some people, this separation can provide maximum support by bringing together people who are similar.)

Personally, I'd love to see a movement throughout Twelve Step organizations to reinterpret "closed" to mean "open to anyone with an addiction, but closed to everyone else." After all, since the Twelve Steps are the same for all types of addictions, in meetings addicts can make their own private translations to suit their own addictions.

You may be wondering why I'm saying all this. Here's why: If Overeaters Anonymous or Food Addicts Anonymous meetings are not available in your area, I strongly encourage you to go to a Twelve Step meeting that is not centered around recovery from an appetite disorder. (Here's a tip if you think you'll feel like an outsider: Say nothing but your name for the first few meetings. Soon you will be recognized and welcomed.)

For years, there were no eating recovery meetings in my area. The best meeting around was an AA meeting, so I asked the AA group to include me, which they did, and the partnership has benefited us all.

The one potential disadvantage to attending a Twelve Step group for a different addiction is that your trigger foods may be sitting around. Many groups provide no food or drinks, others offer coffee or tea, but some will have sweets or snacks as well.

Your library, grocery, and church may have Twelve Step meeting lists posted, and these usually indicate whether meetings are closed or open. To locate Twelve Step groups in your area, see Appendix B.

### Twelve Step Programs Specifically for Overeaters

*Overeaters Anonymous (OA)*

OA was the first offshoot from AA for people with eating disorders. Because of its longevity, it has more groups, so you may find it easier to locate an OA meeting than other types of eating recovery meetings.

OA doesn't define abstinence, which is both an advantage and a disadvantage. The advantage is that you can fit the abstinence you've defined for yourself into OA without any problem. The disadvantage is that a lot of people who attend OA haven't become abstinent yet and, thus, are still using food as a drug.

This means that some of these folks will be suffering from a central characteristic of addiction—unmanageability. At meetings, they may focus on what isn't working rather than on how they are using sobriety to change their lives. Also, unlike people at AA, people in OA often disappear once they get sober. Therefore, you'll find a smaller percentage of people with long-term sobriety at OA meetings.

Now and then someone in OA wants to run a stricter ship, insisting on a single food plan or adherence to a specific set of eating guidelines. This desire has led to splinter groups such as CEA-HOW, FAA, and GreySheeters Anonymous (which will soon be explained). That these factions develop is an indication of just how desperately we food addicts want something to work. It also demonstrates how seductive it is to try to control our addiction.

You don't need to involve yourself in the arguments brought out by these factions. In fact, stay out of them. You know what your food plan needs to be because you built it using an organic, evolving process that you evaluated. Attend meetings to hear and share recovery messages, to get rid of what's eating you, and to use support.

You can make OA work for you, especially if you go online to find a variety of meetings and resources.

### Food Addicts Anonymous (FAA)

Food Addicts Anonymous meetings have more of an AA feel than OA meetings do. FAA clearly defines abstinence and focuses closely on recovery. Members recognize recovery as a lifelong process, so there are folks at meetings with years of recovery. Thus meetings have a tautness and direction that OA meetings sometimes lack.

FAA defines abstinence as refraining from sugar, wheat, and flour. As a result, it is very likely to be in at least partial alignment with your own eating map. (Ignore parts that don't align. For example, if wheat isn't a trigger food for you, sit silently while others in the room talk about its allure and dangers. Don't argue with them, but don't take their words to heart, either. What they're saying is totally true for them, but not for you.)

The Big Three are FAA's official abstinence foods. All forms of sugar, all forms of wheat, and all forms of flour are discouraged. However, sometimes there's also an unofficial abstinence in FAA that may not match your requirements. For example, at some meetings, nuts, cheese, and certain fresh fruits may be denigrated.

Some people—including some health professionals—may even believe (incorrectly) that the foods that trigger them trigger all other people as well. Thus you may find a certain food demonized in one program and accepted in another.

You know my stand. You need to eat according to your own personal thresholds for each of the Big Three foods that trigger you.

With regard to foods not within the Big Three, gradually remove these personal trigger foods from your eating map. Other foods can stay on your map, no matter what people at FAA may insist. I'll say more on this in Chapter 35.

Remember, abstinence purely for the sake of abstinence is a setup that eventually will lead to relapse. Abstinence has no moral purity. You become abstinent from certain foods for your own health and well-being, not because it makes you more righteous or virtuous.

You have to believe in the addictive power of the foods you are eliminating. You have to know without doubt that they will spur your eating and distract you from recovery. Then you can be faithful to your own eating map.

Here's the paradox of trying to follow someone else's food plan. If you eat a food restricted by the plan, even though you know clearly that you are neither triggered nor soothed by it, you'll feel unnecessary guilt. Then you either hide the fact that you ate forbidden food from the people at your recovery meeting (also a setup because openness and honesty are important) or you reveal what you've done and feel unnecessarily defensive.

I propose being honest. Find out if your meeting has room for you to follow your own eating map. Explain that it is one that is the result of careful observation and discernment. Mention this book, if you need backup. If you're asked to forgo your own eating map and adopt the eating regimen of the group (which is unlikely but possible), find another meeting.

As you continue to more accurately define the limits of your own unique eating map, stick to your guns about which foods are appropriate for you. Surrender to recovery, acknowledge your powerlessness over your trigger foods, pay attention to your reaction to marginal foods, and keep talking to your sponsor.

Continue to use the Body Signals Chart each day during withdrawal. An unexplained rise in appetite or eating is your signal that either stress or a food has stimulated you. Talk with your recovery partner to figure out which.

### Compulsive Eaters Anonymous-HOW (CEA-HOW)*

Compulsive Eaters Anonymous is quite different from the previous two Twelve Step options. CEA requires all of its members to follow a very specific eating plan. This plan includes three daily meals that are sugar- and flour-abstinent and strictly weighed and measured. The only items allowed in between these meals are sugar-free gum, sugar-free soda, and noncaloric beverages. Members are required to make four support calls a day and go to three meetings a week. These are not suggestions, but requirements. New members must have thirty days of abstinence in CEA before they can talk at a meeting without first being vetted by their sponsor.

I've learned from my clients and from my own experience that sustaining abstinence is only possible if you get used to making support calls every day. Since we tend to be unaware of when we need help, requiring four daily phone calls is a great idea. Most folks have a resistance to calling and need help breaking it, so making four daily calls a rule can be useful.

Still, there are some problems with making something a requirement rather than a choice. First, it means that the impetus for self-care is coming from outside of yourself rather than from inside. Second, it sets up a compliance/defiance dynamic and creates unnecessary guilt if legitimate circumstances prevent you from following the rules. Also, some people will want to rebel against a program that's so tightly governed.

However, the big issue that keeps me from recommending CEA-HOW is its insistence on exactly three meals a day, without real food snacks in between. I understand this structure may be a relief for many people. But if someone has poorly working satiety chemicals, this three-meal schedule prevents natural satiety from building up. It also sets up triggering dips in blood sugar and NPY accumulation if a meal is unavoidably delayed.

It's important to make a distinction among the various factors that stimulate appetite. In CEA, some of the rules that help with certain facets of addiction ignore other equally important causes of appetite surges. A successful eating map takes all appetite and satiety factors into account.

---

*Honesty, Openness, and Willingness

*GreySheeters Anonymous (GSA—but not Girl Scouts of America)*

Years ago, OA offered food plans. In fact, OA had a wonderful little pamphlet called *Dignity of Choice,* which provided eight food plans members could use as eating guides. The strictest of these plans was called Grey Sheet because during the 1960s, this plan was printed on gray paper, which was the cheapest to print on at the time.

OA stopped using the Grey Sheet plan because nutritionists vetted it and found it lacking. Then OA stopped dispensing any food plan, reasoning that providing food plans violated the Twelve Traditions.

GSA may be viewed as either a tough love station or as a compulsive place. The food plan—yes, GreySheet—is the only one allowed, and members are required to eat three weighed and measured GreySheet meals a day, with nothing in between except water, coffee, tea, or diet drinks. Everything is tightly structured. Sponsors and meeting leaders have to have a period of GSA-defined abstinence. You can only get a GreySheet from a sponsor.

A strict structure does help some people. They find peace in the simple meals, clear guidelines, and tight boundaries. If this works for them, then more power to them. I'm in favor of anything that works.

Still, I'm always attending to what works in the long term. I'm aware that GreySheeters have members with impressive long-term abstinence. I wonder, though, about the number of people who ultimately fall away.

The strict structure has a little taste of the same fervor that sometimes causes ministers of very strict religions to secretly sin. We addicts need structure, but we need intelligent structure. There's a world of difference between structuring eating and trying to control eating. We already know that control measures rarely work, so if a program ventures into territory that uses control and submission rather than surrender, my internal alarm rings. Surely there are some folks that just can't—and shouldn't—keep a program like this going. When they leave, do they feel like failures? Are they treated like outcasts?

The following issues also bother me:

If members must adhere to three meals a day, with no nutrition in between, then they have nothing to fall back on when a meal is unavoidably delayed. That means they have to white-knuckle the appetite surge that is inevitable when they do eat.

Plus, as you know, three meals a day isn't the way to rebuild your body's natural satiety. In a sense, GSA members have to work against their own bodies' resources for managing eating.

Another source of worry concerns the between-meal drinks. Members can have water, diet soda, black tea, and black coffee. That's it. But carbonated drinks may cause bone loss in postmenopausal women. Diet drinks sweetened with aspartame or Equal can cause health risks. Caffeinated drinks promote insulin release and hunger. Thus, restricting between-meal drinks to these choices causes people to fight their own body chemistry. That is not a prescription for success.

Are GreySheet proportions and choices adjusted for a pregnant or nursing member? I'm not sure about the answer to this question, but I hope so.

I have enough concerns here to recommend that you try other Twelve Step programs first.

### Eating Disorders Anonymous (EDA)

Eating Disorders Anonymous focuses primarily on recovering from anorexia and bulimia. In some instances, its thrust is opposite of what you need.

EDA promotes balanced eating, which is perfect for nonfood addicts. However, this approach doesn't work for food addicts. We can't be moderate with our main trigger foods, just as alcoholics can't drink two glasses of wine and then stop.

## Other Support Programs

### Church-Based Programs

Church-based programs are not Twelve Step programs. Their focus is on weight management rather than on recovery from food addiction. There are dangers in putting weight loss in the forefront. The biggest danger is the thinking that, with the right attitude, even an addict can control her eating. That's just not so.

Another common misconception found in these groups is that members have to pay attention only to their appetite disorder for a certain number of weeks; then the problem will be fixed, and they can eat as they please. Again, this isn't so. Recovery from any kind of addiction is a lifelong commitment.

A weight-loss program that doesn't address food addiction can wake your sleeping giant, allowing it to take over your mind.

One other drawback of some church-based programs is that they may not recognize some foods as addictive. If you join such a program, be clear that you are already following a carefully researched eating map tailored specifically for you that you will continue to follow. If you are told that you must follow the program's own one-size-fits-all eating plan, then it's not a good program for you. (Of course, the church that sponsors the plan, and its minister and congregation, may nevertheless be wonderful.)

If you are Christian, you may find real benefit in a church-based program. You may find fellowship, support, tips, recipes, Bible study, and prayer, all of which can be greatly helpful.

However, if you do join such a program, it's important to resist the temptation of viewing successful members as spiritual people and unsuccessful members as spiritual lightweights.

### Secular, Nonreligious Recovery Programs

If the idea of acknowledging any kind of spiritual source turns you off completely, consider secular recovery programs such as LifeRing and Rational Recovery. These programs promote sobriety through meetings and fellowship but leave all spiritual matters out of the recovery process. The great majority of these groups are geared toward alcoholics and drug addicts, but they do offer a model for nonspiritual sobriety.

In general, I recommend Twelve Step programs or church-based programs over nonspiritual ones. I'd suggest going with LifeRing or Rational Recovery only if you have a real aversion to spirituality or the thought of any kind of higher power.

• • •

*Opening*

*Today's Agenda*

Discuss the following questions:

- Shall I expand my support network? Why or why not? If not now, when?

- What type of support group am I drawn to?

- What are my fears or worries about each type of group?

- Do we want to go to a meeting together?

*Closing*

# 29

# Decreasing Life Stress

**Tracks A and B rejoin us here.**

Do you eat more when you're stressed?

Of course, most of us do.

Here's how to stop: Reduce the stress in your life.

❦ HA. IF ONLY IT WERE THAT SIMPLE.

Maybe you've heard the observation that every decision you've ever made has brought you to where you are right now. At first, I didn't like hearing that, but as I thought about those words, I realized they were true. Then I found hope, knowing I could make new decisions and take myself in a new direction.

You can too.

Sometimes stress just happens in our lives, but many times, we create the stress that dogs us. Your challenge is to discern when the stress you experience in life is self-imposed.

There are many different types of stress. The following stressors are common among addicts.

■ **BLACK-AND-WHITE THINKING**

You have to do something completely or not at all (e.g., you must clean the entire house or you clean nothing); you see yourself as all good or all bad; you see other people as either wonderful or terrible.

■ **PERFECTIONISTIC THINKING**

You must do everything perfectly. If you don't do something perfectly, you think you blew it. If you can't do something perfectly, you don't even want to bother trying.

■ **SELF-ABUSE**

You push yourself too far, work too hard or too long, or exercise too much or too strenuously. You don't rest enough and don't listen to your body when it tells you to stop or slow down.

■ **DEPRIVING YOURSELF**

You skip medications or vitamins, or you make yourself wait before you meet basic needs like thirst, sleep, hunger, and going to the bathroom.

■ **ISOLATING YOURSELF**

You back away from people when you need to be with them. This includes not talking when you need to talk, not asking for a hug when you need comfort, and declining an invitation when you need social connection.

■ **OVERSTIMULATION**

You say yes to too many invitations, do too much in general, and stay around too many people for too long.

■ **CARETAKING OTHERS**

You give more to others than you give to yourself and sacrifice your needs to meet someone else's.

■ **NOT KEEPING GOOD BOUNDARIES**

You do not set or maintain limits with intrusive people or in difficult situations. You allow people to treat you badly, rather than tell them to stop or let them know how their actions make you feel.

■ **POOR PLANNING**

You fail to take your snacks with you. You don't store food supplies. You over-schedule yourself and don't give yourself enough time to get to appointments or meetings. You keep your schedule in your head instead of recording it.

■ **PROCRASTINATION**

You put off renewing your license, paying a bill, balancing your checkbook, canceling an appointment, or accepting an invitation.

■ **SHORT-TERM THINKING**

You pay attention to immediate results rather than long-term consequences, which means you may buy things impulsively, avoid an argument that will only worsen without communication, or say yes to someone when you'd rather say no.

■ **BEING AROUND MEAN PEOPLE**

You stay in the presence of people who are abusive, mean, thoughtless, discourteous, rude, critical, unkind, threatening, or violent.

■ **MISPERCEIVING THREAT**

You equate another person's disappointment, natural anger (but not rage), busy schedule, unavailability, or refusal as a threat. (Trauma survivors may have a sensitive "threat button" that can cause an innocent question or mild look from someone to ignite an internal response of terror or rage. If this feeling is acted out, it may push away people and opportunities.)

■ **NOT ASKING FOR OR ACCEPTING HELP**

You don't turn to others when you need them. This avoidance makes things even tougher when something—a feeling or situation—is too hard for you to handle by yourself.

These same stressors are listed on the next page. For each one that rings true for you, put a check in the appropriate box. If you don't relate to an item, then don't check anything.

| Stressor (source of stress) | Do occasionally | Do fairly often | Do very often |
|---|---|---|---|
| Black-and-white thinking | | | |
| Perfectionistic thinking | | | |
| Self-abuse | | | |
| Depriving yourself | | | |
| Isolating yourself | | | |
| Overstimulation | | | |
| Caretaking others | | | |
| Not keeping good boundaries | | | |
| Poor planning | | | |
| Procrastination | | | |
| Short-term thinking | | | |
| Being around mean people | | | |
| Misperceiving threat | | | |
| Not asking for or accepting help | | | |

You already know that stress pushes up your norepinephrine levels, which leads to hypervigilance, an external focus, reactivity, misperception of threat, and an enhanced need to be soothed. The more you can tone down the stressors, the more you will enhance your health and peace of mind.

Here's a process you can use:

**Reducing Stressors**

1. Look back over the list and check the stressor that looks easiest to change.

2. Decide whether or not you are truly powerless over that stressor.

3. If you are powerless over it, jump to number 9.

4. List all of the good reasons for reducing this stressor.[1] What draws you to making a change in this situation? Write down the elements in your life that will help you make this change.

5. List the obstacles to changing this stressor. What blocks you from making a change in this situation? Be as specific as you can. Include fears, concerns about the opinions of others, family reactions, and so on.

| Motivators/Helps | Blocks/Obstacles |
|---|---|
| | |
| | |
| | |
| | |
| | |

6. In your list of obstacles, pick the easiest one to change.

7. Decide one thing you can do to reduce the strength of number 6.

8. Do it and notice what happens.

9. If you are powerless, say, "I am powerless over (the stressor), and it makes my life more unmanageable."

10. Say, "I am coming to the belief that a power greater than myself can restore my sanity."

11. Say, "I am willing to turn my life and my will over to the care of this Higher Power."

12. Notice what happens.

As you have probably realized by now, the Twelve Steps can be used for any situation or problem that has you stuck. If nothing else works to reduce your stressors, use the Twelve Steps. If that still doesn't make a difference, you need more help. Talk to your recovery partner or your support group, or try a therapy group or one-to-one counseling. Support can be the lever that moves a rock that is impossible to move by yourself.

*Most rocks can be moved,*
*With a big enough lever.*

## External Stressors

Stresses that hit with a bang from the outside, especially those that are un-expected, carry the greatest risk for causing relapse (losing sobriety and abstinence). This proves the value of maintaining your commitment to two daily calls to your recovery partner and a couple of meetings each week. Your safety net will keep you from falling back into the temptations of food.

I hesitate to list these external stressors because just reading the list may arouse anxiety. I suggest you place a bookmark here and wait to cover the following material until your next meeting with your recovery partner. At that point, you can read the next few pages aloud together. If difficult feelings arise, process them using focused talking (SHARP) and effective listening. Then recommit to supporting each other daily for an extended period of time.

**STEP 22**

Reduce the stress in your life.

### Threats to Your Well-Being and Safety

Your husband saying he's thinking of leaving you; your boss leaving you a threatening message; a near-brush with death; a severe weather event such as a hurricane or earthquake; receiving scary medical news; an attack from a political enemy—such events can make you fear for your life or your sur-vival.

When something like this happens, your body mobilizes instantly for your survival. After a period of shock that may last seconds or weeks, your animal body moves into high gear, gathering all of your resources to prepare you to fight or survive any way you can.

Partly due to the depletion of internal chemicals, and partly due to a true need for nourishment and a boost to your blood sugar, you'll eventually be hungry, even ravenous (particularly if you skipped a meal while in survival mode). Your worn-out brain may make impaired judgments, which means you might pick food items that you normally would never choose.

Even if you've had a long run of making excellent food choices and following your eating map, in this immediate post-threat phase, you may load up on unhealthy foods without even thinking about it. You may be barely conscious of what you are eating.

If such a threat occurs, get as much help as you can. Call anyone and everyone who is good in a crisis, particularly those closest to your heart. The important thing is getting the care you need. Throw away any guilt you feel about the eating you did while you were too distracted to remember your program. Just get back to following your map as soon as possible. Your recovery partner will help.

### Abuse

The human body has centuries of experience honing its response to threat. A comprehensive defense system automatically locks in when you are in an abusive situation. You will be vigilant. Your focus will be geared toward pleasing or appeasing the person causing the threat rather than following your own inner voice (which will speak too softly for you to hear).

If you are in an ongoing situation of abuse, you will need to use all the support available to stay in recovery. Talk frequently to your recovery partner and go regularly to support group meetings. Consider group therapy or one-to-one counseling.

Remember that your effort neurotransmitter, norepinephrine, will stay in continuous action while you are warding off threat. Therefore, you will have an ongoing stimulus to eat. Sometimes there's a reciprocal relationship between abuse and food addiction. The only way a person can tolerate the climate of abuse is to find comfort and solace through eating.

If you are in an ongoing abusive situation, I encourage you to consider what it is costing you to remain there. The situation won't get better, you know. Unchecked abuse always worsens. The longer you wait, the harder it will be to extricate yourself, and, meanwhile, the life that is your true path stays vacant.

By pursuing recovery, you give yourself a valuable gift. Your support system will expand, your thinking will get clearer, your fortitude will increase, and you'll find strength in yourself that you forgot you possessed.

As long as you are in an abusive situation, your body chemistry will be working against satiety, so it will be more of a challenge to keep on your eating map. Still, it is worth the effort, because every day you are successful with your program is a day you have been good to your body. Above all, if you slip with your abstinence, just get right back onto the program and keep going.

Sometimes it might seem impossible to work a recovery program while living with abuse, but I want you to know that it can be done. I was living in an abusive situation when I first entered recovery. I went to support meetings, got a sponsor, and started a decade of abstinence, all while living with abuse. Eventually, my abstinence gave me the strength and clarity that made it possible to pack up and leave. In fact, my support group carried boxes out of the house for me and gave me a place to stay while I grieved.

Recovery may be the lever that lets you pry yourself free.

*Parenthood*

A whole category of humankind is routinely deprived of its basic needs for years. I'm talking about mothers (and sometimes fathers) of infants. These parents experience interrupted sleep, and they put off their own meals to care for their children. Not even their rest is self-determined, but occurs around their child's schedule. They may spend long periods of time without adult company, and their focus is entirely outside of themselves.

It's no wonder that many young mothers and child care workers gain weight. Constant deprivation puts them in perpetual need for relief, and the relief most readily available is sweet or starchy food.

Plus, ghrelin levels rise when we get insufficient sleep. (Remember, ghrelin is the chemical that causes you to feel hungry.) When ghrelin increases, you are stimulated to eat. So, mothers of infants, who suffer from interrupted and curtailed sleep, are naturally prompted to eat more.

If you're a young mother, you absolutely must have help. You don't want to abuse yourself or resent your children. No good comes from either situation.

Reduce the stress of parenting by asking for and using the help of the extended family members whom you consider safe. Take breaks when you can, spend time with adults, and use community resources. If money is tight, create a baby-sitting co-op where you and other parents can take turns watching each other's children.

## A Simple Solution?

Obviously, the most effective way to prevent relief-seeking eating is to take good care of yourself and to protect yourself from abusive or threatening situations as much as possible. It may sound simple, but I know it isn't.

Expand your resources. Find books, support groups, therapy groups or providers, or classes that will help you make new decisions for your improved life.

And remember to regularly eat plenty of tryptophan, the all-important ingredient for serotonin production and stress relief.

• • •

## Support Meeting 16

*Opening*

*Today's Agenda*

1. Discuss which stressors in your life are self-imposed. Fill out the stressors chart and discuss what you learn from this.

2. Do the reducing stressors exercise on page 269.

3. Read aloud the sections called "Threats to Your Well-Being and Safety," "Abuse," and "Parenthood." If any of the information in these sections triggers fear or anxiety, use focused talking and effective listening to move through these hard feelings. Be sure to get enough support so that you won't eat unwisely after the meeting.

4. Talk about the true threats or external stressors in your life. Over the next weeks, consider expanding your support network so that these stressors are reduced.

*Closing*

# 30

# Weighty Warnings

✂ YOU'RE ALMOST ready to choose your diet, but first, I want to warn you of the dangers ahead.

As you know, weight, like eating, is a side effect of appetite disorder. You didn't set out to gain weight. Any extra weight you carry is a consequence of your appetite demanding more food than your body uses. The very foods that called out to your food addiction are the same foods that promoted weight gain.

This isn't to discount how safe we can sometimes feel behind the shield that weight gives us. The fear that some of us feel as our bodies lose pounds must, of course, be dealt with or that fear alone will send us back to the cupboard. You'll have a chance to deal with this issue in your support meeting guidelines at the end of this chapter.

Meanwhile, you'll have to help yourself keep track of the real causes of overeating, or you run the risk of being pulled into a diet mentality, and you know what that's like.

### The Eight Deadly Dangers of Focusing on Weight

1. Fixating on the bathroom scale

2. Distracting yourself from the present moment

3. Comparing your appearance or progress with others

4. Obsessing over food, meals, calories, exchanges, units, pounds, inches, clothing sizes, or appearance

5. Activating norepinephrine, the effort neurotransmitter that leads to eating

6. Focusing on externals and ignoring what's going on inside you

7. Believing that eating is bad and skipping meals is good

8. Putting a time frame on your progress (for example, expecting yourself to lose so many pounds in a particular length of time)

## The Paradox

Many programs tell you that if you want something to change, you need to set a goal and work toward it. Yes, you want your weight to change, but if you make weight loss your goal, you'll slip into one or more of the Deadly Dangers. Then, instead of moving toward your goal, you'll move away from it.

You don't really need me to tell you this. You've already done this experiment yourself. (How many times *have* you proved that it doesn't work to focus on weight loss?)

The way to avoid this paradox is to stay focused on the *cause* of weight gain, which you now know is appetite disorder. A weight-loss program can work *if* your goal is to continue recovering from your appetite disorder. Always put your recovery first and maintain a recovery perspective.

The good news is that by focusing on recovery, you'll have plenty of signs that you are progressing toward your goal:

- Improved appetite indicators on your Body Signals Chart
- Smaller portion sizes
- Fewer addictive symptoms
- Better feelings about yourself
- Greater acceptance of your body

> **MY GOAL**
>
> To continue my recovery from appetite disorder

Another way you can tell that your program is helping you is that you stop *gaining* weight. This is a fantastic success. Think about what it means. If, typically, you gain five pounds a year (which, by the way, works out to only an ounce and a half a week), then a year from now, it's the same as if you've lost five pounds. Five years from now, you will have prevented yourself from having to lose twenty-five pounds. That is a great accomplishment.

I notice—and I've heard many other women say the same thing—that when I'm abstinent and following my eating map, my body automatically feels better and smaller. And the minute I eat a food that's not on my map, I feel bigger and heavier.

### Sleight of Mind

The magic trick you have to pull is this: While you're on a diet, pretend you're not on a diet. Think of it as a refinement of your eating map, a guide that you are using while you are recovering from your appetite disorder.

Thinking this way takes some serious discipline, especially for those of us who have a well-worn track that slides us into that deadly diet mentality.

Do not go there. Keep bringing your mind back to the healthy reality that you are on a program of recovery from an appetite disorder. The eating plan you choose to follow is being guided by the advice of a specific expert. You will follow some of that person's advice, but not all of it. Your recovery comes first.

**STEP 23**

Keep priorities clear. Put recovery first.

· · ·

## Support Meeting 17

*Opening*

*Today's Agenda*

1. Do the following exercise:

   Imagine that you are walking down a road. You come to a place where the road splits. There's an arrow that points toward each path. One arrow reads: This Way to Sanity, Health, and Well-Being. The other arrow reads: Lose Weight.

   In your mind, turn toward one of the branches in the road. How does it feel to go that direction?

   Now, turn toward the other branch. How does it feel to go that way?

   Discuss what you noticed and felt. Pay attention to what happened in your body (e.g., did it tighten or relax, did you feel stress or lightness?).

2. Discuss one or more of the following:
   - Plans for keeping my priorities clear
   - Emergency plans should I slip into a diet mentality
   - The things that could sabotage me, and how I can avoid them

3. Share with your recovery partner any fears you have about being thinner.
   - Explore what the fear is and where it comes from. Then bring yourself back to the present. List the skills you have now that you didn't have in the situation that caused you to fear being smaller. List the ways you can now protect yourself and get help.
   - Then switch roles.
   - Use effective listening and focused talking each time.

*Closing*

**Stepping Forward**

Here are the steps that you'll come across in the remaining chapters.

Step 24: Analyze diet plans to find the best fit for you.

Step 25: Select your ideal diet plan.

Step 26: Start your diet.

Step 27: Handle the issues that arise with your recovery partner.

Step 28: Determine your degree of fat temperance, while continuing to eat healthy oils.

Step 29: Accepting that relapse is a natural aspect of addiction, handle slips wisely.

Step 30: Keep your recovery going.

# 31

# Diet Plan Analysis

❧ YOU HAVE earned this next step. By now, your mind is clearer, your appetite disorder is in recovery, and you may well have more energy.

Remember how you got here. You changed one aspect of eating, one week at a time, until you'd taken care of most of the causes of your appetite disorder. In the first week, you kept a record of the signals your body gave you when you ate the old way. This gave you a baseline against which you measured the changes you implemented in the following weeks.

Remember, an appetite disorder can be caused by any or all of the following:

1. Extreme fluctuations in blood sugar and insulin

2. An NPY/PYY imbalance

3. A serotonin deficiency

4. Serotonin delivery problems

5. Food addiction

6. Excessive norepinephrine

7. Ghrelin spikes after meals or insufficient intake of good fats

**STEP 24**

Analyze diet plans to find the best fit for you.

With eating changes one, two, and three, you tackled the first three causes of your appetite disorder. Then, if needed, you went through the critical process of addressing number five.

(If you had trouble with serotonin delivery [cause number four], manifesting in depression or other symptoms even after your tryptophan intake increased, I hope you consulted with a health care professional and, if advised, began the search for your best treatment or medication.)

If you found signs of cause five, food addiction, either in your Body Signals Charts or in your behavior, you made decisions about the attitude you would carry, the support you would use, and the abstinence you would begin.

After giving your brain time to adjust to a clean environment, you tackled cause number six by reducing stress. We'll address cause seven in Chapter 35.

By taking all of these steps, your appetite disorder is well on its way to being managed. You deserve several pats on the back, daily.

You will now decide which diet plan you want to follow. The plan that will work best for you depends in part on the causes of your appetite disorder.

In the next section, you'll find some of the most popular, widely used diets and their characteristics. Then in later chapters, you will use the data you collected on your Body Signals Charts to determine which diets can work for you, and which ones can't.

Hopefully, you'll choose a diet that is a good match for your body chemistry. However, no matter how good the fit, each diet plan contains some advice that won't be appropriate for you if you are to stay in recovery from your appetite disorder.

Whenever a conflict occurs between a diet's directions and your recovery needs, *always* choose your recovery first. Your ability to stay on a diet depends on staying in recovery from your appetite disorder. If you lose your recovery, you'll lose the power of choice that enables you to follow the diet.

If you do lose an aspect of your recovery, put down the diet book, come back to this book, and leaf through each chapter until you discover the piece of recovery you let go of. Start there, fix that step, and then continue through this book until you're sure you've picked up all the reins again.

Then pause. Stay focused *just on recovery* for a month before returning to the diet.

Even then, work closely with your recovery partner to look at what the diet triggered and how to keep that from happening again. You might reread Chapter 30 every few weeks, just to remind yourself of the attitude that keeps a diet from stealing your brain.

## Characteristics of a Workable Diet

For any diet to work, it must meet four criteria:

1. It must be chemically sound and appropriate for your physical makeup.

2. It must be sustainable.

3. It must not set up a rebound of eating or weight gain, either during or after the diet.

4. It must support you in changing your relationship with food *permanently* and recognize that certain practices must be sustained throughout your life. It's even better if the diet recognizes the power of food addiction and promotes some simple, ongoing practices that support recovery. (If it doesn't, you must see to that yourself.)

Now, let's measure some of the most common diet plans against these standards.

## Diets That Promise, "Lose ___ Pounds/Inches in ____Days"

These diets sound so good. What could be better than ridding ourselves of a lifelong problem in just a weekend? Such diets may be legitimate and have good tips, but the come-on sets us up to think we can fix our appetite disorder fast and then go back to our old ways.

We are vulnerable to the seductive shout of a temporary fix. We want so much for this solution to be the truth that we can be easily tempted to turn our back on the facts.

The most important success factor you carry is your attitude. If a diet's seductive marketing yanks you off your bearings, you'll lose your way.

Whenever you see such a headline, remind yourself of the reality. Call your recovery partner for a reality fix. You might even commiserate with her about how rotten it is to have a chronic condition that requires ongoing vigilance.

"Lose ____ Pounds/Inches in ____ Days" Diets

| Criteria | Fails | So-So | Succeeds |
|---|---|---|---|
| 1. Chemically sound | | ? | |
| 2. Sustainable | ✔ | | |
| 3. No rebound eating | | ? | |
| 4. Supports permanent change | ✔ | | |

## Liquid Fasting Diets

About twenty years ago, when hospitals and medical centers burst out with controlled fasting programs, women flocked to their doors. Because hospitals or doctors were running these programs, women trusted them.

Though fasting was somewhat difficult for some women to adjust to at first, many felt liberated by not having to deal with food every day. In fact, many of the problems inherent to dieting—such as having to eat, handle, or prepare food several times a day—were relieved for fasters. Four times a day, they mixed their special shake, drank it, rinsed the glass, and were done.

To immunize them from the temptation of exposure to food or food smells, professionals gave liquid fasters a little chemical help from a new group of appetite suppressants. These drugs were considered safe metabolism boosters that would help burn fat. Many contained fenfluramine: Pondimin, Redux (dexfenfluramine), and fen-phen, all of which are off the market today due to dangerous side effects.

Women and men dropped pounds by the ton and everyone was thrilled. Providers were raking in the bucks, and insurance companies liked the time-limited nature of the programs.

The plan was to reintroduce patients to eating at a measured rate once they'd fasted down to their advised weight. This is not what happened. For all the holiday eating they'd missed, for all the treats they'd bypassed, for all the lunches they didn't have with friends, for all the buildup of NPY, these fasters had a deficit. They wanted a reward for their sacrifices.

Plus, they felt safe. They believed that their new, slim bodies would give them a grace period of eating without consequences.

For many, as soon as they had any food, they experienced rebound appetite that wouldn't quit. Chemically, it was impossible to follow the clinic's plan for realimentation (reintroducing ordinary food). The body's own defense against starving went into powerful gear as soon as real food appeared in the tummy.

You probably already know the ending to this story. Within five years, 95 percent of the fasters regained the weight they lost, and then some.

Plus, there was also a problem with patients needing more and more of the appetite suppressant. They were commonly started at low doses, but soon patients would need higher doses for the suppressant to work. This should have been a red flag. Fenfluramine was following the same course that amphetamines had taken years before.

Even after statistics about the long-range weight boomerang began to be published, the programs continued and people still tried them. How did we get a population of people who were so desperate about their weight that they would endanger their health, risk addiction, and pay big money for a long shot?

It shows how frantic we are to escape the prison of food tyranny, that we'll risk high stakes on a method with a 5 percent success rate.

And before you think that this type of dieting is a thing of the past, know that every year or so another company appears with a liquid fasting or semi-fasting program.

**Liquid Fasting Diets**

| Criteria | Fails | So-So | Succeeds |
|---|---|---|---|
| 1. Chemically sound | ✔ | | |
| 2. Sustainable | ✔ | | |
| 3. No rebound eating | ✔ | | |
| 4. Supports permanent change | ✔ | | |

Liquid diets fail on all four criteria necessary for weight loss to last.

### Low-Carb Diets/Atkins[1]

These diets work very well for the person who has become insulin resistant, and who, therefore, has a body quick to store calories and slow to burn fat. The nice thing about these diets is, after the first few bullet-biting days, one's appetite falls off, energy increases, and weight does begin to decrease.

The problem is that before long, carb cravings start building, to the point that an apple or a potato seems worth its weight in gold.

So, even though these diets are very effective in terms of weight loss, they aren't sustainable. Eventually carb cravings overpower the dieter—and once she starts eating carbs, it's unlikely she'll be able to return to the diet.

**Low-Carb Diets/Atkins**

| Criteria | Fails | So-So | Succeeds |
|---|---|---|---|
| 1. Chemically sound | | | ✔ |
| 2. Sustainable | ✔ | | |
| 3. No rebound eating | ✔ | | |
| 4. Supports permanent change | | ✔ | |

### The Negative Calorie Diet[2]

Eat all you want and lose weight! Now that you are diet-wise, what is the problem with this claim?*

The premise of this diet is that certain foods use so many calories during digestion that they burn up some stored fat in the process. Therefore, the more you eat of these foods, the more you burn your own calories. Obviously, a limited number of foods meet this criterion, so the nutritional soundness of this diet is in question. The diet seems to be long on theory and short on scientific proof.

---

* If any food that is recommended is one of your trigger foods, then eating all you want of that food will set you up for cravings, and you will eat outside of the plan.

Negative Calorie Diet

| Criteria | Fails | So-So | Succeeds |
|---|---|---|---|
| 1. Chemically sound | ✔ | | |
| 2. Sustainable | ✔ | | |
| 3. No rebound eating | ✔ | | |
| 4. Supports permanent change | ✔ | | |

## The Zone Diet [3]

This well-researched diet balances insulin and hormone levels and has proven successful for many. The theoretical basis for the diet is that some foods promote insulin release and, thus, fat storage. By eating the right combination of nutrients at each meal, you will keep your insulin levels steady and also promote fat-burning hormones.

Earlier versions of this diet used "food blocks" as a way of measuring servings. This method was complicated, so later versions of the diet were simplified, using a quickly grasped one-two-three technique for measuring quantity.

I like this plan because the theory is sound and because it recommends five meals or snacks a day. Still, the Zone needs a bit of tweaking to keep it from triggering your appetite disorder. (I'll discuss these tweaks in the next chapter.)

Remember that you must still avoid your trigger foods—no matter how earnestly the diet lauds them.

The Zone is available free online at www.zonediet.com. For a fee, you can get access to additional help and information.

Zone Diet

| Criteria | Fails | So-So | Succeeds |
|----------|-------|-------|----------|
| 1. Chemically sound | | | ✔ |
| 2. Sustainable | | | ✔ |
| 3. No rebound eating | | | ✔ |
| 4. Supports permanent change | | | ✔ |

## The Fat Flush Plan [4]

This diet plan is my favorite. It is comprehensively researched and very precise. It takes into account a broad range of factors that affect weight gain and loss. Many of the techniques used in this plan are painless and easy to incorporate.

In this system you eat five or six small meals a day, so the plan is closely aligned with what you are already doing.

Plus, the author understands that wheat, sugar, and refined carbohydrates can trigger a response in the body that lowers serotonin levels. Unlike most other diet programs, hers takes these interactions into account. Furthermore, she understands that aspartame (e.g., Equal and NutraSweet) works against weight loss.

The intention of this diet is to repair your liver. Since the liver is the organ that calls the shots when it comes to burning fat cells, you want your liver on your side. By following an eating plan that brings health to your liver, the liver will reward you by increasing your metabolism and using your fat cells as fuel.

This approach addresses the causes of weight rather than the act of eating itself, exactly what is needed. The plan is designed to fix the causes of fat storage and to repair the system as a whole, rather than look at just one part of the picture.

This approach also makes it easy to avoid a diet mentality. You can focus on repairing your liver and burning fat instead of on losing weight.

Fat Flush Plan

| Criteria | Fails | So-So | Succeeds |
|---|---|---|---|
| 1. Chemically sound | | | ✔ |
| 2. Sustainable | | | ✔ |
| 3. No rebound eating | | | ✔ |
| 4. Supports permanent change | | | ✔ |

## The Flavor Point Diet [5]

In the diet sweepstakes, this is my first runner-up. This diet takes into account every major factor that promotes disordered appetite except food addiction and serotonin deficiency. This plan is about losing weight by changing what you eat and when you eat it. This diet also recognizes that appetite, more than hunger, drives excessive eating. Meals are interesting and varied, each one faithful to the flavor point principle, a novel and clever way of promoting ongoing satiety.

The plan has two phases. The first lasts four weeks, and the second two weeks. After that, you are to follow the flavor principles for the rest of your life. One strength of the plan is that it provides daily menus for the entire, initial six-week period, long enough to establish a systematic food practice that you can perpetuate.

Advice is specific, listing recommended brands and food sources. The plan also recognizes that you have other things to do in life besides diet, so it includes specific shopping lists for a week, including, as much as possible, already prepared ingredients so that you don't have to do a lot of chopping, cleaning, and grating. The plan includes three meals and three snacks a day, so it closely aligns with the program you are already following.

But although there is reference to the addictive properties of some foods, and even an understanding of the opioid chemicals involved, this information is not followed up by recommending the special precautions that seriously food-addicted people need to take. Hence, the biggest danger in this diet is that food addicts will disregard the parameters they have set for themselves.

The other aspects of appetite are well researched and explained, including the influences of NPY and ghrelin and the decrease in satiety as new flavors and foods are added. So you must not be lulled into thinking you won't respond addictively to the little dangers that lurk in this otherwise quite excellent food plan.

Flavor does matter, but remember, food addicts often do other things while eating addictively. Instead of savoring their food, they may read, work, play computer games, or watch TV. Food addicts are after the addictive chemicals in the foods they crave and the soothing that those chemicals bring about. Therefore, it will be important to continue building the brain connections that value comfort from human sources.

**Flavor Point Diet**

| Criteria | Fails | So-So | Succeeds |
|----------|-------|-------|----------|
| 1. Chemically sound | | | ✔ |
| 2. Sustainable | | | ✔ |
| 3. No rebound eating | | | ✔ |
| 4. Supports permanent change | | | ✔ |

## The South Beach Diet[6]

I don't need to tell you that the South Beach Diet is highly popular and has received a lot of attention. Originally formulated for heart patients, it attempts to address the problems of earlier low-fat, high-carb diets. The diet is based on certain principles that involve how various foods impact the body. Instead of requiring you to measure calories or ounces, it provides scads of delicious meals keyed to each of the diet's three phases.

Phase 1 provides a quick start that helps to eliminate cravings and is a perfect plan for abstinence. It provides for six meals or snacks a day, all of which are devoid of most common food triggers, and the nutrition is excellent, so your body will be fortified.

Because previous heart-healthy diets were hard to sustain, the author created a diet with enough variety and interest to enable dieters to stay with it.

Phase 1 is well designed, but not sustainable beyond a few weeks—which is why Phase 2 is just ahead with more variety.

Unfortunately, Phase 2 backfires for most food addicts because it reintroduces some common trigger foods. Thus, this diet creates a dilemma. Food addiction problems creep back in during Phase 2, but sustaining Phase 1 beyond a few weeks is difficult. Obviously, if Phase 2 causes problems, the more lenient Phase 3 causes even more.

I have mixed (though mostly good) feelings about this diet. On the one hand, it's a lovely diet plan with lots of great food ideas. On the other hand, Phases 2 and 3 can trigger many appetite disorders unless they are carefully modified.

If you decide to follow this diet, I strongly recommend you use either the online program (www.southbeachdiet.com) so that you can easily substitute foods that fit your abstinence, or have your recovery partner go through the book version with a black marker and cross out all trigger food suggestions in Phases 2 and 3. (Also, of course, follow the suggestions in the next chapter for altering the diet to fit your personal profile.)

The South Beach Web site offers membership at a nominal fee and provides a slick way to plan daily or weekly meals with a shopping list you can edit based on your own kitchen supplies. It also has online groups and a buddy system.

So, this diet succeeds with the first three criteria we've discussed and makes it with the fourth *if* it's appropriately modified. Plus, I have to say that the tone of the book is wonderfully friendly. Instead of coming across as a food Nazi, the author sounds like a forgiving uncle, who knows dieting is hard and has tried his best to make things simple. He understands that life will draw us off our eating plan occasionally, and his attitude is, "Of course that happens, just return to Phase 1 and get back on track."

A minor problem with this diet is that some of the recipes are time intensive, but with practice, it's possible to streamline many of them. (For example, many recipes call for chopped onion, so rather than chopping part of an onion every day, you can chop a whole onion in a food processor and dip from your supply throughout the week.)

South Beach Diet

| Criteria | Fails | So-So | Succeeds |
|---|---|---|---|
| 1. Chemically sound | | | ✔ |
| 2. Sustainable | | | ✔ |
| 3. No rebound eating | | ✔ * | |
| 4. Supports permanent change | | | ✔ |

\* Unless you are careful to avoid your trigger foods in Phases 2 and 3, in which case, it succeeds.

### High-Carb, Low-Fat Diets/Pritikin Principle [7]

The Pritikin diet introduces the idea of caloric density. Foods with a low concentration of calories per pound, such as fruits and vegetables, have a low calorie density and form the basis of meals and snacks. High-density foods, such as dried or processed foods, are to be avoided. Thus oatmeal, rich in fiber and water, has 280 calories per pound, while a granola bar carries a walloping 2,140 calories per pound.[8]

The Pritikin Principle is easy to understand, and the formulas that guide meal selection are fairly easy to remember. The book is worth reading if for no other reason than the change in perspective it offers. Food addicts tend to justify eating with a mental negotiation that goes something like this: "Corn chips are made from corn, right? So eating corn chips is just like eating corn on the cob, only without the butter. That can't be bad for me, and after all, it isn't wheat." The Pritikin diet blows this reasoning out of the water. It points out that, while fresh corn carries 490 calories per pound, corn chips stomp in at 2,450 calories per pound.

The diet is excellent for preventing hunger. The recommended quantities of vegetables create filling meals and snacks. The plan promotes frequent, small meals, and the emphasis on adding rather than subtracting foods is a very appealing idea.

Still, suggestions that are perfectly sensible for other people are deadly for food addicts. For example, here's how you would turn a pasta meal into a low-density meal. You would pile vegetables on top of the pasta, and then cut the serving in two. What if you wanted corn chips? Instead of eating a pound of corn chips, you would add half a pound of guacamole mixed with salsa and tomatoes; then you would eat a half pound of corn chips instead of a whole pound.

Eat just half? Cut the serving in two? Ha! Any self-respecting food addict knows that she can make these additions and then proceed to eat the whole thing anyway. Besides, even half a pound of unsalted tortilla chips plus a quarter pound of guacamole rings in at more than 1,215 calories. Imagine what would happen if a food addict tried to follow this advice and couldn't stop with the half serving. She could well plow into upwards of 2,430 calories!

This is a high-carb, low-fat diet. Pasta and bread are recommended on a regular basis. Supplemental oils are not recommended, based on the supposition that the natural oils in the vegetables you consume will be enough. Diet soda is included as part of a snack nearly every day. These ideas are not helpful for food addicts.

The final problem for food addicts is that fullness doesn't stop their eating. If low-density foods are added to a high-density meal—salad ahead of pizza, for example—a food addict will happily eat the salad first, and then eat just as much pizza as if the salad hadn't been there.

This diet depends, in part, on a consciousness of fullness. The stomach is treated as a sort of attic. Once it's full of salad, less room is supposedly available for high-density foods.

However, food addicts, especially those under stress, may not be tuned in to the internal cues that translate as fullness. The assumption behind this diet—that fullness is all that's required to stop eating—leaves out appetite-driven eating that can operate despite fullness.

If you read the Pritikin book, stay clear about the difference between appetite and hunger, as well as satiety and fullness. The book will sometimes use these words interchangeably.

If you are a food addict, *do not* follow the menu plans. Too many of them have at least one or more foods that will trigger appetite and eating. For a food addict, this diet is very likely to create an inevitable eating rebound.

Based on the problems caused for food addicts, this diet is rated as follows. If you are not addicted to food, all check marks move one space to the right.

High-Carb, Low-Fat or Pritikin Diet

| Criteria | Fails | So-So | Succeeds |
|---|---|---|---|
| 1. Chemically sound | | ✔ | |
| 2. Sustainable | | ✔ | |
| 3. No rebound eating | ✔ | | |
| 4. Supports permanent change | | ✔ | |

## Low-Fat–Vegetarian/Ornish Plans[9]

Dean Ornish is another physician who entered the diet fray sideways, a result of seeking answers for heart disease. His was the first hopeful voice that sang the message that heart disease could be reversed. He also was among the first to add a spiritual dimension to health-gaining efforts.

I respect his work very much, and I've also seen how following his diet has played out for food addicts. So I have to state this warning: If you are a food addict, wait until you are completely comfortable in your recovery before attempting this diet. Give your recovery at least one full year and surround yourself with support before starting this diet.

This plan is an excellent option for vegetarians whose appetite disorder has been managed by eating changes one, two, and/or three, and for those who eat due to stress, but who *are not* food addicts. If you fall into those categories, the rating for this diet is indicated by a check mark. If you are a food addict, the rating is indicated by a dinner plate.

Low-Fat–Vegetarian or Ornish Plans

| Criteria | Fails | So-So | Succeeds |
|----------|-------|-------|----------|
| 1. Chemically sound | | 🍽 | ✔ |
| 2. Sustainable | | 🍽 | ✔ |
| 3. No rebound eating | 🍽 | ✔ | |
| 4. Supports permanent change | | 🍽 ✔ | |

🍽 Dinner plate symbol indicates ratings for food addicts.

## Eat Right 4 Your Type[10] (Blood Type Diet)

This is another fine plan that explains why some diets, such as grapefruit-intensive or food-combining diets, work so well for some and bomb for others. If a diet accidentally works well with your chemical makeup, you'll do well on it. If not, you haven't a prayer.

This is an easy diet to learn. For each blood type, all foods are separated into three lists: preferred foods, neutral foods, and foods to avoid. It's simple to photocopy your lists and use them to make wise food choices. And when you're out with friends or otherwise eating in public, you won't have to feel different.

When this diet came out, I created a questionnaire for my clients. They identified what foods they ate and which ones they avoided. When I compared their lists by blood type, I was intrigued to discover that my normal-weight clients naturally ate from the preferred list for their blood type, and avoided the foods on the foods-to-avoid list. What was more intriguing was that my overweight clients did *exactly the opposite.*

Strictly speaking, this isn't a diet, but a way of eating, a guide to eating foods that work for you chemically. Still, this program passes the first three criteria with flying colors. It doesn't trigger rebound eating because you don't have to eliminate any food group—you just avoid certain foods within each group.

However, a food addict must remember that she doesn't have the power of choice over her trigger foods. Even if this diet considers a food to be neutral, if it's a trigger food for her, she's got to remove it from her neutral list and place it on her foods-to-avoid list.

So if you choose this diet, have your recovery partner go through the book with a black marker and cross out all of your trigger foods in the preferred and neutral lists for your blood type.

Eat Right 4 Your Type (Blood Type) Diet

| Criteria | Fails | So-So | Succeeds |
|---|---|---|---|
| 1. Chemically sound | | | ✔ |
| 2. Sustainable | | | ✔ |
| 3. No rebound eating | | | ✔ * |
| 4. Supports permanent change | | | ✔ |

\* If you stay away from trigger foods.

## Mediterranean[11]/Sonoma[12] Diets

We'll probably never see a book entitled *The American Diet* because most of our best-selling foods are obtained through a car window. Not so for the Mediterranean region. Here we find unabashed, boisterous enjoyment of fresh, wholesome foods that are attractively served and savored adagio. The book covers alone call us to a simpler time.

The struggle for purveyors of this type of eating is how to make their book distinctive from the explosion of other diets following these same principles. Two sets of authors that do a good job are cited here. This is not to rule out the others.

If the Ornish Plan and the Pritikin Principle seem austere, the Mediterranean style of eating may fit you better. The biggest hitch is the inclusion of breads and wheat. If you're not addicted to wheat or bread, no problem. If you are, tread carefully. Both diets have many scrumptious meal and food ideas. You can easily follow many of the suggestions as long as you respect your personal tolerance level for wheat and flour products.

The Mediterranean Diet analyzes the components of Mediterranean eating and explains the science of why it's healthy. The Sonoma Diet uses a clever trick to help you manage portions. This trick is quite handy for appetite disordered eaters who've lost all touch with appropriate serving sizes. The Sonoma way is a great alternative to weighing and measuring.

No sugar, no refined grains, the Sonoma Diet is divided into three waves. These correspond to the three phases of the South Beach and Fat Flush plans and are similar in principle and purpose: to separate you from addictive foods, get rid of your cravings, and give you some immediate success.

Remember that just reading or thinking about addictive foods can trigger your appetite. If the bread suggestions in either diet are too tempting and cause cravings, switch to a different diet.

**Mediterranean and Sonoma Diets**

| Criteria | Fails | So-So | Succeeds |
|---|---|---|---|
| 1. Chemically sound | | | ✔ |
| 2. Sustainable | | | ✔ |
| 3. No rebound eating | | ✔ * | |
| 4. Supports permanent change | | | ✔ |

\* As long as you stay away from the wheat breads and flour products if you are addicted to them.

### 3-Hour Diet [13]

The 3-Hour Diet makes an art form out of eating at appropriate intervals. The creator of this diet clearly understands the interplay of appetite and satiety chemicals, which he calls the starvation protection mechanism.

This is the perfect plan for you if your appetite disorder was completely resolved by eating changes one and two. Some of the suggestions are not helpful for food addicts. If you are a food addict, you would do better choosing a different plan.

This diet does suggest many helpful techniques for reducing stress and includes charts to facilitate menu planning and conscious eating.

**3-Hour Diet**

| Criteria | Fails | So-So | Succeeds |
|---|---|---|---|
| 1. Chemically sound | | iOii | ✔ |
| 2. Sustainable | | iOii | ✔ |
| 3. No rebound eating | iOii | ✔ * | |
| 4. Supports permanent change | | | iOii ✔ |

iOii Dinner plate symbol indicates ratings for food addicts.

\* As long as you stay away from the wheat breads and flour products
   you are addicted to.

### The Schwarzbein Principle [14]

Here we have, finally, the sugar addicts' diet. Besides the brilliantly simple and memorable explanations of healthy versus dangerous foods, at last a diet author understands sugar addiction. Taking a whole body/whole life perspective, the author unfolds a plan backed with sugar abstinence. Whole grains are allowed, so be careful to stay above the personal level at which you're triggered.

Schwarzbein Principle Diet

| Criteria | Fails | So-So | Succeeds |
|---|---|---|---|
| 1. Chemically sound | | | ✔ |
| 2. Sustainable | | | ✔ |
| 3. No rebound eating | | ✔ * | |
| 4. Supports permanent change | | | ✔ |

\* As long as you stay away from the wheat breads and flour products
if you are addicted to them.

## Weight Watchers

This diet club had great success when it began because it addressed all four criteria very well (based on the knowledge at the time). It was a limited-carb, limited-fat food plan that called for lots of vegetables and tasty, filling, easy meals that fit most people's chemical makeup.

Weight Watchers also introduced the idea of a support group for dieters. Even though these groups focused a great deal on menus and food preparation, they were motivational, uplifting, and encouraging. Weight Watchers also provided dieters (mostly women) a community that helped them feel supported.

The regular weigh-in was a problem. Women did what they could to manipulate it, such as not eating or drinking beforehand. This set them up for extreme hunger after a meeting. The focus on scale numbers and the resulting rewards or loss of face created a focus on appearance and comparisons with others.

Then Weight Watchers changed. Because the program was so successful, a big company bought it. That company then put out a huge line of frozen meals under the Weight Watchers brand. These foods were loaded with appetite triggers. Women who had been successful in the program and who trusted the Weight Watchers name naturally trusted the foods. They ate them, thinking they were doing the right thing for their bodies, and then had cravings or weight gain in consequence.

The sweetener aspartame and the flavor enhancer MSG (and related glutamates) were some of the villains in these frozen foods. These additives made the products taste delicious, but may have also promoted fat storage—the kind of fat that is resistant to weight loss. The trick this played on members was that (1) as a result of eating these "diet" foods, they sometimes wanted more food afterward; (2) they thought the resulting weight gain was their fault; and (3) they had an even greater need for the diet club.

Many of these "diet" foods also contained a variety of sugars. Food addicts who ate them had their appetites triggered by the combined action of these sugars. (In many cases, the Weight Watchers foods were diet foods in only one sense: Each portion contained a limited and controlled number of calories.)

This company was a fantastic marketer. So it drew in women with promises of being able to eat whatever they wanted while feeling virtuous about being on a diet. I'm not accusing the company that owns Weight Watchers of deliberately setting up dieters to fail. Like many organizations and people (including many health professionals), the company may be simply unaware of the addictive properties of sugars for some dieters or of the effects of aspartame and MSG on eating and weight gain.

However, you are now informed. You can benefit from Weight Watchers, as long as you either stay away from its foods or read the ingredients lists very carefully.

The Weight Watchers meetings, fellowship, and support remain excellent. Many of its food tips and techniques are helpful. If you can go to meetings and stay loyal to your own eating map, then this program can work for you. (Just remember, never eat any prepared foods that contain sugars, MSG, or aspartame.)

Weight Watchers Diet

| Criteria | Fails | So-So | Succeeds |
|---|---|---|---|
| 1. Chemically sound | | | ✔ |
| 2. Sustainable | | | ✔ |
| 3. No rebound eating | ✔ * | | |
| 4. Supports permanent change | | | ✔ |

\* Unless you read ingredients lists and select your foods very carefully.

## Online Programs

Many of the diets mentioned here offer online programs that provide additional meal options, shopping lists, and support. Be forewarned, this support tends to focus on losing weight, which is not helpful for you, since you need to stay away from a diet mentality.

Be wary of online programs that aren't associated with a sound, long-term, effective system. Some online options are quite strange. Buyer beware.

## Future Diets

The day after this book is published, three new diets are bound to appear, each heralding an end to all dieting and each claiming to render all previous diets obsolete. Proceed with caution. You now know to study any diet carefully, to check it against the four criteria in this chapter, and to *always* put your recovery first.

If a diet is getting a lot of attention, check my Web site for information about it at www.annekatherine.org.

## Men and Women Are Different

Not surprisingly, some diets appeal more to men, and others to women. For this reason, it's not always a good idea for heterosexual couples to follow the same diet. A diet must both fit your chemical profile and be appealing if it is to be sustained.

Men seem to thrive on the Zone, Pritikin Principle, and Ornish plans. Women seem to respond more to the Fat Flush and Mediterranean plans. Both genders respond to the South Beach Diet. The Flavor Point Diet is too new for us to know, but I suspect it will appeal highly to women.

. . .

**Support Meeting 18**

### *Opening*

### *Today's Agenda*

Discuss the following:

After reading this information on diets, I am (pick all that apply):

- Triggered into a diet mentality (go back to the previous chapter and use the tools in it to shift your thinking)

- Feeling _____

- Thinking I'd better stay with my recovery program for another _____weeks/months before beginning any diet

- Feeling ready to begin a diet

I am leaning toward trying the _____ diet plan because _____.

### *Closing*

# 32

# Your Personalized Diet

IN THE previous chapter, diets were rated according to four criteria that compared their general overall effectiveness. In this chapter, those same diets will be rated in terms of the degree to which they either promote or prevent relief from appetite disorder.

As you know, appetite disorder has seven primary causes. A diet that is a perfect solution to the weight gain caused by imbalanced NPY and PYY may be entirely wrong for a food addict. The diet you choose must match your profile.

As you gathered data from your Body Signals Charts, you began to identify which of the seven causes of appetite disorder were affecting you.

Based on your analysis of these charts, fill in the following table:

| Causes of My Appetite Disorder | Yes | No |
|---|---|---|
| 1. Fluctuations in blood sugar and insulin | | |
| 2. NPY/PYY imbalance | | |
| 3. Serotonin deficiency | | |
| 4. Serotonin delivery problems | | |
| 5. Food addiction | | |
| 6. Excessive norepinephrine | | |
| 7. Ghrelin spikes* or oil hunger | | |

* We're not ready yet to deal with this one.

**How Well Does Each Diet Address Each Cause?**

In the chart on the next page, a check mark means that this particular diet addresses the listed cause of appetite disorder. A check mark with a plus symbol ✔ + means that the diet deals with this cause particularly well. An **X** means that the diet in question actually makes the cause of appetite disorder worse. If the box is blank, that diet neither deals with nor worsens that cause.

Note that cause four, serotonin delivery problems, is not included in this chart, because this cause of disordered eating can't be addressed through a diet. It *can,* however, be effectively countered through medication, as well as through some forms of alternative treatment, such as homeopathy.

> **STEP 25**
>
> Select your ideal diet plan.

Now compare your list of causes with those addressed by each diet. You'll want to choose a diet that has as many check marks as possible for the causes that affect you.

For example, if the only cause of your appetite disorder is blood sugar fluctuations, then eating change one should have cleared that up. Therefore, any diet with a check mark in the first column will work for you. In this instance, you may find the Zone or the 3-Hour Diet especially helpful.

On the other hand, if you have a food addiction, any diet with an **X** in the food addiction column will only increase your appetite. Choose a plan with a check mark in column five on the next page and as many check marks as possible in the other columns. In this instance, the Fat Flush or Schwarzbein diets may work especially well for you.

---

Remember to check with your doctor before starting the diet you choose.

You are the expert on your body, and you and your doctor together are the experts on your medical history.

---

FIGURE 15

### Specific Diets and the Causes of Appetite Disorder That They Address

| Diet | 1. Fluctuations in blood sugar and insulin | 2. NPY/PYY imbalance | 3. Serotonin deficiency | 4. Serotonin delivery problems | 5. Food addiction | 6. Excessive norepinephrine | 7. Ghrelin spikes or oil hunger |
|---|---|---|---|---|---|---|---|
| Liquid Fasting | X | X | | | X | | |
| Lose __ Pounds/Inches in __ Days | | | | | X | | |
| Negative Calorie | | | X | | X | | ✔ |
| Low-Carb/Atkins | | | | | X | | X |
| Zone | ✔+ | ✔+ | | | | | ✔+ |
| 3-Hour | ✔+ | ✔+ | | | | ✔ | |
| Fat Flush | ✔ | ✔ | ✔+ | | ✔+ | ✔ | ✔ |
| Flavor Point | ✔ | ✔+ | | | | | ✔ |
| South Beach | ✔ | ✔ | ✔ | | ✔/X* | | ✔ |
| Mediterranean/Sonoma | ✔ | ✔ | ✔ | | ✔** | ✔+ | ✔ |
| Schwarzbein | ✔ | ✔ | ✔ | | ✔+ | ✔+ | ✔ |
| High-Carb, Low-Fat/Pritikin | ✔ | | | | X | ✔ | |
| Low-Fat–Vegetarian/Ornish | ✔ | ✔ | | | X | | |
| Eat Right 4 Your Type | | | | | | ✔ | ✔ |
| Weight Watchers | | | | | X*** | ✔+ | |

   \*   Phase 1 supports abstinence very well, but Phase 2 can seduce you away from abstinence. See page 291 for details.

  \*\*   Take care if you are addicted to wheat or bread.

\*\*\*   Unless you read labels carefully and choose foods that won't trigger eating or weight storage.

### Converting a Chosen Diet to Your Profile

You will need to reconfigure the diet you choose to conform with the changes you have already made, so that the diet doesn't trigger your appetite. I've made this easier for you by providing the list below. For each cause of an appetite disorder, I've listed both the recommended diets and the alterations you must make to protect your satiety.

*If your appetite disorder was entirely resolved by eating change one, here are the recommended diets and required modifications:*

- **3-Hour Diet—preferred**

- **Flavor Point Diet—preferred**

- **Zone Diet—preferred**
    - Add one small nonstarch or Zone snack at midmorning.

- Fat Flush Plan

- South Beach Diet
    - Do not eat foods containing MSG, Equal, or NutraSweet.
    - Use stevia instead of NutraSweet or Equal.
    - During the maintenance phase, continue to have snacks at midmorning and midafternoon.

- Ornish Plan

- Eat Right 4 Your Type
    - Add one small nonstarch snack at midmorning.

- Mediterranean/Sonoma diets
    - Add one snack.

- Pritikin Principle
    - Eliminate diet drinks from snacks.

*If your appetite disorder was entirely resolved by eating changes one and two, here are the recommended diets and required modifications:*

- **Flavor Point Diet—preferred**
  - Either add or retain protein at snack times. (Occasionally, a "weight-loss express" option in this diet allows removal of the protein portion of a snack. Because eating change two helped resolve your appetite disorder, do not take this option.)

- **Zone Diet—preferred**
  - Add one small nonstarch or Zone snack at midmorning.

- **3-Hour Diet—preferred**
  - Stick with 50/50 snacks.

- Fat Flush Plan
  - Add protein to protein-free snacks. (Eat 50/50 snacks.)

- South Beach Diet
  - Do not eat foods containing MSG, Equal, or NutraSweet.
  - Use stevia instead of NutraSweet or Equal.
  - During the maintenance phase, continue to have snacks at midmorning and midafternoon.

- Ornish Plan
  - Be sure each snack has sufficient protein.

  *If you have cravings after meals, change diet plans.*

- Mediterranean/Sonoma diets
  - Add one snack.
  - Be sure each snack includes 50 percent protein.
  - Eliminate breads, crackers, and wheat/flour items from snacks.

- Eat Right 4 Your Type
  - Add one small 50/50 snack at midmorning.
  - Add protein to, and remove starch from, the midafternoon snack.

- Pritikin Principle
  - Eliminate diet drinks from snacks.
  - Add protein to snacks.
  - Eliminate breads, crackers, and wheat/flour items from snacks.
    *If you have cravings after meals, change diet plans.*

*If your appetite disorder was entirely resolved by eating changes one, two, and three, here are the recommended diets and their required modifications:*

- **Fat Flush Plan—preferred**
  - Add protein to protein-free snacks (50/50).
  - Occasionally, have turkey at meals—or add turkey to a protein-free snack—so that you have three servings of tryptophan each week. This diet discourages milk, so your primary turkey substitutes are sesame seeds, tahini, sesame butter, and pumpkin seeds.

- **South Beach Diet—recommended**
  - Do not eat foods containing MSG, Equal, or NutraSweet.
  - Use stevia instead of NutraSweet or Equal.
  - During the maintenance phase, continue to have snacks at midmorning and midafternoon.

- Flavor Point Diet
  - Maintain 50/50 snacks.
  - Add one serving of turkey the first week, two servings of turkey the second and third weeks, and one more serving the fourth week. From then on, the planned meals leave you with a deficit of one tryptophan serving each week, so add 380 mg of tryptophan through your other food choices.
  - Whenever the plan offers a choice between yogurt or cottage cheese and something else, choose the dairy option unless you supplement your tryptophan some other way.

- Zone Diet
  - Add one small nonstarch or Zone snack at midmorning.
  - Use turkey or some other source of tryptophan as your protein three times a week.

- 3-Hour Diet
  - Stick with 50/50 snacks.
  - Include a source of tryptophan three times a week.

- Pritikin Principle
  - Eliminate diet drinks from snacks.
  - Add protein to snacks.
  - Eliminate breads, crackers, and wheat/flour items from snacks.
  - Maintain your tryptophan intake every other day.
  - Add protein to protein-free meals.

    *If you have cravings after meals, change diet plans.*

- Ornish Plan
  - Be sure each snack has sufficient protein.
  - Get your tryptophan from milk.

- Mediterranean/Sonoma diets
  - Add one more daily snack.
  - Be sure each snack includes 50 percent protein.
  - Eliminate breads, crackers, and wheat/flour items from snacks.
  - Get tryptophan from any source three times each week.

- Eat Right 4 Your Type
  - Add one small 50/50 snack at midmorning.
  - Add protein to, and remove starch from, the midafternoon snack.
  - Blood types O, A, and AB: Get your tryptophan from turkey rather than milk.
  - Blood type B: Get your tryptophan from either turkey or low-fat milk.

*If your appetite disorder was entirely resolved by eating changes one, two, three, and four, here are the recommended diets and their required modifications:*

- **Fat Flush Plan—preferred**
  - Add protein to protein-free snacks (50/50).
  - Occasionally, eat turkey at meals—or add turkey to a protein-free snack—so that you bring your tryptophan intake to three servings a week. This diet discourages milk, so your only substitutes for turkey are sesame seeds, tahini, sesame butter, and pumpkin seeds.
  - If you are addicted *only* to high-fat foods, you may follow the plan without any modification except the addition of turkey.
  - If you are addicted to sugar, you may find the fruit smoothie too sweet for your morning meal, and it may trigger a day of hunger and cravings. If this happens even *once,* substitute a different breakfast and try the smoothie as a snack. If you have cravings, emptiness, or hunger afterward, remove it from your eating map.

  Phase 2: Substitute a bread that's above your abstinence line for wheat toast (see page 217).

  Phase 3: Follow precisely the diet's plan for adding carbs. If you react to a carb with cravings or hunger, remove it from your eating map. Don't eat crackers. (Their small size makes it too easy to quickly consume enough to trigger appetite, even if the flour is above your abstinence line.)

- **Schwarzbein Principle—preferred**
  - Maintain two daily 50/50 snacks.
  - Protect your tryptophan level.
  - Take care to eat only the grains, breads, and flours that are above your abstinence line.

- Flavor Point Diet
  - Maintain 50/50 snacks.
  - Add one serving of turkey the first week, two servings of turkey the second and third weeks, and one serving the fourth week.

From then on, the planned meals leave you with a deficit of one tryptophan serving each week, so add 380 mg of tryptophan through your other food choices.

- Whenever the plan offers a choice between yogurt or cottage cheese and something else, choose the dairy option unless you supplement your tryptophan some other way.
- If you are abstinent from bread, wheat, or flour, substitute a grain option that is above your abstinence line.

- Zone Diet
  - Add one small nonstarch or Zone snack at midmorning.
  - Include turkey or some other tryptophan source as your protein three times per week.
  - Avoid any trigger foods that the diet recommends.

- Mediterranean/Sonoma diets
  - Add one more daily snack.
  - Be sure each snack includes 50 percent protein.
  - Get tryptophan from any source three times each week.
  - Do not eat grain or bread snacks during Wave 2.
  - Do not do Wave 3. It is not recommended for bread, wheat, or flour addicts.

- Eat Right 4 Your Type
  - Add one small 50/50 snack at midmorning.
  - Add protein to, and remove starch from, the midafternoon snack.
  - Blood types O, A, and AB: Get your tryptophan from turkey rather than milk.
  - Blood type B: Get your tryptophan from either turkey or low-fat milk.
  - Blood type A: Move wheat and corn from the neutral list to the avoid list.
  - Blood types B and AB: Move wheat from the neutral list to the avoid list.
  - Avoid any trigger food, even if the diet considers it a neutral food.

- South Beach Diet

I don't recommend this diet past Phase 1 for your form of appetite disorder, unless you are addicted only to high-fat foods. Otherwise, Phase 1 is ideal for getting through withdrawal, but after two or three weeks, I strongly recommend switching to a different diet. If you insist on staying with the South Beach Diet into Phase 2, here are the changes you must make:
  - Do not eat foods containing MSG, Equal, or NutraSweet.
  - Use stevia instead of NutraSweet or Equal.

During the maintenance phase, continue to have snacks at midmorning and midafternoon.
  - If you are addicted *only* to high-fat foods, you may follow Phases 1 and 2 without any modification except those noted above.

If you are addicted to sugar, you may find the breakfasts of fruit smoothies start you off with too much sugar on an empty stomach. Substitute breakfasts from Phase 1 if, *even once,* after a fruit smoothie breakfast you are hungry, have cravings, or are focused on food.
  - When a meal or recipe recommends wheat bread, substitute a food that is above your abstinence line.
  - Ignore the diet's recommendations for bread and crackers. Don't get seduced by Phase 2 recommendations such as "eat four crackers." This will trigger your food addiction.
  - Even though the maintenance plan eliminates the morning and afternoon snacks, you must continue having both.

**Eating Change Five**

We won't discuss eating change five until after you've completed your diet. Eating change five has to do with the fats or fatty foods you are addicted to. If you are addicted both to sweets or starches *and* to fats or fatty foods, then you are already handling enough abstinence for now with eating change four.

Once you begin your diet, the diet itself will have recommendations for the amount of oil or fat you can eat. Most of the diets recommended in this chapter are savvy about the types of oil that should be eaten daily.

After you've completed your diet, you can continue to incorporate your diet's suggestions about oil intake, and that can suffice for eating change five. Or, if you have a tendency to crave fatty foods and/or fats, such as butter, cream, or sour cream, then, at that time, take Step 28 in Chapter 35.

And finally, if you are not at all addicted to sweets and starches, but are addicted to fats and fatty foods, you were already directed to skip ahead to Step 28 before moving on to Step 18. In your case, the best diet is the Zone Diet. It is particularly adept at preventing the hunger and appetite that is prompted by cause seven—ghrelin spikes or oil hunger. If you decide to go with the Zone Diet, use the modifications listed below.

*If your appetite disorder was entirely resolved by eating changes one, two, and three, and you are addicted to fats and fatty foods only and not to sweets or starches, then these are the diet recommendations for you:*

- **Zone Diet—preferred**
    - Add one small nonstarch or Zone snack at midmorning.
    - Include turkey or some other tryptophan source as your protein three times per week.
    - Avoid any trigger foods that the diet recommends.

- Flavor Point Diet
    - Maintain 50/50 snacks.
    - Add one serving of turkey the first week, two servings of turkey the second and third weeks, and one serving the fourth week. From then on, the planned meals leave you one serving of tryptophan low each week, so add 380 mg of tryptophan through your other food choices.

- Whenever the plan offers a choice between yogurt or cottage cheese and something else, choose the dairy option unless you supplement your tryptophan intake some other way.

- Ornish Plan
  - Be sure each snack has sufficient protein.
  - Get your tryptophan from milk.

- Pritikin Principle
  - Eliminate diet drinks from snacks.
  - Add protein to snacks.
  - Maintain your tryptophan intake every other day.
  - Add protein to protein-free meals.
    *If you have cravings after meals, change diet plans.*

- 3-Hour Diet
  - No changes needed.

*If your appetite disorder was entirely resolved by eating changes one, two, and three and by reducing stress, and you are not addicted to any foods, then these are the recommended diets and modifications for you:*

- **Mediterranean/Sonoma diets—preferred**
  - Add one snack.
  - Be sure each snack includes 50 percent protein.
  - Get tryptophan from any source three times each week.

- **Flavor Point Diet—preferred**
  - Maintain 50/50 snacks.
  - Add one serving of turkey the first week, two servings of turkey the second and third weeks, and one serving the fourth week. From then on, the planned meals leave you one serving of tryptophan low each week, so add 380 mg of tryptophan through your other food choices.
  - Whenever the plan offers a choice between yogurt or cottage cheese and something else, choose the dairy option unless you supplement your tryptophan some other way.

- **Schwarzbein Principle—preferred**
  - Maintain two daily 50/50 snacks.
  - Protect your tryptophan level.

- **Weight Watchers—preferred**
  - Do not eat foods containing MSG, Equal, or NutraSweet.
  - Use stevia instead of NutraSweet or Equal.
  - Protect your tryptophan level.

- **Fat Flush Plan—preferred**
  - Add protein to protein-free snacks (50/50).
  - Eat turkey occasionally at meals—or add turkey to a protein-free snack—so that you have tryptophan three times a week. This diet discourages milk, so your primary substitutes for turkey are sesame seeds, tahini, sesame butter, and pumpkin seeds.

- **3-Hour Diet—preferred**
  - Stick with 50/50 snacks.
  - Include a source of tryptophan three times a week.

- **Pritikin Principle—preferred**
  - Eliminate diet drinks from snacks.
  - Add protein to snacks.
  - Maintain your tryptophan intake every other day.
  - Add protein to protein-free meals.

- **Eat Right 4 Your Type—preferred**
  - Add one small 50/50 snack at midmorning.
  - Add protein to the midafternoon snack.
  - Blood types O, A, and AB: Get your tryptophan from turkey rather than milk.
  - Blood type B: Get your tryptophan from either turkey or low-fat milk.

- South Beach Diet
  - Do not eat foods containing MSG, Equal, or NutraSweet.
  - Use stevia instead of NutraSweet or Equal.
  - During the maintenance phase, continue to have snacks midmorning and midafternoon.

- Zone Diet
  - Add one small nonstarch or Zone snack at midmorning.
  - Include turkey or another tryptophan source as your protein three times per week.

- Ornish Plan
  - Be sure each snack has sufficient protein.
  - Get your tryptophan from milk.

• • •

### Opening

### Today's Agenda

1. Choose your diet. Plan to check with your doctor about your choice.

2. With the help of your recovery partner, make the changes to your chosen diet plan that will keep your abstinence going.
   - Cross out (or have your recovery partner cross out) all foods your diet allows that you are abstinent from.
   - If the diet allows only a certain number of calories, exchanges, or units a day, plan to spread them out so that you are still eating five or six meals a day. For example, remove some of the foods from lunch and eat them for your midafternoon snack.
   - Cross out any sweeteners and any foods that contain aspartame (Equal or NutraSweet).
   - Remember that your snacks still have to be 50 percent protein and 50 percent complex, nonstarch carbs. No matter what the diet says, don't have any starchy foods for your snacks.
   - Even acceptable starches must be eaten as part of a meal—never for a snack—so that they don't trigger your dormant appetite disorder.

3. Do a reality check. Did reading this chapter trigger your diet mentality? If so, go back to Chapter 30 and get back into a recovery frame of mind.

### Closing

# 33

# Starting Your Diet

✌ CONGRATULATIONS! YOU'VE created your own personalized eating map; you've made important changes in your eating; and you've discovered and addressed most of the causes of your appetite disorder. At last you're ready to begin your diet.

| You've checked with your doctor, right? |
| :---: |

Unlike in the past, you're now well positioned to succeed with whatever diet you've chosen. You've built a foundation of self-knowledge, understanding, and changes in what and how you eat. This foundation will provide profound support for you while you diet.

You'll still also need the support of live, caring human beings. Continue to check in with your recovery partner at least twice a day through daily vitamin calls and evening relief calls; meet with her at least once a week; and call on her in times of crisis or high stress. Regularly attend support group meetings if you can. Keep encouraging (and reminding) the people you live with to support you in the ways described in Chapter 25, and thank them regularly for their efforts.

It's unlikely that you ever made it to the maintenance stage during past dieting efforts—or if you did, you probably weren't able to remain on the diet. This was because you didn't treat your appetite disorder first.

But this time is different; you don't have that problem.

**STEP 26**

Start your diet.

You've been treating your appetite disorder, and you know to put your recovery first.

Just remember to stay faithful to your abstinence and keep eating those regular 50/50 snacks. Your own self-designed eating map will make it possible to sustain the diet you've selected until you've reached the weight you want (as long as you keep getting and giving support).

Also remember that you are now following two simultaneous plans for improving your health and vitality: your personalized eating map and a weight-loss program. If you do stray from your diet, for whatever reason, continue to follow your eating map. This will keep your appetite disorder from creeping back.

And remember, diet or no diet, every day that you stay with the foods on your eating map is a day that supports your body, your health, and your well-being. (You may even lose weight just from following your map, whether or not you're also following a diet plan.)

It's not that unusual for people to fall off their diets now and then, even with a personalized eating map and good support from others. If this happens to you, don't waste even a second blaming yourself or getting caught up in guilt. Just stay true to your eating map, your abstinence, and your recovery. If need be, put the diet aside for a few days, or weeks, or a month—but continue to stay abstinent and follow your map. Then, when you feel you're ready, go back to the beginning of the diet and start again.

And if you decide to forget about dieting altogether, that's truly okay too—so long as you keep following your eating map.

Here's the important thing to remember: Even if you do stray from your diet, you haven't failed. As long as you keep your abstinence, you're succeeding brilliantly because you're continuing to do good things for your health and your body. (Remember, a diet is an extra benefit on top of your abstinence. Simply staying abstinent and in recovery is a significant achievement.)

And if you do lose your abstinence temporarily, call your recovery partner. Talk about the situation with her. Then go back to following your eating map.

## About Weighing and Measuring
Your diet may require you to weigh and measure portions. Go ahead. Some recovery programs also incorporate the act of weighing and measuring

into ongoing abstinence. That's fine; do it.

But what about after you've lost the weight you wanted to lose? Should you continue to weigh and measure past the end of the diet?

Possibly. On the one hand, it's helpful to be reminded meal after meal what portions look like. Even if the dragon that is the addicted part of your brain has been napping, it may pop an eye open when you eat marginal foods and say, "Portion, smortion, forgettabout it." Under the addicted brain's influence, your portions of such foods may start to grow.

Also, weighing and measuring can be a tremendous relief. Because it's easy for some of us to feel guilty about eating anything, knowing we've had a correct portion feels good. If you think weighing and measuring will continue to be helpful, keep doing it.

However, weighing and measuring can also be tedious. Not to mention, carrying scales and measuring cups everywhere we go removes our anonymity.

Once you are in a comfortable routine of eating every two or three hours and avoiding trigger foods, you will probably find that your portions naturally get smaller. Satiety chemicals will kick in, and you won't need to weigh or measure what you eat.

On the other hand, once you're naturally eating less, it may be a good idea to measure portions now and then to make sure you are eating *enough*, particularly if you undereat nonstarchy vegetables.

Over the long term, it's a good idea to weigh or measure the foods you are most likely to overeat—at least at those times when you would be inclined to eat the most. For example, if you're really tempted to overeat on weekends, then measure your portions from Friday night through Sunday night. However, if you start pushing down food into the measuring cup so that it'll take more, this is a signal that you are clinging to food—and a warning that you need support. Call your recovery partner.

### More Tips for Successful Dieting

■ **VARY YOUR MEALS**

Remember way back in Chapter 3, where I described how we become satiated to a specific food or dish once we've eaten a certain amount of it? Well, the same thing can happen when you eat one particular food too often. If you eat the exact same healthy food, dish, or meal day after day, you will soon get sick of it. (That's satiety.) Because you need to be able to eat this food again in the future, don't eat it too often within a short period of time.

## ■ FLAVOR YOUR MEALS

It's okay for your meals to be flavorful and tasty. Use herbs and spices to keep foods interesting. If the foods on your eating map start seeming dull, you'll be sorely tempted to break your abstinence.

## ■ ENJOY YOUR MEALS

Savor them. It's good to enjoy your food. You get to eat. You are supposed to eat. It's okay to like your food.

Put a pause in your meals. Try pausing for a couple of minutes in the middle of each meal. This gives your satiety a chance to catch up with you. If I do something to interrupt my eating—go outside and breathe, go over and pet the cat, stand up and pull the dead leaves off a plant—I often find that by the time I return, I've lost my appetite. That means satiety has kicked in, and I can stop eating and put the rest of the food in the fridge (and now I have a future snack all prepared).

## ■ PUT YOUR FOOD ON A PLATE

Having food on a plate lets you see the exact size of your portion. It also allows you to separate yourself from the carton or serving bowl. Even takeout should be transferred to a plate and not eaten out of the container.

## ■ SIT DOWN TO EAT

Eating while you stand confuses your body. Standing keeps your body alert, makes you eat too fast, and may keep you close to the food supply, thus encouraging grazing. Besides, sitting is more comfortable.

## ■ EAT AT THE TABLE

Restore the healthy association of sitting down at a table to eat. Let your meal be a small bubble of time devoted to nourishment and pleasure. Then get up when you are done. By doing so, you emphasize to yourself that a meal has a clear beginning and end, reinforcing a healthy attitude toward eating. (If you have negative associations with eating at a table, use the Converting a Negative Association exercise on page 148.)

### ■ TRICK YOUR BRAIN

Pay it back for tricking you. Cut servings into pieces, if possible. Eight pieces look to your brain as if you are getting more food. Use small plates so that the food fills it.

### ■ WHENEVER POSSIBLE, EAT WITH UTENSILS

Slowing down your eating helps satiety to catch up, and it takes longer to eat with a fork than with fingers. Chopsticks work even better.

We need mechanical means to slow eating because our rate of eating, unless we pay attention with every bite, is influenced by our serotonin levels and our degree of hunger. Because you've been following your eating map, your eating rate may have slowed automatically.

· · ·

## Support Meeting 20

*Opening*

*Today's Agenda*

1. Discuss the following:
   - The day I'm starting my diet plan
   - My degree of commitment to making the daily vitamin call and the evening relief call
   - Signs a diet mentality has grabbed my brain
   - What I can do to protect myself from a diet mentality
   - What I can do to restore my recovery mentality

2. Answer the following questions:
   - Which of the tips for successful dieting sound easy to incorporate?
   - Which tips will require breaking an old habit?
   - Are any of these old habits somehow connected to a negative association? If so, pick the tip that sounds easiest to change and do the Converting a Negative Association exercise.

*Closing*

# 34

# Bumps in the Support Road

꙳ SOONER OR LATER, you and your recovery partner are going to have an issue with each other. You're human, aren't you? The two of you won't always have the same perspective or way of doing things.

Remember too that as the addictive chemicals drain out of your body, you'll feel more vulnerable in the early stages of your recovery. When that fat shield starts melting, you may also feel more exposed. As a result, while you're adjusting, you may misunderstand your recovery partner, misinterpret something she says, have communication problems, or feel she suddenly resembles your sister, mother, or someone else who controlled, hurt, or abandoned you in the past.

Or, you may do something that she reacts to. In your terminally crabby state, you might snap at her, without thinking or meaning to.

To help you sort these problems out, I've provided a few helpful tools. Please read on. I assure you, this turbulent period will pass, and you'll both begin to feel much stronger.

**Preventing Problems**

- Keep this book on hand (each of you) as a close resource.

- Proceed through the book at your own pace.

- Allow each other to spend more time with a certain step, if needed.

- Recognize that it's okay for the two of you to be out of sync. For example, each of you can be working on a different step at the same meeting. At one meeting you might talk about the topics at the end of Chapter 10, while your partner talks about the topics at the end of Chapter 14.

- Process the steps and discussion questions in this book in your own way. For example, if you tend to talk about thoughts and your recovery partner tends to talk about feelings, that's okay.

- Keep phone calls brief. Daily vitamin calls should be no longer than three minutes, evening relief calls no more than ten minutes, and help calls no longer than ten or fifteen minutes.

- Never turn support calls into a social chat.

- Always respect each other's time boundaries, both in terms of when to call and how long any call should last.

- When leaving voice mail messages, respect your recovery partner's privacy, especially if someone else has access to her voice mail. (For example, if she told you something personal, don't refer to it when you leave a message that her mate can hear.)

- Show up for support meetings on time.

- End support meetings on time.

- Never turn support meetings into social occasions. Stick to the agenda and end the meeting before doing anything social. (If you want to add some social time and your recovery partner doesn't, don't push for it. And if your recovery partner asks to add social time and you'd rather not, simply say, "Let's just stick to the meeting," and hold your ground.)

- Watch for your own competitive tendencies. If you notice yourself trying to one-up your partner, catch yourself and stop. If appropriate, admit the error and apologize.

- Never sacrifice your own needs for your partner's emergency. You may be able to spare two minutes for a help call, but don't go longer if doing so will make things worse for you. If necessary, set a specific future time to talk. For example, "I can't talk now, but I can certainly talk for ten minutes this afternoon. How about three o'clock?"

**Principles before Personalities**

This concept comes from one of the traditions of Twelve Step programs, and it's a wise practice.

Naturally, we'll occasionally feel angry or irritated with our recovery partner. Putting principles before personalities can protect you from sabotaging yourself in such a situation. This concept means that you give more importance to the principle of focusing on recovery than on any personality conflict.

When we put principles before personalities, regardless of whether our anger or irritation is legitimate—and regardless of who may be right and who may be wrong—we give our recovery a big boost. While we get to feel whatever we feel, we can't always trust our perceptions, which can be easily manipulated by our appetite disorder or food addiction, especially early in our recovery.

Picture this. After three months of working together, your recovery partner persists in asking you how you are when you make a support call. You are committed to the support call script. You never vary it. When she stretches its boundaries, it drives you crazy.

First, good for you that you are following my advice so closely. Technically, you've got a reasonable point—your recovery partner is varying from the official script. But let's check to see what else could be going on under the radar. When your partner does this, what do you feel like doing? Do you feel like yelling at her, pounding the phone into the wall, quitting support calls, or ending the recovery partnership?

And what would happen next if you actually did one of those things? Your daily source of support would disappear. And then there would come a point when you'd need either her support—which would be gone—or your favorite food to help you get through a stressful situation.

So what part of your psyche would be pleased if you got back into the food? The addictive part of your brain. Remember, the addictive brain is sneaky. It would love to fan the flames of discord just to rope you back in.

You're making a difficult change. You're learning to conduct your life in a new way—and doing it with the frayed nerve endings that result from withdrawal. Of course you're going to be touchy occasionally, especially within the first three weeks, and possibly at certain times throughout the year. (Perhaps due to subtle associations with changes in light or season, this touchiness seems to peak at predictable intervals, usually on the monthly anniversary of your first to third day of abstinence. Cravings also intrude at these times.)

The whole process can manifest in crankiness, confusion, or a tendency to feel victimized. Like your initial withdrawal, these feelings will pass, but while in the midst of this period, your perceptions may be a little off, and minor things may bother you disproportionately to their importance.

Think of it this way. Imagine that you are treading water in the middle of the ocean. You are getting weaker and weaker. A boat comes by and offers help. Are you going to reject that help if the boat is the wrong color? What if one of the rowers speaks poor English or the boat has hard seats? Sure, you could jump back in the water, but then where would you be?

**STEP 27**

Handle the issues that arise with your recovery partner.

Trying to recover by yourself is like treading deep water. It's only a matter of time before your appetite disorder or food addiction sucks you under. You need the lifeboat and the help of other rowers. If these people bother you sometimes, go ahead and feel bothered. But don't push these important people away.

Nothing is more crucial than preventing yourself from drowning in the addiction.

Here are some questions to ask yourself when issues arise between you and your recovery partner.

1. Could your feelings be the result of withdrawal?

    a. Is it an anniversary time?

    b. Are you feeling a bit victimized? (If so, this is a red flag that you really do need support right now.)

2. Would it make a difference if you set clearer or firmer boundaries with your partner?

    a. What new or different boundaries do you need to set?

    b. If your partner has ignored a past boundary, make it stronger. Remind her, be more emphatic, and provide a consequence if she violates it again.*

---

\* You may want to read one of my books on the subject: *Boundaries: Where You End and I Begin* or *Where to Draw the Line: How to Set Healthy Boundaries Every Day.*

3. Are any of the feelings you are having toward your partner based on an assumption or projection rather than real data?

   a. For example, ask your recovery partner, "Are you mad at me?" or "Did I do something to bother you?"

   b. Don't assume your partner feels negatively toward you unless she says so directly—and never act on a presumption that you haven't checked out.

## Presumption vs. Reality

Point three is so important. Let's look at it in more detail.

Whenever you're unsure about what your recovery partner is thinking or feeling—or if you think she's having negative thoughts or feelings about you—you can clear everything up quickly by saying these two simple sentences:

"I'd like to check out something with you. Are you _____ at me or thinking _____ about me?"

Here are some examples:

1. "Jean, I want to check out something. When I told you I wanted to eat another celery stick, I figured you thought I was weak. Were you thinking that?"

   "Heavens no. I was thinking I wanted to eat another celery stick too."

2. "Marilyn, when I called you that fourth time yesterday, I felt like I was bothering you. Was I?"

   "I know I sounded irritated. At the moment the phone rang, I was lifting a heavy box, and I was irritated that I had to put it back down to get the phone. I would have been irritated if anyone had called right then. And I suppose I could have just let the phone ring, but I didn't."

3. "Sylvia, sometimes when we talk in the evening, you sound like your attention is elsewhere—or like maybe you wish you were somewhere else. Is that true, or am I imagining it?"

"Oops. Okay, it's confession time. Sometimes I'm watching the twins when we talk. While I'm listening to you, I'm also making sure they aren't getting into trouble. So there are moments when I'm paying more attention to them than to you. Would you rather we make our evening support calls later, after the little ones are in bed? Or, how would you feel if we kept the same time, but I could just say, 'There go the twins,' hang up, and then call you back ASAP?"

### Principles: Checking Presumptions

The following is a guide the two of you can use when the presumption problem occurs.

Presumer:  State your presumption and ask if it's accurate.

Responder:  Validate or invalidate the presumption. Give context for your reaction if her presumption is accurate.

P:  Take the context into account. Consider whether you'd have the same feeling if you were in her situation. Notice how you feel now that you know what was really going on. Appreciate her for being honest.

R:  Appreciate her for checking out a presumption.

Both:  Validate that you are doing a difficult thing, that the road will occasionally be bumpy, and that you both provide a lot of support for each other.

### Dissolving Discord

When you feel angry, irritated, or discouraged by something your partner does or says, handle the situation as quickly as you can. The longer you wait, the fuzzier the details will become, and the harder it will be for both of you to zoom in on the particulars.

The temptation is to focus on what the other person has done. This causes you to direct your attention away from yourself, which eventually only causes the situation to escalate. The path through dissention lies inside us. That's where we find what the perceived injury means to us, how it affects our participation in the relationship, and what our needs are. By communicating these things, we create a foundation that allows us to empathize with each other and resolve conflicts peaceably.

We all make mistakes. Most of the time, when people make a mistake that hurts someone else, it is unintentional and not meant personally. The mistake results from their own patterns.

Still, if we suffer consequences from another person's words or actions, particularly if those words or actions are repeated after we've set a boundary about them, then we have to take care of ourselves.

If the relationship gives you something, try saving it by using the script below. Relationships that can tolerate conflict become stronger and, over time, quite valuable.

Here's a process for quickly resolving conflicts:

1. Briefly refer to what happened—the bare bones, not a play-by-play.
2. Express how you felt about the situation. Be as specific as you can and start your sentences with "I" rather than "You." ("I felt angry and confused," rather than "You upset me.")
3. Emphasize your feelings more than her behavior so that the focus is on your inner process.
4. Express the consequences her action had on you and on your interaction and relationship with her.
5. Look inside yourself to find out what human need got touched in this situation. Express this.
6. Let the person respond, and listen mindfully.

The process might look something like this:

"Tia, can we talk about something that's been bothering me?"

"Okay, shoot."

"When you were late to our meeting for the third time, I felt irritated. Your lateness has an impact on me because I end up sitting here waiting when I could be getting something else done."

"Merrill, I understand your irritation. I feel irritated too when I'm waiting for someone who's late. And I know you have a lot to do too."

"I do, Tia, and I feel disregarded when you're late. It affects my attitude toward you during the meeting. I don't feel as generous about listening. I feel myself drawing back."

"You know, this is an ongoing problem for me. I'm late for lots of things, so it's not about you."

"Thanks, Tia, but we still need to do something about it. I know that I need the meetings, and I'd like to continue them with you, because once you're here, you're very present. But I don't want to keep wasting time. I'd like to have future meetings at my house. Then if you're late, I can be getting something done and I won't resent it so much. And if I have to leave the house after waiting twenty minutes for you, I will."

"Hey, that works, Merrill. But what if we decide on this? If I mend my ways and get to a month of meetings on time, I'd like us to talk about coming back here to meet."

"Fair enough."

When someone raises an issue with *you*, here are some tips to help you move the discussion toward rapid resolution:

1. Listen mindfully.

2. Acknowledge and accept her feelings.
   a. Remember, the other person gets to feel whatever she feels. "Don't feel that way" and "How can you possibly feel like that?" are phrases virtually guaranteed to increase the conflict.
   b. Say something like, "I can see how worried you are about this" or "This scares you, doesn't it?"
   c. Keep in mind that feelings are internal experiences such as anger, loneliness, despair, shock, delight, and relief. Saying, "I feel you owe me an apology" is expressing a thought or opinion, *not* a feeling. (Most sentences that start with "I feel you" or " I feel that" are thoughts or opinions.)

3. If you can understand or share in her reaction, say so. For example, "I can see why you'd feel that way," or "I'd probably feel the same way in those circumstances myself," or "I hate it when people do that same thing to me."

4. If you agree that what you did caused a problem, own up to it. For example, "I do make an awful lot of noise stomping the snow off my boots. I keep forgetting that your husband works the night shift. Please tell him I'm sorry that I woke him up." And if what you did seems to be a pattern in your life—like Tia's repeated lateness—then look at that pattern carefully later, when you've got some time for self-examination.

5. If you don't agree that what you did was a problem—or if you believe you didn't do what your recovery partner says you did—then say so, calmly and straightforwardly, perhaps while acknowledging her feelings once again. For example: "You have every right to be angry at someone who's repeatedly late. But I've figured out the problem. My watch is three minutes slow, and the clocks in your home are ten minutes fast," or "I can completely understand your feelings, given what you thought I was doing, but I want you to know what was really happening with me, because it is different than you thought."

6. If you've made a mistake, accept or negotiate an appropriate consequence, or suggest one of your own. For example, "Let me make a sign right now that says, 'Shhh!,' and let's post it on your front porch by the boots. And if I do forget again, I'll write your husband a note of apology."

7. Even if you feel you've done nothing wrong, it's still okay to discuss a potential resolution. For example, "Tell you what. You set your clocks back ten minutes. I'll set my watch ahead by five. That should get me here on time."

Here's what both parties should do to dissolve any discord that crops up:

- Continue to listen mindfully.
- Remember to check out any presumptions you start making.
- Designate a boundary if one is needed.
- Forgive each other.
- Think about what you gain from your relationship.

## Delayed Reactions

Sometimes we don't realize we're irritated with someone until a couple of days after an incident happens. If we weren't in a lifeboat in the middle of the ocean, we'd probably withdraw from the friend, at least until we felt we could get together and work it out.

But you *are* in a lifeboat. There's nowhere to go unless you can walk on water.

Agree with your partner *in advance* that you will still give each other mutual support, even if an issue shows up. There's always a chance that your addictive brain is blowing smoke to lure you to jump out of the boat.

That way, even if you don't like each other for a while, you can still paddle, watch for sharks, and share the much-needed nourishment of recovery. Meanwhile, if you like, you can both start looking for other boats.

Remember too that any dispute with your recovery partner is probably temporary and may well blow over in a week or two or four. But, together, the two of you are making changes that can last a lifetime—changes that can prevent diabetes, strengthen your health, give you more energy, and lighten your heart. To make those changes happen and stick, you need a dependable, well-meaning, trustworthy partner in the same boat.

Committing to your recovery partner to check out presumptions and resolve conflicts honestly and peacefully is Step 27.

• • •

*Opening*

*Today's Agenda*

Discuss one or more of the following:

- Your willingness to commit to checking out your presumptions

- Your willingness to commit to resolving conflicts peaceably and honestly

- Your willingness to keep calling and asking for support, even if you are upset

- Your willingness to keep listening and giving support, even if you are angry

*Closing*

# 35

# Refining Your Abstinence

❦ THROUGHOUT THIS book I've occasionally mentioned ghrelin spikes as a cause of appetite disorders, though I haven't yet fully explained them. Now that you have the previous chapters under your belt, it's time to discuss how ghrelin and oils affect your eating.

As long as you are on your diet, you probably won't be troubled with ghrelin spikes, which show up as a quick rise in hunger within an hour after eating.

But when you are done with your diet and are maintaining your weight, your health, and your recovery by following your eating map, you may find yourself gradually consuming more fatty foods. This is no surprise, really; fats taste good to most people.

Strangely enough, eating a lot of fat at once can *cause* hunger. Studies with animals show that a high-fat meal can cause a rise in ghrelin, the body chemical that signals hunger.[1] If you are still using the Body Signals Chart to observe your eating and appetite, a ghrelin spike shows up as a rise in hunger during or just after a meal.

Some people are perpetually hungry. If a lack of serotonin isn't the cause, a lack of healthy oils can be. In this case, the remedy is to eat heart-healthy oils daily.

So, oil or fat, too little or too much, can cause hunger. If you aren't eating enough healthy oil daily, add that to your eating map. If you are eating too much fat, it's time to temper your intake.

What's the difference between a genuine bodily need for oil and an addictive craving? Take one to three teaspoons of an essential fatty acid blend of omega-3 and/or omega-6 oil. If, afterward, the craving is relieved, you needed oil. However, if you are still craving a fried or fatty food, your addiction has awakened. In this case, it's trying to pull you back into the addictive cycle with fat as the trigger. Go to the next chapter—right now, please—and come back here when the danger of relapse has been averted. Then read on.

If you aren't tempted to eat more fat, great. You can skip most of the rest of this chapter. You might, however, want to review the good fat/bad fat continuum below to remind yourself how different fats affect your health.

## Your Fat Temperance

You shouldn't be abstinent from fat because fat abstinence isn't good for you. You need good fats to keep your body running well. Furthermore, certain vitamins and minerals are fat based, so you need to eat the foods that carry them. Plus, if you aren't eating enough of the fats that your body needs, you can become fat-hungry.

FIGURE 16

**Fats**

**Healthy**

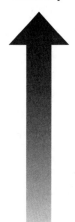

Omega-3 fatty acids
*(Salmon, soybeans, walnuts)*

Monounsaturated fats
*(Olive oil, peanut oil, nuts)*

Polyunsaturated fats
*(Vegetable oil, margarine, salad dressing)*

Saturated fats
*(Meats, whole milk, cream, cheese, butter, coconut oil)*

Trans fats
*(Shortening, fried foods, fried snack foods, some margarine)*

**Bad**

Even if a type of fat is healthy for the human body, a form of it can still be addictive to you. For example, peanut butter made from 100 percent peanuts is a monounsaturated food that lowers bad cholesterol (LDL). But for some people, peanut butter is a pistol trigger.

You'll have to be discriminating about how to get the fats you need for your health. Even when you eat good fats, you'll still have to get them from foods that don't trigger your eating.

You're probably thinking, *Yikes! Will this ever be simple?* No, I'm sorry; it won't. Abstinence is a living, breathing, ongoing process.

You'll need to figure out where to draw your own line at fat temperance.

Look at the oil can below. Draw a line across the can at the point above which you think you can safely eat fats and oils without being triggered. (Assume you are safe in eating omega-3 oils. These rarely trigger appetite.)

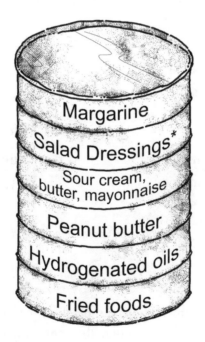

---

* If you're already abstinent from sugar or wheat, watch for these ingredients in salad dressing.

## Eating Change Five

For the next month, continue eating foods above the line and abstain from the foods below it. Also be sure to eat the super-good fats, those with omega-3 fatty acids.

Watch what happens during this month. If your satiety and fullness improve, you've drawn your line in the right place.

If you still have cravings for fat and have to struggle against hunger, you have probably drawn your line too low (or possibly too high). Be sure you are eating enough foods that have good fats. Draw a new line and see what happens during the next month. Keep making adjustments as necessary, one month at a time, until the cravings go away. When they do, you've found your own fat temperance line.

You may need to make decisions about some of the following foods and add them to the appropriate level on your oil can:

- Potato chips
- Corn and tortilla chips
- Other vegetable chips
- Cream (and half-and-half)
- Cream cheese
- Cheese
- Fried poultry skin
- Vegetables cooked in fat
- Avocados
- Nuts
- Fatty meats (ribs, bacon, ham)

**STEP 28**

Determine your degree of fat temperance, while continuing to eat healthy oils.

## Your Oil Can

After a month of experimentation, the blank oil can on the following page may be useful. If you need to rearrange the items on your can to make a more accurate hierarchy for yourself, do so. The more addictive a fat or fatty food is for you, the farther toward the bottom of your can it should be.

• • •

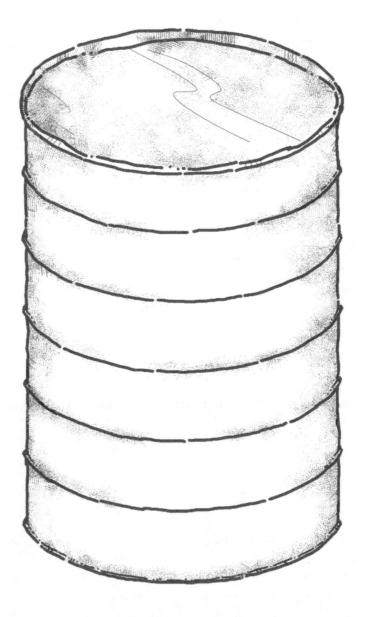

## Track C (Ongoing Abstinence)

**Your Personalized Eating Map:**

☐ Eat every two to three hours, for as long as you are awake.

☐ Eat snacks that are 50/50 protein and complex carbs.

☐ Do not eat flour, wheat, sugar, or simple carb snacks.

☐ Take 50/50 snacks with you wherever you go.

☐ Eat the equivalent of four ounces of turkey three times a week. You may substitute tryptophan from another source.

☐ When your stress level goes up, increase your tryptophan intake.

☐ Follow your current ongoing abstinence/temperance, which includes (check any that apply):

    ☐ Sugar

    ☐ Wheat

    ☐ Flour

    ☐ Fats and fatty foods

☐ Maintain daily and weekly support so that you are getting comfort and relief regularly.

## Support Meeting 22

*Opening*

*Today's Agenda*

1. Talk frankly with your recovery partner about the fats you crave that need to become part of your abstinence. Decide where you will draw your temperance line.

2. Agree to support each other faithfully this week. Fat withdrawal starts on the first day of temperance and usually gets better by the fifth day.

3. Protect your nose. Stay away from the smell of frying food, which is a powerful trigger.

*Closing*

# 36

# Handling Slips

YOU'VE GIVEN yourself a great treasure: sobriety. Your entire body, from your brain to your toes, will benefit every day that you remain in recovery from your appetite disorder.

Now the challenge is to keep your recovery going.

Those of us who are recovering not just from an appetite disorder but from a food addiction lead challenging lives. More than any other type of addict, we are stalked by the dragon of addiction. Our addictive substance is everywhere, and we have to deal with it often.

You are riding on a set of tracks. In one direction is recovery. In the other direction is relapse. At any given moment, you are moving either toward recovery or relapse.

Here's the difficult news: The ground is not even. It slopes in the direction of relapse. So if you do nothing, you will be pulled toward relapse, and it will gain momentum quickly.

You can protect yourself from relapse in the following ways:

- Make daily vitamin calls and evening relief calls to your recovery partner.
- Meet weekly with your recovery partner.
- Continue to encourage and accept support from the people you live with.
- Attend support group meetings. (This is optional but highly recommended.)
- Protect your abstinence zealously.

**STEP 29**

Accepting that relapse is a natural aspect of addiction, handle slips wisely.

• Protect yourself from appetite triggers by following your eating map.

• Call for support whenever you are stressed.

• Increase your exposure to healthy forms of comfort.

• Be aware of the symptoms of relapse, so you can catch yourself when you are about to slide backward.

FIGURE 17

**Symptoms of Relapse**

• Food cravings

• Feeling stubborn about not doing recovery activities

• Avoiding your feelings

• Skipping meetings

• Feeling resistant to using support

• Going to places of temptation (food courts, bakeries, smorgasbords, buffets)

• Pushing the boundaries of your abstinence

• Eating marginal foods

• Focusing on weight, size, appearance

• Comparing yourself to others

• Feeling defensive when you are invited to do recovery-related things

• Making excuses to skip meetings

• Starting a fight with your recovery partner

• Judging your recovery partner

• Judging your support group

• Feeling depressed

Whenever you start eating outside the boundaries of your eating map, you are heading for relapse.

A slip is always a signal—a signal that your mind is about to be hijacked by the addiction and that you need more support.

Go reach out and get that support—*immediately.*

The actions required at this critical moment are actually simple. But your attitude may have already started to shift, and a part of you may not want to stop the slide. It's the subtle shift in attitude that makes it seem like a lot of trouble to make a phone call or that may tell you that you are too busy for a meeting.

These thoughts are not rational. They are the voice of addiction. How can a five-minute call seem less practical than succumbing to the type of eating that will put your health at risk?

If you see any sign of relapse, the best thing you can do for yourself is to immediately pray for a willingness to stay with your recovery.

### *The Prayer of Willingness*

If you begin to sense a slip, stop for just one minute. Ask yourself the following questions:

- Am I willing to be willing? *(I may not be willing to make a call, but am I willing to have this stubbornness inside of me altered somehow?)*

- Am I willing to pray for willingness? If so, pray:

   "Dear _____ , please grant me willingness. Please save me from my addiction. Make me willing to be willing. And it is so."

- Am I willing to say the first three steps of recovery out loud?
   *Here's the short version:*

   > I can't do it.
   > But my Higher Power can.
   > I'll let Her/Him.

- Are you willing, now, to call your recovery partner or a recovering friend?

**Life after Relapse**

Here's the important thing for food addicts to remember about relapse: It happens to all of us. When it happens to you, don't run away. Don't hide your head in shame or despair.

Instead, come back.

Come back to meetings, come back to your recovery partner, come back to abstinence.

Call a support meeting with your recovery partner, and, with her, look through the chapters on stress, support, and abstinence. (Chapters 18, 22, 26, and 29.) Talk about any signs of relapse you see in yourself. Use focused talking (SHARP, page 176) to get to the bottom of the issue.

Strengthen your efforts toward recovery. Go to more meetings, work the steps, and expand your spiritual practices.

Once you have practice returning from relapse, you will be able to take any future relapses seriously, but without shame.

There's no shame in relapse. Any addiction is powerful, and relapse is just a part of it.

We want so much to believe that we can conquer an addiction once and for all, that we can live our lives without having to do these extra things to keep from being taken over again. Many of us have to test this belief a few times before we really accept the reality that we need to work an ongoing program to stay out of trouble.

But it's not that bad a trade when you think about it. For an average of just fifteen minutes a day and an additional three hours per week, you can keep your recovery—and all its benefits—moving forward.

> *There's no shame in relapse.*
> *Any addiction is powerful, and relapse is just a part of it.*

Time Investment: Ongoing Recovery

| Minutes | Activity | Daily | Weekly |
|---|---|---|---|
| 3 | Daily vitamin call | ✔ | |
| 10 | Evening relief call | ✔ | |
| 5 | Help call | ✔ | |
| 60 | Support meeting 1 | | ✔ |
| 60 | Support meeting 2 | | ✔ |
| 60 | Weekly snack bag preparation | | ✔ |

• • •

# 37

# Keep Going

❧ YOU'RE HOME FREE. All you have to do now is keep yourself in recovery. It's simple, but not easy.

Anytime you feel bogged down, come back to this book. Reread the chapter that speaks to your situation. Do the suggested practices. Go deeper than before.

I promise you: If you stay with this program, using the tools to advance yourself through each gate and passageway, your life will expand into glory and joy.

My own life is marked by a great divide—the land of dead ends and wrong turns before my recovery from my appetite disorder, and the world of friendship and fulfillment that I've inhabited since my recovery began.

Welcome.

**STEP 30**

Keep your recovery going.

· · ·

# Appendices

# Appendix A

# Meeting Format

This appendix offers a detailed format for a recovery meeting. Whether that meeting is a group of fifty or just you and your recovery partner, please follow this format.

My experience is that we all need frequent reminding of the nature of our disorder and of the higher goals we hold for our lives. That awareness permeates all of the text that follows.

Appetite disorders, and food addiction in particular, are so subtle that without routine rituals, they will slowly take us over. For that reason, I suggest that you read aloud at every meeting the opening remarks provided here.

Other excellent openings are "How It Works" (pages 58–60, 4th ed.) in the Big Book of *Alcoholics Anonymous,* "Our Invitation to You" in *Overeaters Anonymous,* and "Who Is a Food Addict?" in *The Steps to Recovery* by Food Addicts Anonymous.

Be sure to open and close the meeting on time. Meetings may last from sixty to ninety minutes.

## Opening

Good morning. We have come together because each of us has made some important decisions about reversing a problem that has controlled our lives for quite a while—an appetite disorder. This problem is not our fault; it's a condition that stems from imbalances in the way our brains function.

Fortunately, we can choose to reverse these imbalances, keeping in mind that our appetite/satiety balance will continue to improve as long as we maintain the practices we learn in this program. An appetite disorder is a lifelong condition and reversing it requires ongoing commitment.

Today we'll take another step in building the support that makes it possible to recover from this condition. Support is what makes the difference between genuine recovery and barely getting by. By sharing our stories and connecting to others, we are strengthened to continue our journey toward wholeness.

People who have an appetite disorder are generally vulnerable to pain, unkindness, ridicule, and harsh situations. Therefore, it's crucial to make this meeting a very safe place.

Here are some principles that will increase the feeling of safety in our meeting. Please choose to commit to them.

PRINCIPLE 1:

**PROTECT EACH OTHER'S ANONYMITY**

One definition of anonymity is "the state of blending into a crowd and going unnoticed." Many of us who have an appetite disorder would prefer just that. We do not want to broadcast to others that we have this condition. To follow this principle, we agree that we will not reveal the name or identity of any other member of this meeting.

Please indicate your willingness to follow this principle by either raising your hand or saying, *Yes.*

PRINCIPLE 2:

**KEEP CONFIDENTIAL ALL DISCLOSURES MADE IN THIS MEETING**

Protect each other's privacy by not repeating anything anyone says. We are being entrusted with others' private thoughts. Do not pass on either the content or the meaning of those thoughts to anyone outside the meeting—not even your spouse, best friend, or close family member. By honoring this principle, we create a sacred place, a sanctuary for all members.

Please indicate your willingness to follow this principle by either raising your hand or saying, *Yes.*

PRINCIPLE 3:

**DO NOT GOSSIP ABOUT OTHER MEMBERS**

It is important that we not gossip about one another. We are all safer if we can each trust that the others will not align themselves against us.

The desire to gossip comes from one or more of the following: a power imbalance, indirect anger, unresolved issues, or irritation with someone because they carry traits or behaviors we dislike in ourselves. Eventually, if we stay with the principles of this meeting and continue to practice the skills taught in this book, we'll have the ability to handle the issues that prompt the desire to gossip. Until then, the meeting will stay safe and progress only if each member commits to staying in right relationship with the others by not gossiping.

Please indicate your willingness to follow this principle by either raising your hand or saying, *Yes.*

PRINCIPLE 4:

**WHEN SOMEONE TALKS, LISTEN OPENLY AND RECEPTIVELY**

When other people talk, please join\* in spirit with them.

The members of this meeting have decided that (pick one of the following, which should stay the same each week):

- We will simply listen actively, mindfully, and without comment as each person speaks, as is done in Twelve Step recovery meetings.
- We will listen actively and mindfully as each person speaks. Then other members may, if they choose, offer brief responses of support.

If you decide on the second option, listen in stereo when another person talks. Keep part of your attention on the person. With another part of your attention, notice when you resonate with her experience. Then, when it's your turn to talk, you might start with the part that resonates for you, and then add your own unique experiences.\*

The following are some response styles that *don't* work so well:

- Using "Yes, but"—preparing a rebuttal to whatever's being said
- Teaching—preparing a lecture in response to what is being said
- Explaining—preparing an explanation for the other person's experiences
- Criticizing—preparing a critical, possibly judgmental, response

*As appropriate, add:* Today we will do an activity that requires dialogue. Therefore, this meeting will have two parts: first, a part in which each person who wishes may speak, and, second, a part in which we participate in the exercise or dialogue together. (This is usually done in pairs.)

PRINCIPLE 5:

**WHEN YOU TALK, EXPRESS WHAT IS GOING ON FOR YOU RIGHT NOW**

We tend to focus much of our attention on the past or the future, but it is the present— the here and now—that holds the most fruit for growth.

In this meeting, we talk about what we are experiencing now, in this moment, here in this situation. Notice if you are sad or anxious or irritated. Express your feelings. Paying attention to your own thoughts and emotions, noticing your reactions moment by moment, and clearly expressing how you feel will help you stay in the here and now.

---

\* Attending to a person with the intent of joining at points of resonance comes from the work of Yvonne Agazarian and Systems-Centered Training. For more information about SCT®, see Appendix C.

**Today's Agenda**

This meeting will include *(choose one or more of the following)*:

- Open sharing in which, one at a time, anyone who wishes to speak about their recovery may briefly do so.
- Open discussion on the following topic(s):
- The following dialogue(s) and/or exercise(s):
- Pairing up and helping each other plan or fine-tune our recoveries.

(Bring the agenda portion of the meeting to a close two minutes before the meeting is scheduled to end.)

**Closing**

It is time to bring our meeting to a close. Remember that we've all committed ourselves to the principles of anonymity and confidentiality, and that we will protect the safety of the meeting by not gossiping about each other.

Thank you for being here. Your presence is a service to the rest of us.

We will close with *(choose one or more of the following)*:

- Standing in a circle and holding hands
- The Serenity Prayer
- A shared moment of silence
- Silent prayer
- A reading or prayer

> ### *Serenity Prayer*
>
> *God, grant me the serenity*
> *to accept the things I cannot change,*
> *the courage to change the things I can,*
> *and the wisdom to know the difference.*

# Appendix B

# Support Groups

## Overeaters Anonymous (OA)

www.oa.org
World Service Office
P.O. Box 44020
Rio Rancho, NM 87174-4020
Telephone: (505) 891-2664
Fax: (505) 891-4320

## Food Addicts Anonymous (FAA)

www.foodaddictsanonymous.org
Food Addicts Anonymous World
  Service Office
4623 Forest Hill Blvd., Suite #109-4
West Palm Beach, FL 33415-9120
Telephone: (561) 967-3871
Fax: (561) 967-9815

## Compulsive Eaters Anonymous-HOW (CEA-HOW)

www.ceahow.org
5500 E. Atherton St., Suite 227-B
Long Beach, CA 90815-4017
Telephone: (562) 342-9344
Fax: (562) 342-9346

## Alcoholics Anonymous (AA)

www.aa.org
AA World Services, Inc.
P.O. Box 459
New York, NY 10163
Telephone: (212) 870-3400

## Misery Addicts Anonymous (MAA)

www.miseryaddicts.org

MAA Phone Bridge
To attend phone meetings, call
(641) 497-7400 and enter 622622
(MAAMAA). The meeting schedule
is on the Web site.

# Appendix C

# Resources

**International Association of Eating Disorders Professionals (IAEDP)**

www.iaedp.com

IAEDP is a professional organization devoted to educating, training, and certifying eating disorders therapists. You can use IAEDP's online membership directory to find an eating disorders professional in your area.

International Association of Eating Disorders Professionals Foundation
P.O. Box 1295
Pekin, IL 61555-1295
Telephone: (309) 346-3341
Membership: (800) 800-8126
Fax: (309) 346-2874
E-mail: iaedpmembers@earthlink.net

**Systems-Centered Training (SCT®)**

www.systemscentered.com

Developed by Yvonne Agazarian, SCT is a powerful therapeutic system that brings rapid clarity and integration to any level of human system—the individual, family, group, or organization. Loaded with simple, effective techniques that are easily learned and quickly applied, SCT trains people to separate themselves from the defenses that entrap them. Through a series of special processes we can learn to not take things personally. We can move beyond our defenses into enhanced personal awareness and straightforward interaction.

This Web site has training dates and contact information.

Systems-Centered Training and Research Institute
P.O. Box 2118
Decatur, GA 30031
Telephone: (404) 378-5709
Fax: (404) 378-8970

### National Eating Disorders Association (NEDA)

www.nationaleatingdisorders.org

This organization is dedicated to promoting public understanding of eating disorders and offering access to treatment. At the NEDA Web site you can locate therapists and support groups in your area.

NEDA
603 Stewart St., Suite 803
Seattle, WA 98101
Telephone: (206) 382-3587
Toll-free information and referral helpline: (800) 931-2237
E-mail: info@NationalEatingDisorders.org

### U.S. Department of Agriculture (USDA)

www.MyPyramid.gov

This clever, colorful, and interactive Web site sponsored by the USDA lets you build your own personalized food pyramid and contains activities for kids. However, remember, no matter what the USDA says, you can't eat any foods below your triggering threshold.

# Appendix D

# Articles of Interest

**Food Addiction**

Balon-Perin, S., J. Kolanowski, A. Berbinschi, P. Franchimont, and J. M. Ketelslegers. 1991. The Effects of Glucose Ingestion and Fasting on Plasma Immunoreactive Beta-Endorphin, Adrenocorticotropic Hormone and Cortisol in Obese Subjects. *Journal of Endocrinological Investigations* 14 (11): 919–25.

Georgescu, D., R. M. Sears, J. D. Hommel, M. Barrot, C. A. Bolaños, D. J. Marsh, M. A. Bednarek et al. 2005. The Hypothalamic Neuropeptide Melanin-Concentrating Hormone Acts in the Nucleus Accumbens to Modulate Feeding Behavior and Forced-Swim Performance. *Journal of Neuroscience* 25 (11): 2933–40.

Kelley, A. E., V. P. Bakshi, S. N. Haber, T. L. Steininger, M. J. Will, and M. Zhang. 2002. Opioid Modulation of Taste Hedonics within the Ventral Striatum. *Physiology and Behavior* 76 (3): 389–95.

Levine, A. S., J. E. Morley, B. A. Gosnell, C. J. Billington, T. J. Bartness. 1985. Opioids and Consummatory Behavior. *Brain Research Bulletin* 14 (6): 663–72.

National Institute on Drug Abuse. 1996. The Brain's Drug Reward System. *NIDA Notes* 11 (4). http://www.drugabuse.gov/NIDA_Notes/NNVol11N4/Brain.html

Tuomisto, T., M. M. Hertherington, M. F. Morris, M. T. Tuomisto, V. Turjanmaa, and R. Lappalainen. 1999. Psychological and Physiological Characteristics of Sweet Food "Addiction." *International Journal of Eating Disorders* 25 (2): 169–75.

Wang, G. J., N. D. Volkow, P. K. Thanos, and J. S. Fowler. 2004. Similarity between Obesity and Drug Addiction as Assessed by Neurofunctional Imaging: A Concept Review. *Journal of Addictive Diseases* 23 (3): 39–53.

Zelissen, P. M., H. P. Koppeschaar, J. H. Thijssen, and D. W. Erkelens. 1991. Beta-Endorphin and Insulin/Glucose Responses to Different Meals in Obesity. *Hormone Research* 36 (1–2): 32–35.

## NPY or PYY

Batterham, R. L., S. R. Bloom. 2003. The Gut Hormone Peptide YY Regulates Appetite. *Annals of the New York Academy of Sciences* 994 (June): 162–8.

Batterham, R. L., M. A. Cohen, S. M. Ellis, C. W. Le Roux, D. J. Withers, G. S. Frost, M. A. Ghatei et al. 2003. Inhibition of Food Intake in Obese Subjects by Peptide YY3-36. *New England Journal of Medicine* 349 (10): 941–8.

Batterham, R. L., M. A. Cowley, C. J. Small, H. Herzog, M. A. Cohen, C. L. Dakin, A. M. Wren et al. 2002. Gut Hormone PYY(3-36) Physiologically Inhibits Food Intake. *Nature* 418 (6898): 650–4.

Grove, K. L., P. Chen, F. H. Koegler, A. Schiffmaker, M. Susan Smith, and J. L. Cameron. 2003. Fasting Activates Neuropeptide Y Neurons in the Arcuate Nucleus and the Paraventricular Nucleus in the Rhesus Macaque. *Brain Research, Molecular Brain Research* 113 (1–2): 133–8.

Hung, C. C., F. Pirie, J. Luan, E. Lank, A. Motala, G. S. Yeo, J. M. Keogh et al. 2004. Studies of the Peptide YY and Neuropeptide Y2 Receptor Genes in Relation to Human Obesity and Obesity-Related Traits. *Diabetes* 53 (9): 2461–6.

Kalra, S. P., P. S. Kalra. 2003. Neuropeptide Y: A Physiological Orexigen Modulated by the Feedback Action of Ghrelin and Leptin. *Endocrine* 22 (1): 49–56.

Small, C. J., S. R. Bloom. 2004. Gut Hormones and the Control of Appetite. *Trends in Endocrinology and Metabolism* 15 (6): 259–63.

Williams, G., J. A. Harrold, D. J. Cutler. 2000. The Hypothalamus and the Regulation of Energy Homeostasis: Lifting the Lid on a Black Box. *The Proceedings of the Nutrition Society* 59 (3): 385–96.

# Appendix E

# Body Signals Charts

# Body Signals Chart, Week 1

Date: _____

| CATEGORY | DESCRIPTIONS | BASELINE DATA—NO CHANGES | | | | | | | | | | | | | | | | | | | | | | |
|---|---|---|---|---|---|---|---|---|---|---|---|---|---|---|---|---|---|---|---|---|---|---|---|---|---|
| **Timeline** | Circle Wake-up | 6AM | 7 | 8 | 9 | 10 | 11 | 12PM | 1 | 2 | 3 | 4 | 5 | 6 | 7 | 8 | 9 | 10 | 11 | 12AM | 1 | 2 | 3 | 4 | 5 |
| **Food**<br><br>*Numbers go in this section* | Proteins | | | | | | | | | | | | | | | | | | | | | | | | |
| | Complex carbs | | | | | | | | | | | | | | | | | | | | | | | | |
| | Simple carbs | | | | | | | | | | | | | | | | | | | | | | | | |
| | Fats | | | | | | | | | | | | | | | | | | | | | | | | |
| *Check* | **Equal/NutraSweet** | | | | | | | | | | | | | | | | | | | | | | | | |
| **Drink**<br><br>*Dots go in this section* | Water | | | | | | | | | | | | | | | | | | | | | | | | |
| | Pop | | | | | | | | | | | | | | | | | | | | | | | | |
| | Diet pop | | | | | | | | | | | | | | | | | | | | | | | | |
| | Coffee | | | | | | | | | | | | | | | | | | | | | | | | |
| | Herbal drink | | | | | | | | | | | | | | | | | | | | | | | | |
| | Milk | | | | | | | | | | | | | | | | | | | | | | | | |
| | Juice | | | | | | | | | | | | | | | | | | | | | | | | |
| | Alcohol | | | | | | | | | | | | | | | | | | | | | | | | |
| | Tea | | | | | | | | | | | | | | | | | | | | | | | | |
| *Check* | **Caffeine** | | | | | | | | | | | | | | | | | | | | | | | | |
| **Timeline** | | 6AM | 7 | 8 | 9 | 10 | 11 | 12PM | 1 | 2 | 3 | 4 | 5 | 6 | 7 | 8 | 9 | 10 | 11 | 12AM | 1 | 2 | 3 | 4 | 5 |
| **Fullness** | Stuffed | | | | | | | | | | | | | | | | | | | | | | | | |
| | Comfortable | | | | | | | | | | | | | | | | | | | | | | | | |
| | Empty | | | | | | | | | | | | | | | | | | | | | | | | |
| **Hunger** | Starving | | | | | | | | | | | | | | | | | | | | | | | | |
| | Really hungry | | | | | | | | | | | | | | | | | | | | | | | | |
| | Mildly hungry | | | | | | | | | | | | | | | | | | | | | | | | |
| | Not hungry | | | | | | | | | | | | | | | | | | | | | | | | |
| **Appetite** | Craving food | | | | | | | | | | | | | | | | | | | | | | | | |
| | Food focused | | | | | | | | | | | | | | | | | | | | | | | | |
| | Quiet | | | | | | | | | | | | | | | | | | | | | | | | |
| **Satiety** | Satiated | | | | | | | | | | | | | | | | | | | | | | | | |
| | Not | | | | | | | | | | | | | | | | | | | | | | | | |
| **Energy** | High | | | | | | | | | | | | | | | | | | | | | | | | |
| | Medium | | | | | | | | | | | | | | | | | | | | | | | | |
| | Low | | | | | | | | | | | | | | | | | | | | | | | | |
| **Thinking** | Very sharp | | | | | | | | | | | | | | | | | | | | | | | | |
| | Clear | | | | | | | | | | | | | | | | | | | | | | | | |
| | Cloudy | | | | | | | | | | | | | | | | | | | | | | | | |
| **Blood Sugar Reaction** | Headache | | | | | | | | | | | | | | | | | | | | | | | | |
| | Light-headed | | | | | | | | | | | | | | | | | | | | | | | | |
| | Even | | | | | | | | | | | | | | | | | | | | | | | | |
| | Sugar daze | | | | | | | | | | | | | | | | | | | | | | | | |
| | Sleepy | | | | | | | | | | | | | | | | | | | | | | | | |
| **Mood** | Optimistic | | | | | | | | | | | | | | | | | | | | | | | | |
| | Okay | | | | | | | | | | | | | | | | | | | | | | | | |
| | Depressed | | | | | | | | | | | | | | | | | | | | | | | | |
| **Stressed?** | Highly | | | | | | | | | | | | | | | | | | | | | | | | |
| | Mildly | | | | | | | | | | | | | | | | | | | | | | | | |
| | No | | | | | | | | | | | | | | | | | | | | | | | | |
| **Seeking Comfort?** | | | | | | | | | | | | | | | | | | | | | | | | | |
| **Timeline** | | 6AM | 7 | 8 | 9 | 10 | 11 | 12PM | 1 | 2 | 3 | 4 | 5 | 6 | 7 | 8 | 9 | 10 | 11 | 12AM | 1 | 2 | 3 | 4 | 5 |

Duplicating this page for personal use is permissible.

## Body Signals Chart, Week 2

Date: _____

| CATEGORY | DESCRIPTIONS | CHANGE: EAT EVERY 2–3 HOURS | | | | | | | | | | | | | | | | | | | | | | | |
|---|---|---|---|---|---|---|---|---|---|---|---|---|---|---|---|---|---|---|---|---|---|---|---|---|---|
| Timeline | Circle Wake-up | 6AM | 7 | 8 | 9 | 10 | 11 | 12PM | 1 | 2 | 3 | 4 | 5 | 6 | 7 | 8 | 9 | 10 | 11 | 12AM | 1 | 2 | 3 | 4 | 5 |
| **Food** | Proteins | | | | | | | | | | | | | | | | | | | | | | | | |
| | Complex carbs | | | | | | | | | | | | | | | | | | | | | | | | |
| Numbers go in this section | Simple carbs | | | | | | | | | | | | | | | | | | | | | | | | |
| | Fats | | | | | | | | | | | | | | | | | | | | | | | | |
| Check | **Equal/NutraSweet** | | | | | | | | | | | | | | | | | | | | | | | | |
| **Drink** | Water | | | | | | | | | | | | | | | | | | | | | | | | |
| | Pop | | | | | | | | | | | | | | | | | | | | | | | | |
| Dots go in this section | Diet pop | | | | | | | | | | | | | | | | | | | | | | | | |
| | Coffee | | | | | | | | | | | | | | | | | | | | | | | | |
| | Herbal drink | | | | | | | | | | | | | | | | | | | | | | | | |
| | Milk | | | | | | | | | | | | | | | | | | | | | | | | |
| | Juice | | | | | | | | | | | | | | | | | | | | | | | | |
| | Alcohol | | | | | | | | | | | | | | | | | | | | | | | | |
| | Tea | | | | | | | | | | | | | | | | | | | | | | | | |
| Check | **Caffeine** | | | | | | | | | | | | | | | | | | | | | | | | |
| Timeline | | 6AM | 7 | 8 | 9 | 10 | 11 | 12PM | 1 | 2 | 3 | 4 | 5 | 6 | 7 | 8 | 9 | 10 | 11 | 12AM | 1 | 2 | 3 | 4 | 5 |
| **Fullness** | Stuffed | | | | | | | | | | | | | | | | | | | | | | | | |
| | Comfortable | | | | | | | | | | | | | | | | | | | | | | | | |
| | Empty | | | | | | | | | | | | | | | | | | | | | | | | |
| **Hunger** | Starving | | | | | | | | | | | | | | | | | | | | | | | | |
| | Really hungry | | | | | | | | | | | | | | | | | | | | | | | | |
| | Mildly hungry | | | | | | | | | | | | | | | | | | | | | | | | |
| | Not hungry | | | | | | | | | | | | | | | | | | | | | | | | |
| **Appetite** | Craving food | | | | | | | | | | | | | | | | | | | | | | | | |
| | Food focused | | | | | | | | | | | | | | | | | | | | | | | | |
| | Quiet | | | | | | | | | | | | | | | | | | | | | | | | |
| **Satiety** | Satiated | | | | | | | | | | | | | | | | | | | | | | | | |
| | Not | | | | | | | | | | | | | | | | | | | | | | | | |
| **Energy** | High | | | | | | | | | | | | | | | | | | | | | | | | |
| | Medium | | | | | | | | | | | | | | | | | | | | | | | | |
| | Low | | | | | | | | | | | | | | | | | | | | | | | | |
| **Thinking** | Very sharp | | | | | | | | | | | | | | | | | | | | | | | | |
| | Clear | | | | | | | | | | | | | | | | | | | | | | | | |
| | Cloudy | | | | | | | | | | | | | | | | | | | | | | | | |
| **Blood Sugar Reaction** | Headache | | | | | | | | | | | | | | | | | | | | | | | | |
| | Light-headed | | | | | | | | | | | | | | | | | | | | | | | | |
| | Even | | | | | | | | | | | | | | | | | | | | | | | | |
| | Sugar daze | | | | | | | | | | | | | | | | | | | | | | | | |
| | Sleepy | | | | | | | | | | | | | | | | | | | | | | | | |
| **Mood** | Optimistic | | | | | | | | | | | | | | | | | | | | | | | | |
| | Okay | | | | | | | | | | | | | | | | | | | | | | | | |
| | Depressed | | | | | | | | | | | | | | | | | | | | | | | | |
| **Stressed?** | Highly | | | | | | | | | | | | | | | | | | | | | | | | |
| | Mildly | | | | | | | | | | | | | | | | | | | | | | | | |
| | No | | | | | | | | | | | | | | | | | | | | | | | | |
| **Seeking Comfort?** | | | | | | | | | | | | | | | | | | | | | | | | | |
| Timeline | | 6AM | 7 | 8 | 9 | 10 | 11 | 12PM | 1 | 2 | 3 | 4 | 5 | 6 | 7 | 8 | 9 | 10 | 11 | 12AM | 1 | 2 | 3 | 4 | 5 |

Duplicating this page for personal use is permissible.

# Body Signals Chart, Week 3

Date: _____

| CATEGORY | DESCRIPTIONS | CHANGE: EAT 50/50 SNACKS | | | | | | | | | | | | | | | | | | | | | | |
|---|---|---|---|---|---|---|---|---|---|---|---|---|---|---|---|---|---|---|---|---|---|---|---|---|---|
| Timeline | Circle Wake-up | 6AM | 7 | 8 | 9 | 10 | 11 | 12PM | 1 | 2 | 3 | 4 | 5 | 6 | 7 | 8 | 9 | 10 | 11 | 12AM | 1 | 2 | 3 | 4 | 5 |
| **Food** <br> *Numbers go in this section* | Proteins | | | | | | | | | | | | | | | | | | | | | | | | |
| | Complex carbs | | | | | | | | | | | | | | | | | | | | | | | | |
| | Flour | | | | | | | | | | | | | | | | | | | | | | | | |
| | Sugar | | | | | | | | | | | | | | | | | | | | | | | | |
| | Fats | | | | | | | | | | | | | | | | | | | | | | | | |
| Check | Equal/NutraSweet | | | | | | | | | | | | | | | | | | | | | | | | |
| **Drink** <br> *Dots go in this section* | Water | | | | | | | | | | | | | | | | | | | | | | | | |
| | Pop | | | | | | | | | | | | | | | | | | | | | | | | |
| | Diet pop | | | | | | | | | | | | | | | | | | | | | | | | |
| | Coffee | | | | | | | | | | | | | | | | | | | | | | | | |
| | Herbal drink | | | | | | | | | | | | | | | | | | | | | | | | |
| | Milk | | | | | | | | | | | | | | | | | | | | | | | | |
| | Juice | | | | | | | | | | | | | | | | | | | | | | | | |
| | Alcohol | | | | | | | | | | | | | | | | | | | | | | | | |
| | Tea | | | | | | | | | | | | | | | | | | | | | | | | |
| Check | Caffeine | | | | | | | | | | | | | | | | | | | | | | | | |
| Timeline | | 6AM | 7 | 8 | 9 | 10 | 11 | 12PM | 1 | 2 | 3 | 4 | 5 | 6 | 7 | 8 | 9 | 10 | 11 | 12AM | 1 | 2 | 3 | 4 | 5 |
| **Fullness** | Stuffed | | | | | | | | | | | | | | | | | | | | | | | | |
| | Comfortable | | | | | | | | | | | | | | | | | | | | | | | | |
| | Empty | | | | | | | | | | | | | | | | | | | | | | | | |
| **Hunger** | Starving | | | | | | | | | | | | | | | | | | | | | | | | |
| | Really hungry | | | | | | | | | | | | | | | | | | | | | | | | |
| | Mildly hungry | | | | | | | | | | | | | | | | | | | | | | | | |
| | Not hungry | | | | | | | | | | | | | | | | | | | | | | | | |
| **Appetite** | Craving food | | | | | | | | | | | | | | | | | | | | | | | | |
| | Food focused | | | | | | | | | | | | | | | | | | | | | | | | |
| | Quiet | | | | | | | | | | | | | | | | | | | | | | | | |
| **Satiety** | Satiated | | | | | | | | | | | | | | | | | | | | | | | | |
| | Not | | | | | | | | | | | | | | | | | | | | | | | | |
| **Energy** | High | | | | | | | | | | | | | | | | | | | | | | | | |
| | Medium | | | | | | | | | | | | | | | | | | | | | | | | |
| | Low | | | | | | | | | | | | | | | | | | | | | | | | |
| **Thinking** | Very sharp | | | | | | | | | | | | | | | | | | | | | | | | |
| | Clear | | | | | | | | | | | | | | | | | | | | | | | | |
| | Cloudy | | | | | | | | | | | | | | | | | | | | | | | | |
| **Blood Sugar Reaction** | Headache | | | | | | | | | | | | | | | | | | | | | | | | |
| | Light-headed | | | | | | | | | | | | | | | | | | | | | | | | |
| | Even | | | | | | | | | | | | | | | | | | | | | | | | |
| | Sugar daze | | | | | | | | | | | | | | | | | | | | | | | | |
| | Sleepy | | | | | | | | | | | | | | | | | | | | | | | | |
| **Mood** | Optimistic | | | | | | | | | | | | | | | | | | | | | | | | |
| | Okay | | | | | | | | | | | | | | | | | | | | | | | | |
| | Depressed | | | | | | | | | | | | | | | | | | | | | | | | |
| **Stressed?** | Highly | | | | | | | | | | | | | | | | | | | | | | | | |
| | Mildly | | | | | | | | | | | | | | | | | | | | | | | | |
| | No | | | | | | | | | | | | | | | | | | | | | | | | |
| **Seeking Comfort?** | | | | | | | | | | | | | | | | | | | | | | | | | |
| **Body Conscious?** | | | | | | | | | | | | | | | | | | | | | | | | | |
| Timeline | | 6AM | 7 | 8 | 9 | 10 | 11 | 12PM | 1 | 2 | 3 | 4 | 5 | 6 | 7 | 8 | 9 | 10 | 11 | 12AM | 1 | 2 | 3 | 4 | 5 |

Duplicating this page for personal use is permissible.

# Body Signals Chart, Week 4

Date: _____

| CATEGORY | DESCRIPTIONS | CHANGE: ADD TRYPTOPHAN ONCE A DAY | | | | | | | | | | | | | | | | | | | | | | |
|---|---|---|---|---|---|---|---|---|---|---|---|---|---|---|---|---|---|---|---|---|---|---|---|---|---|
| Timeline | Circle Wake-up | 6AM | 7 | 8 | 9 | 10 | 11 | 12PM | 1 | 2 | 3 | 4 | 5 | 6 | 7 | 8 | 9 | 10 | 11 | 12AM | 1 | 2 | 3 | 4 | 5 |
| **Food** Numbers go in this section | Proteins | | | | | | | | | | | | | | | | | | | | | | | | |
| | Complex carbs | | | | | | | | | | | | | | | | | | | | | | | | |
| | Flour | | | | | | | | | | | | | | | | | | | | | | | | |
| | Sugar | | | | | | | | | | | | | | | | | | | | | | | | |
| | Fats | | | | | | | | | | | | | | | | | | | | | | | | |
| Check | **Tryptophan** | | | | | | | | | | | | | | | | | | | | | | | | |
| Check | **Equal/NutraSweet** | | | | | | | | | | | | | | | | | | | | | | | | |
| **Drink** Dots go in this section | Water | | | | | | | | | | | | | | | | | | | | | | | | |
| | Pop | | | | | | | | | | | | | | | | | | | | | | | | |
| | Diet pop | | | | | | | | | | | | | | | | | | | | | | | | |
| | Coffee | | | | | | | | | | | | | | | | | | | | | | | | |
| | Herbal drink | | | | | | | | | | | | | | | | | | | | | | | | |
| | Milk | | | | | | | | | | | | | | | | | | | | | | | | |
| | Juice | | | | | | | | | | | | | | | | | | | | | | | | |
| | Alcohol | | | | | | | | | | | | | | | | | | | | | | | | |
| | Tea | | | | | | | | | | | | | | | | | | | | | | | | |
| Check | **Caffeine** | | | | | | | | | | | | | | | | | | | | | | | | |
| Timeline | | 6AM | 7 | 8 | 9 | 10 | 11 | 12PM | 1 | 2 | 3 | 4 | 5 | 6 | 7 | 8 | 9 | 10 | 11 | 12AM | 1 | 2 | 3 | 4 | 5 |
| **Fullness** | Stuffed | | | | | | | | | | | | | | | | | | | | | | | | |
| | Comfortable | | | | | | | | | | | | | | | | | | | | | | | | |
| | Empty | | | | | | | | | | | | | | | | | | | | | | | | |
| **Hunger** | Starving | | | | | | | | | | | | | | | | | | | | | | | | |
| | Really hungry | | | | | | | | | | | | | | | | | | | | | | | | |
| | Mildly hungry | | | | | | | | | | | | | | | | | | | | | | | | |
| | Not hungry | | | | | | | | | | | | | | | | | | | | | | | | |
| **Appetite** | Craving food | | | | | | | | | | | | | | | | | | | | | | | | |
| | Food focused | | | | | | | | | | | | | | | | | | | | | | | | |
| | Quiet | | | | | | | | | | | | | | | | | | | | | | | | |
| **Satiety** | Satiated | | | | | | | | | | | | | | | | | | | | | | | | |
| | Not | | | | | | | | | | | | | | | | | | | | | | | | |
| **Energy** | High | | | | | | | | | | | | | | | | | | | | | | | | |
| | Medium | | | | | | | | | | | | | | | | | | | | | | | | |
| | Low | | | | | | | | | | | | | | | | | | | | | | | | |
| **Thinking** | Very sharp | | | | | | | | | | | | | | | | | | | | | | | | |
| | Clear | | | | | | | | | | | | | | | | | | | | | | | | |
| | Cloudy | | | | | | | | | | | | | | | | | | | | | | | | |
| **Blood Sugar Reaction** | Headache | | | | | | | | | | | | | | | | | | | | | | | | |
| | Light-headed | | | | | | | | | | | | | | | | | | | | | | | | |
| | Even | | | | | | | | | | | | | | | | | | | | | | | | |
| | Sugar daze | | | | | | | | | | | | | | | | | | | | | | | | |
| | Sleepy | | | | | | | | | | | | | | | | | | | | | | | | |
| **Mood** | Optimistic | | | | | | | | | | | | | | | | | | | | | | | | |
| | Okay | | | | | | | | | | | | | | | | | | | | | | | | |
| | Depressed | | | | | | | | | | | | | | | | | | | | | | | | |
| **Stressed?** | Highly | | | | | | | | | | | | | | | | | | | | | | | | |
| | Mildly | | | | | | | | | | | | | | | | | | | | | | | | |
| | No | | | | | | | | | | | | | | | | | | | | | | | | |
| **Seeking Comfort?** | | | | | | | | | | | | | | | | | | | | | | | | | |
| **Body Conscious?** | | | | | | | | | | | | | | | | | | | | | | | | | |
| Timeline | | 6AM | 7 | 8 | 9 | 10 | 11 | 12PM | 1 | 2 | 3 | 4 | 5 | 6 | 7 | 8 | 9 | 10 | 11 | 12AM | 1 | 2 | 3 | 4 | 5 |

Duplicating this page for personal use is permissible.

# Body Signals Chart, Ongoing

Date: _____

| CATEGORY | DESCRIPTIONS | TRYPTOPHAN 3 TIMES A WEEK | | | | | | | | | | | | | | | | | | | | | | |
|---|---|---|---|---|---|---|---|---|---|---|---|---|---|---|---|---|---|---|---|---|---|---|---|---|---|
| Timeline | Circle Wake-up | 6AM | 7 | 8 | 9 | 10 | 11 | 12PM | 1 | 2 | 3 | 4 | 5 | 6 | 7 | 8 | 9 | 10 | 11 | 12AM | 1 | 2 | 3 | 4 | 5 |
| **Food** Numbers go in this section | Proteins | | | | | | | | | | | | | | | | | | | | | | | | |
| | Complex carbs | | | | | | | | | | | | | | | | | | | | | | | | |
| | Flour | | | | | | | | | | | | | | | | | | | | | | | | |
| | Sugar | | | | | | | | | | | | | | | | | | | | | | | | |
| | Fats | | | | | | | | | | | | | | | | | | | | | | | | |
| Check | **Tryptophan** | | | | | | | | | | | | | | | | | | | | | | | | |
| Check | **Equal/NutraSweet** | | | | | | | | | | | | | | | | | | | | | | | | |
| **Fluids** Dots go in this section | Juice | | | | | | | | | | | | | | | | | | | | | | | | |
| | No sugar added | | | | | | | | | | | | | | | | | | | | | | | | |
| | Contains sugar | | | | | | | | | | | | | | | | | | | | | | | | |
| | Artificially sweet | | | | | | | | | | | | | | | | | | | | | | | | |
| Check | **Caffeine** | | | | | | | | | | | | | | | | | | | | | | | | |
| Timeline | | 6AM | 7 | 8 | 9 | 10 | 11 | 12PM | 1 | 2 | 3 | 4 | 5 | 6 | 7 | 8 | 9 | 10 | 11 | 12AM | 1 | 2 | 3 | 4 | 5 |
| **Hunger** | Starving | | | | | | | | | | | | | | | | | | | | | | | | |
| | Really hungry | | | | | | | | | | | | | | | | | | | | | | | | |
| | Mildly hungry | | | | | | | | | | | | | | | | | | | | | | | | |
| | Not hungry | | | | | | | | | | | | | | | | | | | | | | | | |
| **Appetite** | Craving food | | | | | | | | | | | | | | | | | | | | | | | | |
| | Food focused | | | | | | | | | | | | | | | | | | | | | | | | |
| | Quiet | | | | | | | | | | | | | | | | | | | | | | | | |
| **Satiety** | Satiated | | | | | | | | | | | | | | | | | | | | | | | | |
| | Not | | | | | | | | | | | | | | | | | | | | | | | | |
| **Stressed?** | Highly | | | | | | | | | | | | | | | | | | | | | | | | |
| | Mildly | | | | | | | | | | | | | | | | | | | | | | | | |
| | No | | | | | | | | | | | | | | | | | | | | | | | | |
| **Seeking Comfort?** | | | | | | | | | | | | | | | | | | | | | | | | | |
| Timeline | | 6AM | 7 | 8 | 9 | 10 | 11 | 12PM | 1 | 2 | 3 | 4 | 5 | 6 | 7 | 8 | 9 | 10 | 11 | 12AM | 1 | 2 | 3 | 4 | 5 |

Duplicating this page for personal use is permissible.

## Body Signals Chart, Withdrawal

Date: _____

| CATEGORY | DESCRIPTIONS | ADD TRYPTOPHAN ONCE A DAY | | | | | | | | | | | | | | | | | | | | | | |
|---|---|---|---|---|---|---|---|---|---|---|---|---|---|---|---|---|---|---|---|---|---|---|---|---|---|
| Timeline | Circle Wake-up | 6AM | 7 | 8 | 9 | 10 | 11 | 12PM | 1 | 2 | 3 | 4 | 5 | 6 | 7 | 8 | 9 | 10 | 11 | 12AM | 1 | 2 | 3 | 4 | 5 |
| **Food** Numbers go in this section | Proteins | | | | | | | | | | | | | | | | | | | | | | | | |
| | Complex carbs | | | | | | | | | | | | | | | | | | | | | | | | |
| | Flour | | | | | | | | | | | | | | | | | | | | | | | | |
| | Wheat | | | | | | | | | | | | | | | | | | | | | | | | |
| | Sugar | | | | | | | | | | | | | | | | | | | | | | | | |
| | Fats | | | | | | | | | | | | | | | | | | | | | | | | |
| Check | **Tryptophan** | | | | | | | | | | | | | | | | | | | | | | | | |
| Check | **Equal/NutraSweet** | | | | | | | | | | | | | | | | | | | | | | | | |
| **Fluids** Dots go in this section | No sugar added | | | | | | | | | | | | | | | | | | | | | | | | |
| | Contains sugar | | | | | | | | | | | | | | | | | | | | | | | | |
| | Artificially sweet | | | | | | | | | | | | | | | | | | | | | | | | |
| Check | **Caffeine** | | | | | | | | | | | | | | | | | | | | | | | | |
| Timeline | | 6AM | 7 | 8 | 9 | 10 | 11 | 12PM | 1 | 2 | 3 | 4 | 5 | 6 | 7 | 8 | 9 | 10 | 11 | 12AM | 1 | 2 | 3 | 4 | 5 |
| **Fullness** | Stuffed | | | | | | | | | | | | | | | | | | | | | | | | |
| | Comfortable | | | | | | | | | | | | | | | | | | | | | | | | |
| | Empty | | | | | | | | | | | | | | | | | | | | | | | | |
| **Hunger** | Starving | | | | | | | | | | | | | | | | | | | | | | | | |
| | Really hungry | | | | | | | | | | | | | | | | | | | | | | | | |
| | Mildly hungry | | | | | | | | | | | | | | | | | | | | | | | | |
| | Not hungry | | | | | | | | | | | | | | | | | | | | | | | | |
| **Appetite** | Craving food | | | | | | | | | | | | | | | | | | | | | | | | |
| | Food focused | | | | | | | | | | | | | | | | | | | | | | | | |
| | Quiet | | | | | | | | | | | | | | | | | | | | | | | | |
| **Satiety** | Satiated | | | | | | | | | | | | | | | | | | | | | | | | |
| | Not | | | | | | | | | | | | | | | | | | | | | | | | |
| **Energy** | High | | | | | | | | | | | | | | | | | | | | | | | | |
| | Medium | | | | | | | | | | | | | | | | | | | | | | | | |
| | Low | | | | | | | | | | | | | | | | | | | | | | | | |
| **Stressed?** | Highly | | | | | | | | | | | | | | | | | | | | | | | | |
| | Mildly | | | | | | | | | | | | | | | | | | | | | | | | |
| | No | | | | | | | | | | | | | | | | | | | | | | | | |
| Timeline | | 6AM | 7 | 8 | 9 | 10 | 11 | 12PM | 1 | 2 | 3 | 4 | 5 | 6 | 7 | 8 | 9 | 10 | 11 | 12AM | 1 | 2 | 3 | 4 | 5 |

Duplicating this page for personal use is permissible.

# Notes

## Introduction

1. Centers for Disease Control and Prevention, "Overweight and Obesity: U.S. Obesity Trends 1985–2004," Behavioral Risk Factor Surveillance System, PowerPoint Presentation, http://www.cdc.gov/nccdphp/dnpa/obesity/trend/maps (accessed May 8, 2006).

## Chapter 12

1. R. L. Batterham, S. R. Bloom, "The Gut Hormone Peptide YY Regulates Appetite," *Annals of the New York Academy of Sciences* 994 (June 2003): 162–8.

## Chapter 14

1. A. M. Magariños and others, "Chronic Psychosocial Stress Causes Apical Dendritic Atrophy of Hippocampal CA3 Pyramidal Neurons in Subordinate Tree Shrews," *Journal of Neuroscience* 16, no. 10 (May 15, 1996): 3534–40.

## Chapter 17

1. C. Davis, S. Strachan, and M. Berkson, "Sensitivity to Reward: Implications for Overeating and Overweight," *Appetite* 42, no. 2 (April 2004): 131–8.

2. Ibid., 131.

3. C. Colantuoni and others, "Evidence That Intermittent, Excessive Sugar Intake Causes Endogenous Opioid Dependence," *Obesity Research* 10, no. 6 (June 2002): 478–88.

4. R. Spangler and others, "Opiate-Like Effects of Sugar on Gene Expression in Reward Areas of the Rat Brain," *Brain Research, Molecular Brain Research* 124, no. 2 (May 19, 2004): 134–42.

5. M. J. Will, E. B. Franzblau, A. E. Kelley, "The Amygdala Is Critical for Opioid-Mediated Binge Eating of Fat," *Neuroreport* 15, no. 12 (August 26, 2004): 1857–60.

6. M. A. Galic, M. A. Persinger, "Voluminous Sucrose Consumption in Female Rats: Increased 'Nippiness' During Periods of Sucrose Removal and Possible Oestrus Periodicity," *Psychology Report* 90, no. 1 (February 2002): 58–60.

7. R. Z. Goldstein, N. D. Volkow, "Drug Addiction and Its Underlying Neurobiological Basis: Neuroimaging Evidence for the Involvement of the Frontal Cortex," *American Journal of Psychiatry* 159, no. 10 (October 2002): 1642–52.

8. R. Spangler and others, "Opiate-Like Effects of Sugar on Gene Expression in Reward Areas of the Rat Brain," *Brain Research, Molecular Brain Research* 124, no. 2 (May 19, 2004): 134–42.

9. M. Moorhouse and others, "Carbohydrate Craving by Alcohol-Dependent Men During Sobriety: Relationship to Nutrition and Serotonergic Function," *Alcoholism, Clinical and Experimental Research* 24, no. 5 (May 2000): 635–43.

## Chapter 24

1. R. G. Walton, R. Hudak, R. J. Green-Waite, "Adverse Reactions to Aspartame: Double-Blind Challenge in Patients from a Vulnerable Population," *Biological Psychiatry* 34, nos. 1–2 (July 1–15, 1993): 13–17.

2. J. W. Olney and others, "Increasing Brain Tumor Rates: Is There a Link to Aspartame?" *Journal of Neuropathology and Experimental Neurology* 55, no. 11 (November 1996): 1115–23.

3. S. P. Fowler, L. Bonci, "Artificial Sweeteners May Damage Diet Efforts" (65th Annual Scientific Sessions, American Diabetes Association, San Diego, CA, June 10–14, 2005); Abstract 1058-P. cited T. L. Davidson, S. E. Swithers, "A Pavlovian Approach to the Problem of Obesity," *International Journal of Obesity and Related Metabolic Disorders* 28, no. 7 (July 2004): 933–55.

4. Russell Blaylock, *Excitotoxins: The Taste That Kills* (Santa Fe, NM: Health Press, 1997).

## Chapter 26

1. Food Addicts Anonymous, *The Steps to Recovery* (West Palm Beach, FL: Food Addicts Anonymous, 1996).

## Chapter 29

1. Derived from Kurt Lewin's force fields. Martin Gold, ed., *The Complete Social Scientist: A Kurt Lewin Reader* (Washington, DC: American Psychological Association, 1999).

## Chapter 31

1. Robert C. Atkins, *Dr. Atkins' New Diet Revolution* (New York: Avon Books, 2002).

2. Neal Barnard, *Foods That Cause You to Lose Weight: The Negative Calorie Effect* (New York: Avon Books, 1999).

3. Barry Sears, *The Zone: A Dietary Road Map to Lose Weight Permanently, Reset Your Genetic Code, Prevent Disease, Achieve Maximum Physical Performance* (New York: HarperCollins, 1995).

4. Ann Louise Gittleman, *The Fat Flush Plan* (New York: McGraw-Hill, 2002).

5. David L. Katz and Catherine S. Katz, *The Flavor Point Diet: The Delicious, Breakthrough Plan to Turn Off Your Hunger and Lose the Weight for Good* (Emmaus, PA: Rodale, 2005).

6. Arthur Agatston, *The South Beach Diet: The Delicious, Doctor-Designed, Foolproof Plan for Fast and Healthy Weight Loss* (New York: St. Martin's Press, 2003).

7. Robert Pritikin, *The Pritikin Principle: The Calorie Density Solution* (Alexandria, VA: Time-Life Books, 2000).

8. Ibid., 33.

9. Dean Ornish, *Eat More, Weigh Less: Dr. Dean Ornish's Advantage Ten Program for Losing Weight Safely While Eating Abundantly* (New York: Quill, 2001).

10. Peter D'Adamo and Catherine Whitney, *Eat Right 4 Your Type: The Individualized Diet Solution to Staying Healthy, Living Longer & Achieving Your Ideal Weight: 4 Blood Types, 4 Diets* (New York: Putnam's Sons, 1996).

11. Marissa Cloutier and Eve Adamson, *The Mediterranean Diet* (New York: Avon, 2004).

12. Connie Guttersen, *The Sonoma Diet* (Des Moines, IA: Meredith Books, 2005).

13. Jorge Cruise, *The 3-Hour Diet: How Low-Carb Diets Make You Fat and Timing Makes You Thin* (New York: HarperResource, 2005).

14. Diana Schwarzbein, *The Schwarzbein Principle: The Program: Losing Weight the Healthy Way: An Easy, 5-Step, No-Nonsense Approach* (Deerfield Beach, FL: Health Communications, 2004).

## Chapter 35

1. J. Sanchez, P. Oliver, A. Palou, C. Pico, "The Inhibition of Gastric Ghrelin Production by Food Intake in Rats Is Dependent on the Type of Macronutrient," *Endocrinology* 145, no 11 (November 2004): 5049–55.

# Index

# Meet Anne Katherine

For thirty-three years I've been a therapist, working first in Atlanta and then in the Seattle area. But before that, before graduate school and even college, I was a girl, struggling with weight and eating.

For the first week of my life I didn't eat, and my family was alarmed. At the hospital, my grandmother encountered a minister she knew. She explained that I was dying and asked him to come pray for me.

She led him to my room where he did pray for me, and after that I swallowed nourishment for the first time. That was the last time I had difficulty eating. From then on, eating ran away with me.

As a little girl, I would plot how to earn enough money to walk to the corner grocery and buy candy. I wasn't even ten when I invented the Ritz sandwich—that's white bread spread with mayonnaise, then a layer of Ritz crackers, topped with another piece of white bread. It sounds disgusting now, but back then, this sandwich was a favorite that I made for myself often.

Some people remember childhood events. I also remember foods, like the fried chicken at the Jewel Cafeteria and the hamburgers at the Tennessean, the onion rings at the Double R, and the potato salad at Mac's. I remember banana splits, my first McDonald's hamburger, and ice cream at the locks on the river when I was just a little girl.

My relationship with food ran my life, but I had no consciousness that this was so. I went through college, then grad school, without any awareness that my thoughts and behaviors regarding food were abnormal. Only when my addiction to food was so consuming that it was robbing me of ordinary human experience did I start to wake up. Even then, I didn't know how to stop it. The right words from an honest friend were what finally pointed me to recovery.

My life had been degrading, and like a boomerang, it then turned swiftly in a positive direction. Each successive week of recovery woke me up more. And everything, eventually, changed. I became open to true friendship. I gained the courage to step onto the path that was calling me. I changed states, jobs, lifestyles, and partners. (I kept the friends though.)

The addictive process fascinated me so much that I went back to school to study it. At the time, the idea of addiction was being applied only to alcohol and drug use. My interest lay in researching eating as an addiction.

I was convinced that something particular had driven my eating. It wasn't my choice to be preoccupied with food when I was five or ten years old. Something in my body had responded to something in food. As I became aware of how many others had suffered from the same kind of slavery, I was certain a biochemical process had to be at its root.

My studies led to my first book and at that point, I changed my professional practice, focusing exclusively on treating women with food addiction and binge eating disorder. Over the years, I developed numerous treatment programs, always refining and expanding the process based on unfolding discoveries made through research and observance of what worked—and what didn't work—with my clients.

For ten years, I had almost perfect abstinence from sugar. Then I started pushing the envelope, surprised that I wasn't reacting addictively to sweets. That was great news, so I kept testing my limits and suddenly the addiction had its hands around my throat once again. I found out about relapse and how triggering levels shift based on certain factors. With food addiction recovery, we aim at a moving target.

That sent me back to the medical library, where I began to understand more about how food addiction differs from other addictions and that food addiction recovery has its own unique set of requirements.

I'd love to be the perfect icon of abstinence, but I'm not. I have days and weeks of peace from the addiction and then out of nowhere food starts calling me and I have to struggle to remember to use my tools. This has forced me to invent additional techniques for staying in recovery, to reinforce my safety net.

For me, recovery is a daily process. Every day, I watch for and watch out for my satiety. I support my satiety chemicals that make abstinence easier. I practice the principles of this book and also of traditional recovery. I even make my little dots on the charts, accountable to my own support group in which we all follow the very program in this book.

I don't do any of this perfectly. However, what I do is good enough and allows me to be more available to life experience, more open to intimacy, more present to exploration and joy.

Although I'm no longer seeing clients on an individual basis, I am still leading groups and retreats. You can find out about these at www.annekatherine.org.

My hope is that you find recovery too, recovery that is good enough to show the way to your next steps on your life path and to give you the energy to follow it, so that you can find the joy and intimacy that awaits you.

Your recovery sister,
Anne Katherine

Other Books by Anne Katherine    *Boundaries: Where You End and I Begin*
                                  *Anatomy of a Food Addiction*
                                  *Where to Draw the Line*
                                  *When Misery Is Company*

**Hazelden Publishing and Educational Services** is a division of the Hazelden Foundation, a not-for-profit organization. Since 1949, Hazelden has been a leader in promoting the dignity and treatment of people afflicted with the disease of chemical dependency.

The mission of the foundation is to improve the quality of life for individuals, families, and communities by providing a national continuum of information, education, and recovery services that are widely accessible; to advance the field through research and training; and to improve our quality and effectiveness through continuous improvement and innovation.

Stemming from that, the mission of this division is to provide quality information and support to people wherever they may be in their personal journey—from education and early intervention, through treatment and recovery, to personal and spiritual growth.

Although our treatment programs do not necessarily use everything Hazelden publishes, our bibliotherapeutic materials support our mission and the Twelve Step philosophy upon which it is based. We encourage your comments and feedback.

The headquarters of the Hazelden Foundation are in Center City, Minnesota. Additional treatment facilities are located in Chicago, Illinois; Newberg, Oregon; New York, New York; Plymouth, Minnesota; and St. Paul, Minnesota. At these sites, we provide a continuum of care for men and women of all ages. Our Plymouth facility is designed specifically for youth and families.

For more information on Hazelden, please call **1-800-257-7800.**

Or you may access our World Wide Web site on the Internet at **www.hazelden.org.**

# Other titles that may interest you:

## The Overeater's Journal
EXERCISES FOR THE HEART, MIND, AND SOUL
*Debbie Danowski*

The powerful personal journaling exercises of this book let readers explore the physical, emotional, and spiritual aspects of healing from food obsession or addiction. Softcover, 152 pp.

**Order No. 2036**

## Inner Harvest
DAILY MEDITATIONS FOR RECOVERY FROM EATING DISORDERS
*Elisabeth L.*

These 366 meditations provide daily positive thoughts that offer insight and ideas for meeting the challenges of ongoing recovery from eating disorders. Softcover, 400 pp.

**Order No. 5071**

## Fat Is a Family Affair Second Edition
HOW FOOD OBSESSIONS AFFECT RELATIONSHIPS
*Judi Hollis*

This key resource for people who struggle with eating disorders not only describes the unhealthy dynamics that can exacerbate eating disorders, but also offers strategies for achieving health. Softcover, 320 pp.

**Order No. 2011**

## Locked Up for Eating Too Much
THE DIARY OF A FOOD ADDICT IN REHAB
*Debbie Danowski*

The author gives a gripping account of overcoming the physiological addiction to food and discovering unmet cravings for love and self-acceptance in the process. Softcover, 232 pp.

**Order No. 1932**

# ◼ HAZELDEN®

Hazelden books are available at fine bookstores everywhere.
To order directly from Hazelden, call 1-800-328-9000
or visit www.hazelden.org/bookstore.